Language and Reading Disabilities

Language and Reading Disabilities

Edited by

Hugh W. Catts
University of Kansas

Alan G. Kamhi
University of Memphis

Allyn and Bacon
Boston • London • Toronto • Sydney • Tokyo • Singapore

KH

Executive Editor: Stephen D. Dragin
Editorial Assistant: Elizabeth McGuire
Editorial-Production Administrator: Joe Sweeney
Editorial-Production Service: Walsh & Associates, Inc.
Composition Buyer: Linda Cox
Manufacturing Buyer: Dave Repetto
Cover Administrator: Jennifer Hart

Library of Congress Cataloging-in-Publication Data

Language and reading disabilities / edited by Hugh W.
    Catts, Alan G. Kamhi.
        p.   cm.
    Includes bibliographical references and index.
    ISBN 0-205-27088-3
    1. Reading disability—United States. 2. Children—
United States—Language. 3. Reading—Remedial
teaching—United States. 4. English language—
Composition and exercises—Study and teaching—United
States. I. Catts, Hugh William, 1949–   .
II. Kamhi, Alan G., 1950–   .
LB1050.5.C345   1998
372.43—dc21   98-34364
                                                 CIP

Printed in the United States of America
10   9   05 04

11/22/04

Contents

Preface

During the last ten years, knowledge about reading disabilities has increased tremendously. Evidence has continued to mount in support of the language basis of reading disabilities. This research has shown the importance not only of phonological processes, but of other language processes in reading and reading disabilities. Significant advances have also been made in the early identification, assessment, and remediation of language-based reading disabilities. As a result of these changes, books on reading disabilities have quickly become dated, and ours is no exception.

In our initial conversations about revising the book, we considered simply updating the chapters of the book. However, as we began to discuss how we would revise the various chapters, it became clear that more substantial changes were necessary. With the exception of a few chapters, this is a completely new book with a new title. The book has nine chapters, five of which are written by us. The remaining chapters are contributions by recognized experts in the areas of assessment and remediation of reading and writing disorders.

As with our previous book, we begin by taking the position that reading and spoken language share much in common. In Chapter 1, we present a model depicting the common processes involved in spoken and written language. Although spoken and written language share common processes, there are also important nontrivial differences between the two. Reading and writing are not simple derivatives of understanding and producing spoken language.

Much has been learned in the past decade about how children learn to read. This research is reviewed in Chapter 2, which focuses on the development of reading abilities. In the first part of the chapter, the importance of early exposure to literacy materials and experiences is stressed. Stage theories of reading development are then compared to more current models that emphasize the role of self-teaching mechanisms in learning to read. While it is clear that instruction is critical to learning to read, becoming a proficient reader is largely "self-taught" and based on children's phonological, orthographic, and language knowledge.

Chapter 3 considers the difficult issues involved in defining reading disabilities. We begin by tracing the historic roots of the study of reading disabilities, focusing on how language processes came to play a central role in reading disabilities. We then address the confusions surrounding terminology and provide a brief discussion of prevalence and gender issues. In the next section, the various definitions of reading disabilities and dyslexia are considered; we conclude this section with our definition of dyslexia as a developmental language disorder. Although our definition is similar to other current definitions, we place more emphasis on the developmental nature of the disorder. We view dyslexia as more than a reading disability; it is a disorder that affects the development of spoken and written language and is caused primarily by difficulties in phonological processing. In the final part of the chapter, we contrast dyslexia with a language learning disability.

The distinction between dyslexia and a language learning disability sets the stage for the next chapter, which focuses on the classification of reading disabilities. In this chapter, we review the evidence for individual differences among children with reading disabilities and consider various attempts to subtype poor readers based on these individual differences. We suggest that children should be distinguished on the basis of their word recognition and listening comprehension abilities. In our classification scheme, children with dyslexia are defined as having word recognition problems and normal listening comprehension abilities whereas children with a language learning disability are defined as having deficits in both word recognition and listening comprehension. A third group of children, those with hyperlexia, have normal word recognition abilities with deficient listening comprehension abilities. We think that this classification system will allow practitioners to provide more appropriate intervention for children with reading disabilities.

In Chapter 5, we review the wealth of information about causal factors related to reading disabilities that has accumulated over the last ten years. We first consider extrinsic factors that affect reading, such as early literacy experiences and reading instruction. The remainder of the chapter is devoted to intrinsic causes of reading disabilities, such as genetic, neurological, visual, attentional, and language factors. Although multiple factors interact to cause reading disabilities, language deficits are central to most reading disabilities. Importantly, language deficits are both a cause and a consequence of reading disabilities.

In Chapters 6 and 7, Torgesen and Westby offer recommendations for the assessment and remediation of reading disabilities. In the initial section of his chapter, Torgesen discusses the assessment and instruction of phonological awareness. This discussion is followed by a consideration of assessment and instructional issues related to decoding and recognizing printed words. Most of the information provided is based on Torgesen's vast experience in the study and treatment of reading disabilities. Westby also relies heavily on her clinical experience to provide a comprehensive chapter on intervention strategies for text-level comprehension. She provides numerous suggestions for assessing and remediating problems that underlie deficits in reading comprehension.

In the last two chapters, writing disorders are addressed. In Chapter 8, Scott discusses the writing process and what is known about how children learn to write. She also addresses the writing problems encountered by children with language and reading disabilities. This chapter lays the groundwork for the next chapter in which Westby and Clauser provide an extensive discussion of the philosophies and frameworks for assessing and facilitating written language development. Extensive information is provided about both the products and the processes involved in writing.

Acknowledgments

In our first book, we noted that writing books can strain the best of friendships. Well, our friendship survived another book. Despite our stubborn nature, we managed to work our way through numerous points of contention. While painful at times, hopefully, this process has resulted in a better book. Will we write another book together? Anything is possible, we suppose.

We would like to thank the other contributors to this book. Joe Torgesen, Cheryl Scott, Carol Wesby, and Pat Clauser were gracious enough to take time out of their busy schedules to revise and/or contribute new chapters. Thank you. Special thanks also go to Kathy Fulmer for proofreading the entire book and completing the index. The staff at Allyn and Bacon, particularly Steve Dragin and Liz McGuire, have been very helpful and supportive throughout the writing of the book. We would also like to acknowledge the support we have received from our respective departments at the University of Kansas and University of Memphis.

We'd would also like to formally acknowledge and thank all the people who took the time to share their comments with us and especially thank those people who told us how our work has led to better services for children with language and learning problems. Like most academics who are accustomed to criticism, we were slightly uncomfortable accepting praise and hope that this discomfort did not make us appear too abrupt with anyone. The so-called ivory towers in which academics work are obviously a very different world than the one practitioners and students with language-learning problems live in. Your comments are an important bridge between these worlds.

Acknowledgments are, of course, not complete without the recognition of friends and family. Thanks for giving us the support and encouragement necessary to complete this project. Finally, we would like to dedicate this book to our parents for providing the kind of home environment that instilled in us a lifelong desire to explore the new worlds of people, places, and most importantly, ideas.

Contributors and Affiliations

Editors

Hugh W. Catts, Ph.D.
Department of Speech-Language-
Hearing: Sciences and Disorders
University of Kansas
Lawrence, KS

Alan G. Kamhi, Ph.D.
The School of Audiology and
  Speech Pathology
University of Memphis
Memphis, TN

Contributors

Patricia Clauser, MS, CCC-SLP
Educational Researcher
University of New Mexico
Albuquerque, NM

Cheryl M. Scott, Ph.D.
Department of Speech and
Language Pathology and Audiology
Oklahoma State University
Stillwater, OK

Joseph K. Torgesen, Ph.D.
Department of Psychology
Florida State University
Tallahassee, FL

Carol E. Westby, Ph.D.
Communication Disorders and Sciences
Wichita State University
Center for Family and Community
  Partnerships
University of New Mexico

Language and Reading
Disabilities

Chapter *1*

Language and Reading: Convergences and Divergences

ALAN G. KAMHI   *HUGH W. CATTS*

It is now well accepted that reading is a language-based skill. This was not the case ten years ago when we first wrote this chapter. Ten years ago, the idea that most reading disabilities were best viewed as a developmental language disorder was an emerging one. A developmental language perspective of reading disabilities was the major theme of our original book and continues to be the major theme of the present book. This view rests, in part, on the fact that there are numerous similarities between spoken and written language. Reading shares many of the same processes and knowledge bases as talking and understanding. Reading, however, is not a simple derivative of spoken language. Although spoken language and reading have much in common in terms of the knowledge and processes they tap, there are also fundamental, nontrivial differences between the two. Knowledge of the similarities and differences between spoken language and reading is critical for understanding how children learn to read and why some children have difficulty learning to read. In this chapter, we begin by defining language and reading. This is followed by an in-depth comparison of the processes and knowledge involved in understanding spoken and written language. Other differences between spoken and written language are then discussed.

Defining Language

Definitions of language are broad based and highly integrative. An example of such a definition is offered by the American Speech-Language-Hearing Association (ASHA, 1983, p. 44).

1

Language is a complex and dynamic system of conventional symbols that is used in various modes for thought and communication. Contemporary views of human language hold that: (a) language evolves within specific historical, social, and cultural contexts; (b) language, as rule-governed behavior, is described by at least five parameters—phonologic, morphologic, syntactic, semantic, and pragmatic; (c) language learning and use are determined by the interaction of biological, cognitive, psychosocial, and environmental factors; and (d) effective use of language for communication requires a broad understanding of human interaction including such associated factors as nonverbal cues, motivation, and sociocultural roles.

As reflected in the definition, it is generally agreed that there are five parameters of language. These parameters are described briefly below.

Phonology

Phonology is the aspect of language concerned with the rules that govern the distribution and sequencing of speech sounds. It includes a description of what the sounds are and their component features (phonetics) as well as the distributional rules that govern how the sounds can be used in various word positions and the sequence rules that describe which sounds may be combined. For example, the /ʒ/ sound that occurs in the word *measure* is never used to begin an English word. Distributional rules are different in different languages. In French, for example, the /ʒ/ sound can occur in the word-initial position, as in *je* and *jouer.* An example of a sequence rule in English would be that /r/ can follow /t/ or /d/ in an initial consonant cluster (e.g., *truck, draw*), but /l/ cannot.

Semantics

Semantics is the aspect of language that governs the meaning of words and word combinations. Sometimes semantics is divided into lexical and relational semantics. *Lexical semantics* involves the meaning conveyed by individual words. Words have both intensional and extensional meanings. Intensional meanings refer to the defining characteristics or criterial features of a word. A dog is a dog because it has four legs, barks, and licks people's faces. The extension of a word is the set of objects, entities, or events to which a word might apply in the world. The set of all real or imaginary dogs that fit the intensional criteria becomes the extension of the entity *dog.*

Relational semantics refers to the relationships that exist between words. For example, in the sentence *The Panda bear is eating bamboo*, the word *bear* not only has a lexical meaning, but it also is the agent engaged in the activity of eating. *Bamboo* is referred to as the "patient" (Chafe, 1970) because its state is being changed by the action of the verb. Words are thus seen as expressing abstract relational meanings in addition to their lexical meanings.

Morphology

In addition to the content words that refer to objects, entities, and events, there is a group of words and inflections that convey subtle meaning and serve specific grammatical and pragmatic functions. These words have been referred to as *grammatical morphemes*. Grammatical morphemes modulate meaning. Consider the sentences *Dave is playing tennis, Dave plays tennis, Dave played tennis,* and *Dave has played tennis.* The major elements of meaning are similar in each of these sentences. The first sentence describes an action currently in progress, whereas the next sentence depicts a habitual occurrence. The last two sentences describe actions that have taken place sometime in the past. What differentiates these sentences are the grammatical morphemes (inflections and auxiliary forms) that change the tense and aspect (e.g., durative or perfective) of the sentences.

Syntax

Syntax refers to the rule system that governs how words are combined into larger meaningful units of phrases, clauses, and sentences. Syntactic rules specify word order, sentence organization, and the relationships between words, word classes, and sentence constituents, such as noun phrases and verb phrases. Knowledge of syntax enables an individual to make judgments of well-formedness or grammaticality. For example, all mature English speakers would judge the sentence *The boy hit the ball* as well formed and grammatical. In contrast, the sentence *Hit the boy ball the* would be judged as ungrammatical. It should be apparent that knowledge of syntax plays an important role in understanding language.

Pragmatics

Pragmatics concerns the use of language in context. Language does not occur in a vacuum. It is used to serve a variety of communication functions, such as declaring, greeting, requesting information, and answering questions. Communicative intentions are best achieved by being sensitive to the listener's communicative needs and nonlinguistic context. Speakers must take into account what the listener knows and does not know about a topic. Pragmatics thus encompasses rules of conversation or discourse. Speakers must learn how to initiate conversations, take turns, maintain and change topics, and provide the appropriate amount of information in a clear manner. Different kinds of discourse contexts involve different sets of rules (Lund & Duchan, 1993; Schiffrin, 1994). The most frequent kinds of discourse children encounter are conversational, classroom, narrative, and event discourse.

Defining Reading

Reading, like language, is a complex cognitive activity. Gates (1949), for example, defined reading as "a complex organization of patterns of higher mental processes . . . [that] . . . can and should embrace all types of thinking, evaluating, judging, imagining, reasoning, and problem-solving" (p. 3). A view of reading that emphasizes higher-level thinking processes is a broad view of reading (Perfetti, 1986). Thinking guided by print is another way to characterize a broad view of reading. Reading ability defined in this way is associated with skill in comprehending texts. Although this is a widely accepted view of reading, particularly among practitioners, there are both practical and theoretical problems with this broad definition.

 The basic problem is that with a broad definition of reading, a theory of reading necessarily becomes a theory of inferencing, a theory of schemata, and a theory of learning

(Perfetti, 1986). Another problem is that every one of the higher-level thinking processes listed by Gates, for example, can be achieved by individuals who cannot read. For this reason, Gough and his colleagues (Gough & Tunmer, 1986; Hoover & Gough, 1990) proposed what they called a "simple" view of reading. The central claim of the simple view is that reading consists of two components, decoding and comprehension. Decoding refers to word recognition processes that transform print to words. Comprehension, which refers to linguistic (listening) comprehension, is defined as the process by which words, sentences, and discourses are interpreted (Gough & Tunmer, 1986). Also included within this component are higher-level thinking processes. Decoding and linguistic comprehension are both important in this model. Decoding in the absence of comprehension is not reading, just as comprehension without decoding is not reading.

Gough's simple view of reading has appealed to many researchers and practitioners. Some researchers, however, prefer restricting the definition of reading to just the decoding component (e.g., Crowder, 1982). One advantage of this narrow view of reading is that it delineates a restricted set of processes to be examined (Perfetti, 1986). Crowder (1982), who advocates a decoding definition of reading, made the following analogy between the "psychology of reading" and the "psychology of braille." The psychology of braille does not include such topics as inferences and schema application. These abilities involve broad-based cognitive-linguistic processes. Crowder argued that it was superfluous to make the study of these higher-level processes part of the study of braille. The study of braille is necessarily restricted to the decoding process, or how a reader decodes braille to language. By analogy, the study of reading should also be restricted to the decoding process.

These different views of reading would necessarily be associated with different levels of literacy. Perfetti (1986), for example, has suggested that basic literacy conforms to a narrow definition of reading, whereas intelligent literacy conforms to the broad definition. Another level of literacy, falling somewhere in between basic and intelligent literacy, would be associated with Gough's simple view of reading. Developmentally, the decoding and simple views of reading are more applicable to children learning to read, whereas the complex thinking definition is more applicable to older children and adults who read to learn.

Models of Spoken and Written Language Comprehension

In a book about language and reading, an understanding of the similarities and differences between spoken and written language is crucial. The sections that follow compare the specific processes and knowledge involved in comprehending spoken and written language. First, however, a brief overview of models of language and reading is necessary.

Models of spoken and written language comprehension have often been divided into three general classes: bottom-up, top-down, and interactive. Bottom-up models view spoken and written language comprehension as a step-by-step process that begins with the initial detection of an auditory or visual stimulus. The initial input goes through a series of stages in which it is "chunked" in progressively larger and more meaningful units. Top-down models, in contrast, emphasize the importance of scripts, schemata, and inferences that allow one to make hypotheses and predictions about the information being processed. Familiarity with the content, structure, and function of the different kinds of spoken and written discourse enables the listener and the reader to be less dependent on low-level perceptual information to construct meanings.

Reliance on top-down versus bottom-up processes varies with the material being processed and the skill of the reader. Bottom-up processes are presumed to be necessary when reading isolated, decontextualized words, whereas top-down processes facilitate not only word recognition but also discourse-level comprehension. Top-down processes are especially important when reading partially illegible material, such as cursive writing.

Many language and reading theorists (Butler, 1984; Duchan, 1983; Perfetti, 1985; Rumelhart, 1977; Stanovich, 1985) have advocated interactive models in which both bottom-up and top-down processes contribute to reading and language comprehension. An interactive model of reading comprehension, for example, would acknowledge that individuals must have proficient word recognition skills as well as higher-level linguistic and conceptual knowledge in order to be good readers. Whereas bottom-up and top-down models emphasize sequential processing, interactive models allow for parallel or simultaneous processing to occur. Later stages could thus begin before earlier stages have been completed. Although more complex than serial processing models, parallel processing models better reflect the types of processing that occur in complex tasks such as reading.

Recent models of language and reading emphasize connectionist parallel distributed-processes. These models are sometimes referred to as "asymbolic" because they are not preprogrammed with rules and do not specify the nature of the representations at various processing levels. Instead, behavioral patterns are achieved by adjusting connections among networks of simple processing units based on feedback about the adequacy of the output from response units. For example, in word recognition, visually presented words activate orthographic units, which activate a set of hidden units, which in turn activate phonological units. A learning algorithm adjusts the weights of units based on the accuracy of the system's output (Plaut, McClelland, Seidenberg, & Patterson, 1996; Rumelhart, Hinton, & Williams, 1986; Seidenberg & McClelland, 1989). A detailed review of parallel processing models of spoken and written language processing is beyond the scope of this chapter. For our purposes, it is sufficient to note that simplistic serial processing models, whether bottom-up or top-down, cannot adequately capture the complex interactions that occur within and between different processing levels.

Comprehending Spoken and Written Language

We have found that the model depicted in Figure 1-1 provides a useful framework for comparing the processes and knowledge involved in comprehending spoken and written language. This model, though unique, shares components with other processing models (Gough & Tunmer, 1986; Thomson, 1984). Although the components of the model will be discussed in a linear, bottom-up fashion, the model should be viewed as an interactive one that allows for parallel processing within and between levels.

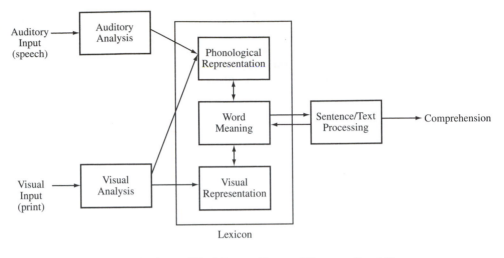

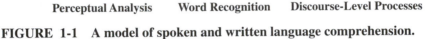

Perceptual Analysis   **Word Recognition**   **Discourse-Level Processes**

FIGURE 1-1   A model of spoken and written language comprehension.

Perceptual Analyses

The input to the perceptual analysis is speech or print. In order for this input to be recognized, it must be detected and analyzed. The sensory mechanisms involved in the detection of speech and print are distinctive; the ear is used to detect speech and the eye is used to detect print. Sensory deficits involving hearing or vision place a child at risk for spoken and written language problems. Children born deaf cannot detect the speech signal through the auditory modality and, as a result, have considerable difficulty developing intelligible speech. Individuals who are blind cannot detect print through the visual modality. Braille, which relies on the tactile modality, is one way to bypass the visual deficit. An intact auditory system provides the blind another avenue to access text material by way of tape recordings.

Once the input has been detected, the segmental and suprasegmental features of spoken and written words are analyzed. In speech the processes underlying phonetic discrimination and phonemic identification are involved. *Phonetic discrimination* refers to the ability to hear the difference between two sounds that differ acoustically and phonetically. For example, the initial *t* in the word *tap* is phonetically different from the final *t* in the word *bat*. Phonetic differences that do not affect meaning are often referred to as *allophonic variations*. If the *t* sounds in the words above were changed to *k* sounds, this would change the meaning of the words. *Tap* would become *cap*, and *bat* would become *back*. The phonetic differences between /t/ and /k/ are thus also phonemic differences because they change the meaning of the word. The task for the young child learning language is to determine which differences between sounds make a difference in meaning.

The language a child is learning determines which phonetic differences are phonemic. In Japanese, for example, the differences between /r/ and /l/ are allophonic. In English, however, the phonetic differences between /r/ and /l/ make a difference in meaning. In French the front rounded vowel /y/ is phonemically different from the back rounded /u/. An American who does not make this distinction will not be able to differentiate between the words *tout* (all) and *tu* (you). These examples are meant to illustrate that learning phonemic categories requires knowledge of the language being learned. The acquisition of phonological knowledge about language necessarily involves higher-level conceptual processes. Low-level perceptual processes, such as detection and discrimination, do not lead to knowledge about phonemic categories. In light of these points, it is important to note that in most listening situations, individuals seldom have to make distinctions between minimal phoneme pairs (e.g., *p/b* in the words *pin* and *bin*) that are common stimuli on tests of discrimination. In many instances, lexical and higher-level language knowledge often eliminate the need for phonemic-level identification.

In reading, just as with speech, discrimination and identification processes are involved. In reading, *discrimination* refers to the ability to see the visual differences between letters. *Identification* requires knowledge of the correspondences between letters and phonemes. For example, the child who confuses the letters *b* and *d* in words such as *bad* and *dad* is often said to have a visual discrimination problem. It is more likely, however, that the child can perceive the visual differences between the letters *b* and *d* but has not learned that the letter *b* is associated with the phoneme /b/ and the letter *d* is associated with the phoneme /d/. In other words, the child has not learned the phoneme-letter correspondences for these two sounds.

To illustrate the difference between a low-level visual discrimination ability and a higher-level conceptual (identification) ability, consider the following analogy. In teaching large classes, it is common to confuse students. Last year, the first author called a girl named Aimee, Anna. Although Aimee and Anna are both 20-something female graduate students, they can be easily differentiated by their physical characteristics, personalities, clothes, and so forth. I have no difficulty differentiating between the two students. The problem I have is associating a particular characteristic or a set of characteristics with a name. The similarity between the two names makes it more difficult to consistently use the right name with the right student. This is similar to the problem children have associating the features of a particular phoneme with the features of a particular letter. When letters and sounds are similar, as is the case for "b" and "d," it is particularly difficult to learn the correct correspondences.

These examples are meant to show that sound or letter confusions are not caused by phonetic or visual discrimination problems. With respect to spoken language, the difficulty is learning which phonetic differences make a difference in meaning. With respect to reading, the difficulty is learning which sounds are associated with which letters. In both cases, what often appear to be discrimination problems are in fact identification problems.

Word Recognition

Reading and spoken language begin to share similar knowledge domains and processes in the word recognition stage. Until this point, the processing of print and speech involves different sensory and perceptual processes. In the word recognition stage, the features identified in the previous perceptual stage are used to access the mental lexicon. The words heard or seen must activate or be associated with previously stored concepts in the individual's mental lexicon. These stored concepts in the mental lexicon represent one's vocabulary. Importantly, the content and structure of the mental lexicon is essentially the same for reading and spoken language. The content of the lexicon includes information about the word's phonological or visual form as well as information about the word's meaning and how the word relates to other words. Consider, for example, the kind of conceptual information that might appear in the mental lexicon for the word *pencil.*

> It refers to an instrument used for writing or drawing; it is a manmade physical object, usually cylindrical in shape; and it functions by leaving a trail of graphite along a writing surface. . . . A pencil is one of a class of writing instruments and a close relative of the *pen, eraser,* and *sharpener* (Just & Carpenter, 1987, p. 62)

The mental lexicon also includes syntactic and semantic information that indicates part of speech (e.g., noun, verb, or adjective) and possible syntactic and semantic roles. For example, the syntactic information about *pencil* might indicate that it is a noun that functions semantically as an instrument ("She wrote the letter with a pencil") or as a patient ("Peggy bought a pencil").

The structure of the mental lexicon has received considerable research attention during the past thirty years. Network models consisting of nodes corresponding to concepts and features have been a popular way to depict the structure of the lexicon (Collins & Loftus, 1975; Collins & Quillian, 1969). Early network models were hierarchical in nature, with the ordering in the hierarchy defined by set inclusion relations. For example, higher-order concepts such as *animal* included lower-order concepts such as *bird* and *sparrow.* Other network models have been referred to as *heterarchical,* reflecting concepts from ill-structured domains (Just & Carpenter, 1987). Although theorists might differ in their portrayal of the content and structure of the mental lexicon, they generally agree that the mental lexicon is the same for language and reading. The way in which word meanings are accessed can differ, however, in spoken language and reading.

In processing speech, word meaning is accessed through a word's phonological representation. The output of the perceptual analysis is a representation of a word's acoustic and phonetic features. These acoustic-phonetic representations of speech input are used by the listener to activate or instantiate a word's phonological representation in the lexicon. This may involve the listener attempting to match acoustic-phonetic representations with phonological representations. Phonological representations are directly linked to a word's meaning because this information is stored together for each word in the mental lexicon.

Phonological representations stored in the mental lexicon can take one of several forms. Words may be represented in clusters (e.g., "it's a" as "itsa"; "did you know" as [dIdʒəno]) or as individual words without discrete syllable or phonemic information. Alternatively, phonological representations might contain syllabic and phonemic segments. Although the nature of phonological representations can differ, it is unlikely that preliterate children represent speech as discrete phonemic segments. Young children represent words either as lexical wholes or by syllables (e.g., rimes and onsets). The gradual shift to phonemic-based representations is influenced by reading as well as children's developing speech perception abilities. Recent studies of young children's speech perception (e.g., Nittrouer, Manning, & Meyer, 1993) have found that there is a gradual shift in the acoustic cues used to make phonological decisions. Nittrouer and colleagues hypothesize that as children gain experience with a native language, they become more sensitive to phonetic structure. In a more recent study, Nittrouer (1996) shows that this shift is related to children's developing phonemic awareness. It seems that early exposure to reading as well as developmental changes in speech perception both contribute to young children's ability to represent speech as discrete phonemic segments.

In contrast to speech, in which there is only one way to access a word's meaning, in reading there are two ways: indirectly, by way of a phonological representation, or directly, by way of a visual representation (see Figure 1-1). Use of a visual representation to access the lexicon is variously referred to as the *direct, visual, look-and-say,* or *whole-word* approach. In accessing the lexicon in this way, the reader locates the word in the lexicon whose visual representation contains the same segmental and/or visual features as those identified in the previous perceptual analysis stage. In other words, a match is made between the perceived visual configuration and a visual representation that is part of the mental lexicon for the particular word.

Word meaning can also be accessed through a phonological representation. With this *indirect* or *phonetic* approach, the reader uses knowledge of phoneme-letter correspondence rules to recode the visually perceived letters into their corresponding phonemes. Individual phonemes are then blended together to form a phonological sequence that is matched to a similar sequence in the lexicon. The phonetic approach is particularly important in the development of reading. The ability to decode printed words phonetically allows children to read words they know but have never seen in print. Reading by the phonetic approach also causes the child to attend to the letter sequences within words. The knowledge gained about letter sequence makes the child's visual representations more precise (see Chapter 2).

Reading by the phonetic route is thus similar to speech recognition in that a word is recognized by way of its phonological representation. There is one important difference, however, in using phonological representations to access meaning in comprehending spoken and written language. In order to successfully use the phonetic route in reading, one must have explicit awareness of the phonological structure of words, specifically, the knowledge that words consist of discrete phonemic segments (Liberman, 1983). These segments are not readily apparent to young children because the sound segments of speech are blended together in the acoustic signal. For example, the word *cat* is one acoustic event; its sound segments do not correspond exactly to its three written symbols. Although preschool children might show some phonological awareness, much explicit instruction and practice is usually required for a child to become efficient in using the phonetic approach.

The recognition that there were two possible routes to word recognition led to the popularity of dual-route models of word recognition (cf. Stanovich, 1991). Although early proponents of dual-route models agreed that there were two routes to word recognition, they differed in assumptions about the various speeds of the two access mechanisms and how conflicting information was resolved. The size of the sound-letter correspondences in the phonological route also differed from model to model (e.g., sound-by-sound, syllables, word level). Discussions of the different variations of these models can be found in Coltheart, Curtis, Atkins, and Haller (1993), Patterson and Coltheart (1987), and Rayner and Pollatsek (1989).

Questions about the nature of the print-to-sound conversion have recently taken a new turn due to the increasing popularity of parallel-distributed processing models that contain no word-level representations or lexicon in the network (Share & Stanovich, 1995). Regardless of how the print-to-sound conversion takes place, there is recent evidence that this conversion is essential for the large numbers of low-frequency words that cannot be recognized on a visual basis (Share & Stanovich, 1995). In contrast, high-frequency words seem to be recognized visually with minimal phonological recoding even in the very earliest stages of reading acquisition (Reitsma, 1990). The more exposure a child has to a word, the more likely a visual approach will be used. The use of the a visual versus a phonological approach to word recognition depends on the frequency of the word rather than the particular reading stage a child is in. More will be said about the development of word recognition skills in the next chapter.

Discourse-Level Processes

Up to this point, we have considered the processes involved in recognizing words. Spoken and written language, however, consists of longer discourse units, such as sentences, conversations, lectures, stories, and expository texts. Psycholinguistic studies carried out in the 1960s and 1970s (cf. Carroll, 1994; Clark & Clark, 1977) explored the role that syntactic, semantic, and world knowledge played in comprehending larger units of spoken and written discourse. By focusing on the independent contribution these different types of knowledge made toward meaning, these early studies were limited in what they could tell us about the interaction of different types of knowledge and whether different discourse types are processed the same way by listeners and readers. Despite these limitations, it is useful to consider how structural, propositional, and situation or world knowledge can be used to construct meaning.

Structural Knowledge
A variety of structural cues are used by listeners and readers in comprehending speech and text. These cues include word order, grammatical morphemes, and function words such as relative pronouns, conjunctions, and modals. Listeners and readers often use syntactic and morphologic cues to figure out the meaning of unknown words. Grammatical morphemes, for example, provide information about word classes. Adverbs are signaled by the inflections -*ly* and -*y*, whereas adjectives are marked by the suffixes -*able* and -*al*. Verbs are signaled by the inflections -*ed*, -*ing*, and -*en*. Nouns are marked by definite and indefinite articles, plural and possessive markers, and suffixes such as -*ment* and -*ness*. The reason why readers are able to make any sense at all out of a sentence like "Twas brillig and the slithy toves did gyre and gimble in the wabe" is that inflections (*y* and *s*) and syntactic markers (*the* and *did*) provide cues about grammatical form class.

Clark and Clark (1977) provide an excellent review of studies that demonstrate the influence syntactic and morphologic knowledge has on sentence comprehension. It has been shown, for example, that listeners use function words to segment sentences into constituents, classify the constituents, and construct meanings from them (e.g., Bever, 1970; Fodor & Garrett, 1967). Consider the two sentences below, one with relative pronouns and one without:

1. The pen that the author whom the editor liked used was new.
2. The pen the author the editor liked used was new.

Fodor and Garrett (1967) found that listeners had more difficulty paraphrasing sentences like (2) than sentences like (1). More recent studies have continued to attempt to prove that the initial segmentation of a sentence (i.e., parsing) is performed by a syntactic module that is not influenced by other kinds of knowledge (e.g., Frazier, 1987).

Propositional Knowledge

Although structural knowledge may play an important role in understanding sentences, memory for extended discourse rarely maintains structural information. The fact that we generally store and remember the gist of what we hear or read suggests that processing resources must be devoted primarily to constructing meaningful propositions. A proposition is an *idea-unit* that consists of a predicate and its related arguments. It is generally agreed that listeners and readers use their knowledge of predicates and their inherent arguments to construct propositions. The predicate *give,* for example, requires three noun phrases or arguments: an agent to do the giving, an object to be given, and a recipient of the object. When listeners hear a sentence like *Alison gave the doll to Franne*, they look for the three arguments entailed by the predicate *give.*

A simple semantic strategy suggested years ago by Bever (1970) is that listeners and readers might use content words alone to build propositions that make sense. For example, if the words *pile, raked, girl, leaves* were presented without any other syntactic information, it would be apparent that two propositions were involved: *The girl raked the leaves* and *the leaves were in a pile.* To show that listeners used content words to build propositions, researchers (e.g., Stolz, 1967) showed that semantically constrained sentences (3) were much easier to paraphrase than semantically unconstrained sentences (4).

3. The vase that the maid that the agency hired dropped broke on the floor.
4. The dog that the cat that the girl fought scolded approached the colt.

It has also been shown that propositional complexity influences processing time. Kintsch and Keenan (1973), for example, showed that sentence (5), which contains eight propositions took significantly more time to read than sentence (6), which contained only four propositions. Note that the two sentences have about the same number of words.

5. Cleopatra's downfall lay in her foolish trust in the fickle political figures of the Roman world.
6. Romulus, the legendary founder of Rome, took the women of the Sabine by force.

Subsequent studies have examined the hierarchical networks of propositions that listeners and readers construct to link propositions within spoken discourse and text. Not surprisingly, researchers have found that the propositions listeners and readers construct are affected by many factors, such as nature of the discourse/text, knowledge of the world, processing capacity, interest level, and so forth.

World Knowledge

Structural and propositional knowledge are crucial for constructing meaning, but an individual's knowledge of the world or what has come to be called *situation model representations* also plays an important role in comprehension. Consider, for example, how world knowledge makes the sentence *Jake ate the ice cream with relish* unambiguous while a similar sentence *Jake ate the sausage with relish* is ambiguous (Just & Carpenter, 1987). We know that relish is normally not eaten with ice cream. Such information is not specific to language; instead, it reflects general knowledge about the tastes of foods to assign with *relish*.

World knowledge can be divided into knowledge of specific content domains and knowledge of interpersonal relations. Specific content domains would include academic subjects such as history, geography, mathematics, and English literature; procedural knowledge such as how to fix a car, tie a shoelace, and play tennis; and scriptlike knowledge of familiar events. Interpersonal knowledge involves such things as knowledge of human needs, motivations, attitudes, emotions, values, behavior, personality traits, and relationships. It should be evident how these kinds of world knowledge play an important role in processing spoken and written language.

Because world knowledge can be so broad, psychologists have focused attention on the situation-specific world knowledge that listeners and readers use to construct meaning (e.g., van Dijk & Kintsch, 1983). The assumption is that as we process discourse, we construct a mental or situational model of the world as described by the discourses.

Models of Discourse Processing

In order to understand larger units of spoken and written discourse, it is necessary not only to construct representations that consider structural, propositional, and situational information, but also to relate these representations to one another. One must also use this information to make inferences about meaning and make decisions about which information should be remembered. Given the variety of knowledge types and cognitive processes involved in discourse processing, no one model can expect to capture all of these facets of discourse processing. It is useful, however, to consider the kinds of models that have been proposed. Although these models deal primarily with how readers construct meaning from texts, their basic principles can be applied to spoken language discourse as well.

Kintsch and van Dijk's (1978, 1983) initial model of text comprehension proposed that multiple levels of representation were needed to construct meanings based on different kinds of knowledge. Three levels of representation correspond to the three knowledge types: structural, propositional, and knowledge of the situation/world.

This initial model of comprehension relied on schema-driven, top-down processing to build the knowledge of the world (i.e., situation model) represention. Kintsch (1988), however, felt that these notions were not adaptive to new contexts and were too inflexible. Studies of these different levels of representation found that when readers and listeners had extensive world knowledge, they attended to and remembered their world knowledge of the situation rather than the information actually in the text. In contrast, when reading expository text or listening to new lecture information, individuals relied primarily on information in the text. Kintsch's more recent models can handle these differences whereas the earlier models could not.

Speech-language pathologists, special educators, and other educators are probably familiar with models of text processing based on scripts and schemas. Although psychologists have moved beyond these notions, they still work well for understanding how children construct meaning for certain prototype forms of discourse such as familiar events and stories. A schema is generally thought of as a structure in memory that specifies a general or expected arrangement of a body of information. Familiar events, for example, are well captured by scripts, which are a particular type of schema. Scripts contain slots for the components of an event, such as the main actions, participants, goals, and typical position of each action. Scripts make it easier to process familiar events by providing individuals with a coherent structure into which they can insert new information. Scripts also allow individuals to add necessary information that might be omitted in spoken or written discourse. For example, familiarity with a restaurant script allows listeners and readers to anticipate some mention of the menu. If no mention of the menu is made, but information about the kind of restaurant is given (e.g., Italian), one can infer the contents of the menu.

Certain types of discourse, such as stories, seem to have a consistent structure or grammar. This was recognized years ago when researchers proposed that stories had a common story grammar or schema. A story schema can be viewed as a mental framework that contains slots for each story component, such as a setting, goal, obstacle, and resolution. Story grammars represent a slightly different characterization of the knowledge of story structures. Story grammars specify the hierarchical relations among the components more directly than a story schema (Mandler & Johnson, 1977; Stein & Glenn, 1979). Story grammars attempt to specify the structural organization of stories in the same way that syntactic grammars specify the structural organization of sentences (Just & Carpenter, 1987, p. 231). The main structural components of a story are a setting and an episode. The setting introduces the characters and the context of the story. Episodes can be further divided into an initiating event, internal response, attempt, consequence, and reaction. Knowledge of the structure and function of stories, like knowledge of scripts, can facilitate comprehension of spoken and written language (Just & Carpenter, 1987; Perfetti, 1985).

Other Metaphors for Discourse and Text Understanding

The notion that multiple sources of knowledge or representations are involved in processing discourse and text is an important one for understanding what is involved in comprehension. There are other notions, however, about comprehension that are important as well. Graesser and Britton (1996) have found that five metaphors capture the essence of the various ways of thinking about text comprehension. The first metaphor, understanding is the assembly of a multileveled representation, has already been discussed. Speech-language pathologists and other educators are familiar with at least two of the other metaphors: Understanding is the process of managing working memory and understanding is inference generation. The two metaphors we may not be familiar with are: Understanding is the construction of a coherent representation and understanding is a complex dynamical system. To these five metaphors, we will add a sixth: Understanding is a metacognitive ability. Although Graesser and Britton apply these metaphors to text understanding, in most cases, they can be applied to spoken discourse as well. Each of these metaphors will be discussed briefly below.

Understanding is the management of working memory. Most psychologists and educators are comfortable with the assumption that comprehension is managed in a limited capacity working memory. Every educator has had first-hand experience with this metaphor. For example, when the demands of comprehension exceed the limitations of working memory, students' comprehension decreases dramatically. Students with low working memory spans often experience difficulty when comprehension components tax working memory. Poor comprehenders have also been shown to have problems suppressing irrelevant information from working memory (Gernsbacher, 1996).

Understanding is inference generation. The ability to construct meaning requires more than interpreting explicit propositions. It involves accessing relevant world knowledge and generating inferences that are needed to make sentences cohere (local coherence) and to relate text to world knowledge (global coherence). Two main types of inferences have been identified (Just & Carpenter, 1987): backward and forward inferences. *Backward inferences* are variously referred to as bridging assumptions (Clark & Clark, 1977), integrative inferences, or connective inferences. Consider the sentences *He walked into the classroom* and *The chalk was gone.* In these sentences, there is no previous mention of *the chalk.* In order to make sense of these sentences, one must infer that the classroom should have chalk in it. More specifically, the inference (or implicature) *The room referred to by a room once had chalk in it* must be added to the representation of the two sentences actually spoken or written. *Forward inferencing* embellishes or elaborates the representation of the currently spoken or read text. For example, given the sentence *The two-year-old was eating ice cream*, a forward inference might be that the child's face was smeared with ice cream.

Inferences can also be distinguished according to whether they are derived from the content of activated world knowledge structures (e.g., scripts and schemas) or whether they are novel constructions that are needed to construct the situation model. Inferences that are generated from existing world knowledge tend to be generated "online." Graesser and Britton (1996) argue that a satisfactory model of text understanding should be able to accurately predict inferences that are quickly or automatically made during comprehension as well as those that are time-consuming. Inferences generated online include those that address readers' goals, assist in establishing local or global coherence, and are highly activated from multiple information sources (e.g., Long, Seely, Oppy, & Golding, 1996). Inferences that are more time-consuming may be caused by minimal world knowledge about the topic or by contradictions, anomalies, or irrelevant propositions in the text. Readers attempt to generate explanations and justifications to resolve the contradictions and anomalies. The process of generating these "elaborative inferences" is necessarily time-consuming and may not be used by readers with low motivation (Graesser & Britton, 1996, p. 350).

Understanding is the construction of coherent representations. The basic notion with this metaphor is that the more coherent the discourse or text, the easier it is to understand. A text is fully connected if every proposition is conceptually connected to one or more other propositions. Some theorists, following Kintsch (1974), believe that noun-phrase arguments are critical for connecting propositions and establishing coherence. More recent research, however, has shown that argument overlap is neither a necessary nor sufficient condition for establishing coherence; instead, it is merely one type of connection (cf. Graesser & Britton, 1996). Other types of connections that have been considered include the connections between predicates of propositions (Turner, Britton, Andraessen, & McCutchen, 1996), causal connections and goals of story characters (van den Broek, Risden, Fletcher, & Thurlow, 1996), and the connections that tie deep metaphors to lexical items and explicit expressions (Gibbs, 1996).

Despite the challenge of identifying the specific types of connections that tie texts together, the "understanding-as-coherence" metaphor makes a large number of predictions about comprehension performance. Most of these predictions are generally intuitive. For example, a proposition has a greater likelihood of being recalled when it has more connections to other propositions in the text, and reading time increases when there is a break in coherence. However, some are counterintuitive. For example, Mannes and St. George (1996) found that there are more connections (or stronger ones) between text and world knowledge if there is a discrepancy between an outline and text content. The discrepancy causes improved problem solving, though recall for the text suffers.

Understanding is a complex dynamic system. As mentioned earlier in this chapter, static, linear models of spoken and written language may be useful to identify specific processes and knowledge domains, but they do not have the flexibility to handle complex dynamic systems such as comprehension. A detailed description of a dynamic text comprehension model is beyond the scope of this chapter (cf. Graesser & Britton, 1996). It is interesting to note, however, that even researchers committed to these models recognize the difficulty involved in testing their psychological plausibility (Graesser & Britton, 1996, p. 347). Despite the difficulty in determining which dynamic model provides the best "goodness of fit," no cognitive theorist has rejected the "understanding is a complex dynamic system" metaphor.

Understanding is a metacognitive ability. Metacognition refers to one's knowledge and control of one's cognitive system (Brown, 1987). Metacognitive abilities have been associated with several aspects of reading, including establishing the purpose for reading, identifying important ideas, activating prior knowledge, evaluating the text for clarity, compensating for failure to understand, and assessing one's level of comprehension (Brown, 1987). Brown added that it is not clear whether all or just certain components of these activities are metacognitive.

The ability to monitor comprehension plays an important role in both spoken and written language comprehension (Dollaghan & Kaston, 1986; Markman, 1977). When faced with a word, sentence, paragraph, or other text element that is not understood, it is necessary to do something to aid understanding, such as ask for clarification or reread the text in question. Individuals who are adept at monitoring their comprehension are more proficient processors of spoken and written language.

Summary

We have attempted in this section to provide a way of thinking about the knowledge and processes involved in understanding spoken and written language. While the emphasis has been primarily on the similarity of knowledge and processes, some important differences in the word recognition processes were acknowledged. In our discussion of discourse comprehension processes, we tended to treat research as if it applied both to spoken and written language comprehension when, in fact, it rarely did. Our assumption here was that a model of comprehension that is sufficiently dynamic, flexible, and multifaceted would apply equally well to spoken and written discourse. Although the six metaphors discussed were meant to illuminate the different aspects of comprehension, perhaps they made a complete muddle of comprehension for some. Graesser and Britton (1996) thought that after reading through their book on text understanding with all its different models and views of comprehension someone might ask, "What is text understanding?" Readers of this chapter might wonder the same thing about our view of comprehension. With a slight modification to include discourse as well as text comprehension, the definition of comprehension Graesser and Britton suggest provides a good answer to the question.

> Text [and discourse] understanding is the dynamic process of constructing coherent representations and inferences at multiple levels of text and context, within the bottleneck of a limited-capacity working memory. (p. 350)

Having emphasized the similarities between spoken and written language up to this point, in the next section we consider some of the differences between the two.

Differences between Spoken and Written Language

Delineating the similarities and differences in the processes and knowledge involved in spoken and written language comprehension only begins to capture the complex relationship that exists between language and reading. Consider, for example, the following question posed by Gleitman and Rozin (1977, p. 2): Why is the more general and complex task of learning to speak and understand less difficult and less variable than what appears to be a trivial derivative of this (i.e., learning to read and write)? These authors proceed to point out two major differences between learning to talk and learning to read. We add a third important difference.

The first major difference is that learning to read requires explicit knowledge of the phonological aspects of speech. To become an efficient reader, one must learn the various correspondences between phonemes and letters. The knowledge that words consist of discrete phonemes is crucial for constructing phoneme-grapheme correspondence rules. Spoken language comprehension also requires analysis of utterances into smaller phonological units. But the analysis of the speech stream by the listener is carried out below the level of consciousness by evolutionarily old and highly adapted auditory perceptual processes (Lieberman, 1973). The human perceptual system is thus biologically adapted to process speech. In contrast, the human visual system is not biologically adapted to process written text. This introduces the second major difference between learning to talk and learning to read: Reading is a comparatively new and arbitrary human ability for which specific biological adaptations do not yet exist.

A third important difference is that almost all humans are reared in environments in which spoken language is the principal means of communication. Thus, not only are we biologically endowed to learn language, but we are socialized to use language to communicate. This is not true for reading. More than 40 percent of the world's adult population cannot read or write at all, and an additional 25 percent do not have sufficient mastery of a writing system for it to be of significant practical use (Stubbs, 1980, cited in Perera, 1984). The principal reason for this high rate of illiteracy is that individuals are raised in environments in which reading has little cultural value.

Perera (1984) points out additional differences between spoken and written language. An understanding of these differences helps to further explain why reading is not a simple derivative of spoken language. The differences discussed in the following sections, however, in no way diminish the language bases of reading and reading disabilities.

In order to emphasize the contrasts between written and spoken language, Perera compared prototypical speech (conversation) to prototypical written language (literature or informative prose). She acknowledged, however, that there is a full range of spoken and written discourse types. Certain discourse types have some characteristics of written language and vice versa. For example, speeches and lectures can be planned much like writing, radio talk lacks a visual dimension and contextual support, and tape recordings are durable.

Physical Differences

Whereas speech consists of temporally ordered sounds, writing consists of marks made on a surface (e.g., paper) in a two-dimensional space. As such, writing is relatively durable; it can be read and reread. Speech, unless it is recorded, is ephemeral. It has no existence independent of the speaker. The durability of writing gives the reader control over how fast or slow to read. Certain texts can be savored, whereas others can be skimmed. The listener, in contrast, is tied to the fleeting speech of the speaker. Missed words or sentences will be lost if clarification is not requested.

Perera (1984, p. 161) noted that readers often have the benefit of a whole range of visual cues, such as running headlines, different-size type, color, and summaries or abstracts. In addition, a device such as the footnote allows the writer to provide additional information without interrupting the main thread of the text. Such devices allow the reader to decide the level at which he or she will read. The listener, in contrast, is completely dependent on the speaker's selection of material. Note, however, that the listener could choose not to listen to the speaker's message.

Situational Differences

The most frequent type of spoken language is face-to-face communication. Conversations are often interactive exchanges between two or more individuals. Questions are followed by answers, requests by responses, and statements by acknowledgments. When a listener does not understand something, a clarification is requested. Careful planning is not the rule in conversational discourse. When speakers pause too long before talking, they will usually be interrupted. Despite this time pressure to speak, misunderstandings are infrequent; when they occur, they are easily resolved by repeating or rephrasing the message. Nonverbal communication acts, such as gestures, facial expressions, and body postures, can help to clarify messages. Speakers and listeners also share the same nonlinguistic setting. People and objects that are visible can be referred to by pronouns rather than by noun phrases (even without prior reference), and many adverbials and prepositions can be expressed by *here, there,* and *like this.*

In contrast, writing and reading are often individual endeavors. The writer receives no prompting about what to write and no immediate feedback on the clarity of the writing. But the writer is generally under less severe time constraints and can thus take more time to search for the best way to express a message. The writer can also correct and revise a text until a final copy is produced. Such care and precision is necessary in writing because there are no contextual and nonverbal cues to aid comprehension. The written text thus has to bear the whole burden of communication, which is one reason why writing is usually more precise than talking.

Functional Differences

One of the earliest needs to generate a writing system was to retain accurate records of property, commercial transactions, and legal judgments. A Chinese proverb holds that "The palest ink is better than the best memory." Writing has enabled the knowledge of centuries to accumulate, thus allowing each new generation to build on the ideas, discoveries, and inventions of the generation or generations before. Many academic subjects, such as history, geography, the physical sciences, and social sciences, owe their very existence to writing (Perera, 1984, p. l64). Another function not served by speech is labeling. Although speech is used to label objects in a referential sense, written labels serve more of an information function. Consider such labels as street names, signposts, nameplates on theaters and public buildings, brand labels, and danger warnings. Written language can also serve a variety of communicative functions, such as relating stories, events, and experiences or sharing information; and making requests. Finally, a specialized function of writing is found in literature. Societies have oral literatures, but oral literatures are restricted to a few types, such as ballads, epic poetry, drama, folk stories, and myths. Essays, novels, diaries, and memoirs are some of the genres that are particular to writing.

Perera has suggested that the most basic uses of writing involve the recording of facts, ideas, and information. Although speech also has an informative function, an equally important function of speech is the role it plays in establishing and maintaining human relationships. A large part of everyday speech with friends, acquaintances, and other individuals serves social-interpersonal functions rather than intellectual ones.

One advantage writing has over speech, according to Perera (1984, p. l65), is that it allows ideas to be explored at leisure and in private. Writing can thus become a means of extending and clarifying one's thinking and ideas. Often in conversation when a controversial topic is raised, there is a tendency for opinions to polarize. Someone who tries to take both sides of a issue might be pressed to select one particular view. In writing, however, one can take time to develop a line of thought, weigh opposing arguments, notice errors in reasoning, and develop new lines of thinking.

Form Differences

The most obvious difference in form is that speech consists of sounds whereas written language consists of letters. As indicated earlier, this would not be so much of a problem if speech sounds (i.e., phonemes) stood in one-to-one correspondence with written letters. Form differences between spoken and written language are not limited to the discrete segments (i.e., phonemes and letters) that make up speech and text. Spoken and written language also differ in how they represent suprasegmental, paralinguistic, and prosodic features. *Paralinguistic features* include pitch and timbre differences that distinguish male and female voices; general voice quality, such as breathiness, hoarseness, or nasality; and the general manner of how an utterance is produced, such as shouted, whispered, or spoken. Perera has pointed out that these features do not usually affect the actual meaning of an utterance; however, they may reflect the speaker's attitude about what is being said.

Prosodic features include intonation, stress, and rhythm. Perera presented four functions of prosodic features: (1) to enable the communicative intent of an utterance to differ from its grammatical form (e.g., *He's lost it* versus *He's lost it?*), (2) to group words into information units, (3) to place emphasis, and (4) to convey the speaker's attitude. These functions differ in the extent to which they can be reflected in writing. Whereas punctuation effectively changes the communicative intent of an utterance, it is not so effective in signaling which words belong together in information units. Italics, underlining, and the use of capital letters are some ways to distribute emphasis throughout a written utterance. But heavy use of these devices in formal writing is usually discouraged. Expressing attitudes in writing is clearly difficult. Perera (1984, p. 178) provided an example of how much attitudinal information is conveyed by prosodic features in the following quote of a journalist who listened to one of the Watergate tapes:

> Once you hear the tapes, and the tone in which he (Nixon) uttered the comments which previously have only been available in a neutral transcript, any last shred of doubt about his guilt must disappear.

Perera goes on to consider the extent to which the writing system represents the segmental and suprasegmental aspects of speech. Among other things, she pointed out that graphemes represent the "citation" (well-spoken) form of words rather than the degraded productions that often occur in fast speech (e.g., compare "did you know" to [dɪdʒəno]). Punctuation can signal the grammatical function of a sentence and mark some prosodic boundaries. The writer, however, has no conventional way to express voice quality, volume, rate of speech, rhythm, and intonational patterns.

Grammatical Differences

Samples of spoken language uncover relatively high frequencies of coordination, repetition, and rephrasing. Conversational discourse is typcally low in lexical density and high in redundancy. Lexical items are spaced out, separated by grammatical words, and a high number of total words are used to convey a relatively small amount of information. Written language, in contrast, is high in lexical density and low in redundancy. This results from the use of grammatical structures that decrease redundancy and increase lexical density.

Perera has suggested that in conversation it is more common to provide small amounts of information at a time. Most written language, by contrast, is more dense lexically as well as propositionally. Conversations, because of their interactive nature, are generally less coherent than writing. Speakers are free to change the subject at almost any point in a conversation. Topics need not be related in any logical way. In writing, however, an overall theme is necessary. Topic changes must be justified and explicitly made. Writing also has prescribed rules for organizing content. These rules cover the use of topic sentences, paragraph structure, and introductory and concluding statements.

Processing Differences

Earlier in this chapter, we talked about top-down processing models, discourse-level comprehension processes, and the higher-level knowledge schemas that contribute to comprehension of spoken and written language. The focus in these sections was on the commonalities between understanding speech and text. There are very important differences, however, in the contribution higher-level processes make to spoken and written language comprehension. The role of higher-level processes or context effects in reading has received considerable research attention and caused much confusion. One reason for this confusion is that researchers often fail to distinguish between the use of context to facilitate word recognition and the use of context to facilitate text comprehension. Context plays an important role in facilitating text comprehension; it plays a very limited role, however, in facilitating word recognition in good readers.

Support for the limited role of higher-level processes in word recognition comes from eye-movement experiments. Research using various eye-movement methodologies has been consistent in finding that the vast majority of content words in text receive a direct visual fixation (Just & Carpenter, 1987, Rayner & Pollatsek, 1989). Short function words are likely to be skipped, but even many of these receive a direct visual fixation. The span of effective visual information during a fixation is thus quite small, meaning that text is sampled in a very dense manner, even when the words are highly predictable (Balota & Chumbley, 1985).

Based in part on evidence from these eye-movement studies, most recent models of reading have expectancy-based, top-down processes functioning after words have been recognized (Seidenberg, 1985; Till, Mross, & Kintsch, 1988). Higher-level contextual information plays more of a role in speech perception or language processing because of the well-documented ambiguity in decontextualized speech. For example, isolated words from normal conversation are often not recognized out of context. This is not the case, however, for written language. Fluent readers can identify written words out of context with near-perfect accuracy. As Stanovich notes (1986), the physical stimulus alone completely specifies the lexical representation in writing, whereas this is not always true in speech. It is more important in reading, therefore, for the input systems involved in word recognition to deliver a complete and accurate representation of words to higher-level processes. Paradoxically, then, poor readers who have difficulty accurately decoding words must rely more on contextual information than good readers who have proficient word recognition skills. We will say more about the use of good and poor readers' use of contextual information in subsequent chapters.

Basic Factors in Reading and Language Development

It should be clear that although there is considerable overlap in the processes involved in spoken and written language, there are also many important differences between the two. These differences explain to a large extent why learning to read is not a simple derivative of learning to talk and understand. In the definition of language given earlier in this chapter, language learning and use were said to be determined by the interaction of biological, cognitive, psychosocial, and environmental factors. Learning to read is also determined by the interaction of these four factors. However, the relative importance or weight of these factors for learning to read is not the same as it is for learning spoken language.

Biological factors are crucial in learning spoken and written language. As indicated earlier, however, one important difference between learning to talk and learning to read is that the analysis of the speech stream is carried out below the level of consciousness by evolutionary old and highly adapted auditory processes. In contrast, the human visual system is not biologically adapted to process written text. By itself, this difference does not necessarily make learning to read more difficult than learning to talk; it does suggest, however, that learning to read requires more attentional resources than learning to talk.

Environmental factors play different but equally important roles in learning spoken and written language. As noted previously, almost all humans are reared in environments in which spoken language is the principal means of communication. Thus, not only are we biologically endowed to learn language, but we are socialized to use language to communicate. It is extremely rare, for example, to find a child who did not develop language because of the absence of environmental input. The case of Genie (Curtiss, 1977) is an example of one of the few documented instances of such a child. As indicated earlier, about 40 percent of the world's adult population cannot read. In most cases, illiteracy is caused by environmental factors. Individuals reared in societies in which reading ability is not of cultural value will probably have little exposure to print and no formal instruction in reading.

Because the biological and social bases of reading are not as strong as they are for spoken language, psychosocial factors, such as motivational and attentional states, often play a more important role in learning to read than in learning to talk. Unless a child has a severe emotional disorder, such as autism, language learning will be relatively unaffected by motivational and attentional states. This is not the case in learning to read because reading requires a considerable amount of motivational and attentional resources. Reading difficulties in individuals with motivational and attentional problems have been well documented (Hallahan, Kauffman, & Lloyd, 1985).

Cognitive factors play a fundamental role in learning spoken and written language because spoken and written language are essentially cognitive achievements. Both rely on basic cognitive processes to encode, store, and retrieve information. In addition, the same store of linguistic and conceptual knowledge is tapped by readers as by speakers and listeners. Metacognitive abilities, however, play a more important role in learning to read than in learning to talk and understand. This is because learning to read requires awareness of the phonological properties of speech, whereas learning to talk requires little if any explicit metalinguistic knowledge. By the time children are able to make explicit metalinguistic judgments—around age 4 or 5—they have progressed through the various developmental language stages.

Summary

It should be clear that there are similarities as well as differences in the knowledge and processes that underlie spoken and written language. The similarities between spoken and written language are most evident in the vocabulary both share. Readers and listeners also rely on common sources of structural, propositional, and world knowledge and have attentional and memory limitations that influence how readily spoken and written language is processed. The most fundamental differences between spoken and written language involve the perceptual and biological/social bases of spoken language and the explicit phonological awareness required to become a proficient reader. Because reading is not a biologically endowed human ability, attention, instructional, and motivational factors play a central role in learning to read. These differences explain to a large extent why learning to read is not a simple derivative of spoken language as well as why some children have difficulty learning to read. In the next chapter, we consider what is involved in becoming a proficient reader.

References

ASHA Committee on Language. (June, 1983). Definition of language, *ASHA, 25,* 44.

Balota, D., & Chumbley, J. (1985). The locus of word-frequency effects in the pronunciation task: Lexical access and/or production? *Journal of Memory and Language, 24,* 89–106.

Bever, T. (1970). The cognitive basis for linguistic structures. In J.R. Hayes (Ed.), *Cognition and the development of language* (pp. 279–352). New York: Wiley.

Brown, A. (1987). Metacognition, executive control, self-regulation and other more mysterious mechanisms. In F. Weinert & R. Kluwe (Eds.), *Metacognition, motivation, and understanding* (pp. 65–116). Hillsdale, NJ: Erlbaum.

Butler, K. (1984). Language processing: Halfway up the down staircase. In G. Wallach & K. Butler (Eds.), *Language learning disabilities in school-age children* (pp. 60–81). Baltimore: Williams & Wilkins.

Carroll, D. (1994). *Psychology of language.* Pacific Grove, CA: Brooks/Cole.

Chafe, W. (1970). *Meaning and the structure of language.* Chicago: The University of Chicago Press.

Clark, H., & Clark, E. (1977). *Psychology and language.* New York: Harcourt Brace Jovanovich.

Collins, A., & Loftus, E. (1975). A spreading activation theory of semantic processing. *Psychological Review, 82,* 407–428.

Collins, A., & Quillian, M. (1969). Retrieval time from semantic memory. *Journal of Verbal Learning and Verbal Behavior, 8,* 240–248.

Coltheart, M., Curtis, B., Atkins, P., & Haller, M. (1993). Models of reading aloud: Dual-route and parallel-distributed-processing approaches. *Psychological Review, 100,* 589–608.

Crowder, R. (1982). *The psychology of reading.* New York: Oxford University Press.

Curtiss, S. (1977). *Genie: A psycholinguistic study of a modern-day 'Wild Child'.* New York: Academic Press.

Dollaghan, C., & Kaston, N. (1986). A comprehension monitoring program for language-impaired children. *Journal of Speech and Hearing Disorders, 51,* 264–271.

Duchan, J. (1983). Language processing and geodesic domes. In T. Gallagher & C. Prutting (Eds.), *Pragmatic assessment and intervention issues in language* (pp. 83–100). San Diego: College-Hill Press.

Fodor, J., & Garrett, M. (1967). Some syntactic determinants of sentential complexity. *Perception and Psychophysics, 2,* 289–296.

Frazier, L. (1987). Sentence processing: A tutorial review. In M. Coltheart (Ed.), *Attention and performance, Vol. XII. The psychology of reading* (pp. 559–586). Hillsdale, NJ: Erlbaum.

Gates, A. (1949). Character and purposes of the yearbook. In N. Henry (Ed.), *The forty eighth yearbook of the National Society for the Study of Education: Part II. Reading in the elementary school* (pp. 1–9). Chicago: University of Chicago Press.

Gernsbacher, M. (1996). The structure-building framework: What it is, what it might also be, and why. In B. Britton & A. Graessner (Eds.), *Models of understanding text* (pp. 289–312). Mahwah, NJ: Erlbaum.

Gibbs, R. (1996). Metaphor as a constraint on text understanding. In B. Britton & A. Graessner, (Eds.), *Models of understanding text* (pp. 215–240). Mahwah, NJ: Erlbaum.

Gleitman, L., & Rozin, P. (1977). The structure and acquisition of reading, 1: Relations between orthographies and the structure of language. In A. Reber & D. Scarborough (Eds.), *Toward a psychology of reading* (pp. 1–53). The proceedings of the CUNY conferences. New York: Wiley.

Gough, P., & Tunmer, W. (1986). Decoding, reading, and reading disability. *Remedial and Special Education, 7,* 6–10.

Graesser, A., & Britton, B. (1996). Five metaphors for text understanding. In A. Graesser & B. Britton (Eds.), *Models of understanding text* (pp. 341–351). Mahwah, NJ: Erlbaum.

Hallahan, D., Kauffman, J., & Lloyd, J. (1985). *Introduction to learning disabilities.* Englewood Cliffs, NJ: Prentice-Hall.

Hoover, W., & Gough, P. (1990). The simple view of reading. *Reading and Writing: An Interdisciplinary Journal, 2,* 127–160.

Just, M., & Carpenter, P. (1987). *The psychology of reading and language comprehension.* Boston: Allyn & Bacon.

Kintsch, W. (1974). *The representation of meaning in memory.* Hillsdale, NJ: Erlbaum.

Kintsch, W. (1988). The role of knowledge in discourse comprehension: A construction-integration model. *Psychological Review, 95,* 163–182.

Kintsch, W., & Keenan, J. (1973). Reading rate as a function of the number of propositions in the base structure of sentences. *Cognitive Psychology, 5,* 257–274.

Kintsch, W., & van Dijk, T. (1978). Toward a model of text comprehension and production. *Psychological Review, 85,* 363–394.

Liberman, I. (1983). A language-oriented view of reading and its disabilities. In H. Myklebust (Ed.), *Progress in learning disabilities* (pp. 81–101). New York: Grune and Stratton.

Lieberman, P. (1973). On the evolution of language: A unified view. *Cognition, 2,* 59–94.

Long, D., Seely, M., Oppy, B., & Golding, J. (1996). The role of inferential processing in reading ability. In B. Britton & A. Graesser (Eds.), *Models of understanding text* (pp. 189–214). Mahwah, NJ: Erlbaum.

Lund, N., & Duchan, J. (1993). *Assessing children's language in naturalistic contexts* (3rd ed.). Englewood Cliffs, NJ: Prentice-Hall.

Mandler, J., & Johnson, N. (1977). Remembrance of things parsed: Story structure and recall. *Cognitive Psychology, 9,* 111–151.

Mannes, S., & St. George, M. (1996). Effects of prior knowledge on text comprehension: A simple modeling approach. In B. Britton & A. Graesser (Eds.), *Models of understanding text* (pp. 115–140). Mahwah, NJ: Erlbaum.

Nittrouer, S. (1996). The relation between speech perception and phonemic awareness: Evidence from low-SES children and children with chronic OM. *Journal of Speech and Hearing Research, 39,* 1059–1070.

Nittrouer, S., Manning, C., & Meyer, G. (1993). The perceptual weighting of acoustic cues changes with linguistic experience. *Journal of the Acoustical Society of America, 94,* S1865.

Patterson, K., & Coltheart, V. (1987). Phonological processes in reading: A tutorial review. In M. Coltheart (Ed.), *Attention and performance* (Vol. 12, pp. 421–447). London: Erlbaum.

Perera, K. (1984). *Children's writing and reading: Analysing classroom language.* Oxford: Blackwell.

Perfetti, C. (1985). *Reading ability.* New York: Oxford University Press.

Perfetti, C. (1986). Cognitive and linguistic components of reading ability. In B. Foorman & A. Siegel (Eds.), *Acquisition of reading skills* (pp. 1–41). Hillsdale, NJ: Erlbaum.

Plaut, D.E., McClelland, J.L., Seidenberg, M.S., & Patterson, K.E. (1996). Understanding normal and impaired reading: Computational principles in quasi-regular domains. *Psychological Review, 103,* 56–115.

Rayner, K., & Pollatsek, A. (1989). *The psychology of reading.* Englewood Cliffs, NJ: Prentice Hall.

Reitsma, P. (1990). Development of orthographic knowledge. In P. Reitsma & L. Verhoeven (Eds.), *Acquisition of reading in Dutch* (pp. 43–64). Dordrecht: Foris.

Rumelhart, D. (1977). Toward an interactive model of reading. In S. Dornic & P. Rabbit (Eds.), *Attention and performance VI.* (pp. 183–221). Hillsdale, NJ: Erlbaum.

Rumelhart, D., Hinton, G., & Williams, R. (1986). Learning internal representations by error propagation. In D. Rumelhart & J. McClelland (Eds.), *Parallel distributed processing: Explorations in the microstructure of cognition* (Vol. 1, pp. 318–362). Cambridge, MA: MIT Press.

Schiffrin, D. (1994). *Approaches to discourse.* Cambridge, MA: Blackwell.

Seidenberg, M. (1985). The time course of information activation and utilization in visual word recognition. In D. Besner, T. Waller, & G. MacKinnon (Eds.), *Reading research: Advances in theory and practice* (Vol 5. pp. 199–252). New York: Academic Press.

Seidenberg, M., & McClelland, J. (1989). A distributed, developmental model of word recognition and naming. *Psychological Review, 96,* 523–568.

Share, D., & Stanovich, K. (1995). Cognitive processes in early reading development: Accommodating individual differences into a model of acquisition. *Issues in Education, 1,* 1–57.

Stanovich, K. (1985). Explaining the variance in reading ability in terms of psychological processes: What have we learned? *Annals of Dyslexia, 35,* 67–96.

Stanovich, K. (1986). Matthew effects in reading: Some consequences of individual differences in the acquisition of literacy. *Reading Research Quarterly, 21,* 360–406.

Stanovich, K. (1991). Word recognition: Changing perspectives. In R. Barr, M. Kamil, P. Mosenthal, & P.D. Pearson (Eds.), *Handbook of reading research,*

Volume II (pp. 418–452). White Plains, NY: Longman.

Stein, N., & Glenn, C. (1979). An analysis of story comprehension in elementary school children. In R. Freedle (Ed.), *New directions in discourse processing* (pp. 53–120). Norwood, NJ: Ablex.

Stolz, W. (1967). A study of the ability to decode grammatically novel sentences. *Journal of Verbal Learning and Verbal Behavior, 6,* 867–873.

Thomson, M. (1984). *Developmental dyslexia: Its nature, assessment, and remediation.* Baltimore: Edward Arnold.

Till, R., Mross, E., & Kintsch, W. (1988). Time course of priming for associate and inference words in a discourse context. *Memory & Cognition, 16,* 283–298.

Turner, A., Britton, B., Andraessen, P., & McCutchen, D. (1996). A predication semantics model of text comprehension and recall. In B. Britton & A. Graesser (Eds.), *Models of understanding* (pp. 33–72). Mahwah, NJ: Erlbaum.

van den Broek, P, Risden, K., Fletcher, C., & Thurlow, R. (1996). A "landscape" view of reading: Fluctuating patterns of activation and the construction of a stable memory representation. In B. Britton & A. Graesser (Eds.), *Models of understanding text* (pp. 165–188). Mahwah, NJ: Erlbaum.

van Dijk, T., & Kintsch, W. (1983). *Strategies of discourse comprehension.* Cambridge, MA: The MIT Press.

Chapter 2

Reading Development

ALAN G. KAMHI　　　*HUGH W. CATTS**

For many years, the focus in learning to read was on what the teacher did or should have done rather than on what happened or should happen in the child (Gibson & Levine, 1975). Beginning in the 1980s, and particularly in the last ten years, considerable progress has been made in understanding the reading acquisition process. This progress has occurred because researchers began to focus on the processes, traits, and skills children need to become proficient readers (Juel, 1991). Progress was not made when the sole focus was on teachers and methods.

This is not to say that research on methods of teaching is unimportant. Teachers need information about which instructional methods work best for particular children and classes. But, as Juel (1991) notes, "the lens through which we view reading instruction should be opened more widely to include not just the method in isolation, but factors that accompany the method" (p. 761). Examples of these factors include time spent reading, the kinds of texts that are read, the social setting for instruction, and patterns of interaction. In order to understand how children learn to read, it is thus important to focus on what children are learning as well as on what teachers or parents are purportedly teaching.

Children's path on the road to proficient reading begins well before they have formal reading instruction in school and continues until they can recognize words accurately and with little effort. Most normally developing readers develop accurate, effortless word recognition skills in the first few years of elementary school. The knowledge and mechanisms that underlie the development of proficient word recognition skills are the focus of the first part of this chapter. The second part of the chapter considers the development of reading comprehension abilities. Because a detailed discussion of the development of all of the factors that contribute to reading comprehension is beyond the scope of this chapter, one of

---

*Like the other chapters in the first part of this book, this chapter was a collaborative effort. The chapter is written in the first person to avoid the cumbersome language that would be needed to relate personal anecdotes about family members.

the main objectives in this section is to show that a simple model or theory of comprehension development is not possible.

Emergent Literacy Period (Birth–Kindergarten)

From birth until the beginning of formal education (age five or six in the United States), children growing up in literate cultures accumulate knowledge about letters, words, and books. In theories of reading development, the period of time before children go to school is usually referred to as the emergent literacy period. How much literacy knowledge children acquire during this period depends on how much exposure they have to literacy artifacts and events as well as their interest and facility in learning. At one end of the continuum are children from low-print homes who have little exposure to literacy artifacts and events. These children begin school with little literacy knowledge. At the other end of the continuum are children from high-print homes who enjoy everything about language and literacy. These children may be at an early stage of word recognition by the time they enter school. How much literacy knowledge children acquire during the emergent literacy period is thus highly variable. Most children will not acquire all of the knowledge discussed in this section, but because some do, it seems important to know what children can learn about literacy, language, and reading before they have any formal instruction.

The term "literacy socialization" has been used to refer to the social and cultural aspects of learning to read. Van Kleeck and Schuele (l987) discuss three specific areas of literacy socialization: (1) literacy artifacts, (2) literacy events, and (3) the types of knowledge children gain from literacy experiences. Most children growing up in middle- and upper-class homes in the United States are surrounded by literacy artifacts from the time of birth. Characters from nursery rhymes decorate walls. Sheets and crib borders often have pictures and writing, alphabet blocks and books might be on the shelf, and T-shirts often have slogans or city names printed on them. In addition to the child's own possessions, homes are filled with items such as books, newspapers, magazines, mail, pens, crayons, and writing pads.

Joint Book Reading

More important than literacy artifacts are the literacy events children participate in and observe and the knowledge they acquire from these events. The most instructionally organized literacy event is joint book reading. In 1985, the Commission on Reading of the National Academy of Education called joint book reading "the single most important activity for developing the knowledge required for eventual success in reading" (p. 23). In some mainstream homes, parents begin reading to their children as soon as babies are born. In some families, mothers may even begin reading to their unborn fetuses. My wife began reading to our unborn children as soon as an audiologist colleague told her that their auditory systems were sufficiently developed. In most mainstream homes, parents are reading to their infants by five to six months, which, not coincidentally, is the time when infants are able to sit up and focus at least some attention on a book. What do babies learn from these interactions with books? They learn many things, as van Kleeck (1995) notes in a recent article. For example, babies learn that books are important to the adults in their world and that lots of talk surrounds books. They may also realize that their parents work hard to get and keep their attention on these curious objects and delight in their slightest attempts to participate. Before babies can even talk, they may be turning pages of books and spending considerable time looking at pictures in books.

Because babies are not understanding much of the language they hear, van Kleeck reasons that we might expect parents to read a lot of rhyming books that de-emphasize meaning. But this does not appear to be the case. Van Kleeck and her colleagues found that fourteen middle-class mothers chose rhyming books less than 10 percent of the time with their 6- to 12-month old infants (van Kleeck, Gillam, Hamilton, & McGrath, 1995, cited in van Kleeck, 1995). Mothers did, however, use a rhythmic, singsong cadence, presumably to get and maintain the infant's attention. Even with babies, parents labeled pictures, actions, events, and related the information in the book to the child's life. The focus for parents is primarily on meaning and comprehension.

As infants get older, parents gradually introduce input that is more cognitively demanding. For example, Snow and Goldfield (1981) showed that parents decreased their labeling and increased discussion of events as their children got older (2;6 to 3;6). As children mature, they are also expected to play more of an active role in the book reading activity. One way children become more active is their ability to respond to so-called "test questions." Heath (1982), for example, found that there were three kinds of information children learn to talk about during book reading routines: (l) *what* explanations, (2) *reason* explanations, and (3) *affective* explanations. Learning to respond to these kinds of questions prepares children for the types of questions they will encounter from teachers and on tests once they enter school.

Children have a lot of help in learning to respond to test questions and provide various kinds of explanations about what they read. Parents who are attuned to the child's developmental level will provide questions and answers that the child can understand. Adults will also modify or scaffold a text to ensure that the child is able to make sense of it. Proficient scaffolders are able to reduce vocabulary and syntactic complexity as well as provide explanations and interpretations that the child understands. As children get older, the process of "sense making" becomes more of a shared enterprise (Heath, 1982; van Kleeck, 1995). One important characteristic of this shared enterprise is that children learn how to ask questions about the texts they are reading. The answers they receive to their questions are a key source for the development of conceptual knowledge and reasoning skills during the preschool years. Another important source for conceptual and reasoning skills is the books themselves, which become more sophisticated and complex as children get older.

Joint book reading not only impacts on children's conceptual and reasoning skills, it also exposes children to specific components of print and book conventions. This exposure inevitably contributes to and facilitates the learning of letter names, shapes, and sounds. In some cases, the literacy artifacts and joint book reading activities may lead preschoolers to the discovery of the underlying alphabetic principle—that words consist of discrete sounds that are represented by letters in print.

One could easily get the impression in this section that joint book reading experiences are all children need in order to learn to read. Despite the common-sense appeal of the importance of joint book reading, there is some controversy in the literature about the impact joint book reading actually has on early reading ability. Scarborough and Dobrich (1994) recently reviewed three decades of research on the influence of joint book reading on language and literacy development. The observed effects in this research were quite variable within and between samples. Demographics, attitudes, and skill levels seemed to make stronger direct contributions to early reading success than joint book reading.

Scarborough and Dobrich's (1994) findings have been challenged in a recent study by Bus, van Ijzendoorn, and Pellegrini (1995). Using a more extensive body of studies and a quantitative analysis, Bus and colleagues found support for the hypothesis that book reading had a direct impact on learning to read. There were hardly any studies with negative effects. Although book reading only explained about 8 percent of the variance in the outcome measures, the effect size of .59 was fairly strong. Importantly, the effects were not dependent on the socioeconomic status of the families. Even in lower class families with (on average) low levels of literacy, book reading had a beneficial effect on literacy skills. Because book reading seems to make the start at school easier, it may be particularly important for children from low socioeconomic families.

I don't think it is surprising that direct effects of shared book reading have been somewhat difficult to prove. It seems that there would have to be some kind of threshold for the beneficial effects of book reading. Scarborough and Dobrich (1994) come to the same conclusion: "It might matter a great deal whether a preschooler experiences little or no shared reading with a responsive partner, but beyond a certain threshold level, differences in the quantity or quality of this activity may have little bearing" (p. 285). There is some empircal support for threshold effects in a study by Stevenson and Fredman (1990). These authors found that reading, spelling, and IQ scores of a sample of 550 13-year-olds were strongly predicted by the frequency with which their parents reported reading to them as preschoolers. However, there was a cut-off point at which children who were read to less than four times a week performed more poorly than children who were read to more regularly.

Another possible confounding factor in joint book reading studies is children's interest or facility in literacy activities. A child (typically a boy) who would prefer playing video games may get little out of joint book reading activities. For such children, it is conceivable that too much shared reading might have some negative consequences because they may develop a negative attitude toward reading and other literacy events. The possibility of the negative effects of book reading is an intriguing one. Scarborough and Dobrich (1994, p. 295) use the notion of broccoli effects to refer to this issue. Will serving broccoli to a child who dislikes it make the child into a broccoli lover or will it serve to reinforce and solidify the child's negative attitude? There is some evidence that negative attitudes can impact on early reading ability. Wells (1985), for example, has found that 11 percent of preschoolers did not like being read to. He also found that preliteracy knowledge scores at age 5 were strong predictors of subsequent reading achievement at ages 7 and 10 (Wells, 1985, 1986). These preliteracy scores were significantly correlated with parental reports of the child's perceived interest in literacy ($r = .45$), the degree of concentration exhibited when engaged in literacy experiences ($r = .56$), and the amount of time spent on literacy activities ($r = .65$).

Importantly, negative attitudes may not have long-term effects on reading achievement. One of my neighbors, who is a school librarian, has a child who did not like to be read to when he was young. She would often come down to my house and see my wife reading to my daughter and wonder what she was doing wrong. She kept trying different approaches to get her son interested in books, but he preferred any activity to reading. He is now 16 and still does not like to read, but preference and ability are two very different things. Although this adolescent prefers not to read, he can read and, in fact, reads quite well. Although his parents and schooling have been unable to instill a favorable attitude toward reading, they have helped him to achieve a high level of literacy. This example suggests that negative attitudes toward joint book reading may not prevent children from becoming good readers, but such attitudes may affect how long it takes these children to achieve high literacy levels.

Studies of precocious readers provide additional evidence for the important role early attitudes and motivation have on learning to read. Scarborough and Dobrich cite several studies showing that precocious readers preferred literacy-related toys and that the greater amount of instruction provided by parents was prompted by the child's desires rather than the parents' pre-set goals. My older daughter, Alison, was one of these highly motivated children. She loved everything to do with literacy. In addition to the usual literacy events and artifacts, one of her favorite activities was doing reading workbooks filled with "phonics" activities. She loved playing the phonological awareness "games" that Hugh and I used in our studies. I got so tired of the games, especially on long car rides, that I sometimes wished Alison could be more like my neighbor's child who never tired of playing video games. But Alison's interest in literacy activites paid off; she was reading by age five.

A positive attitude and motivation to read play important roles in how much preschool children learn about the form of printed language. Most parents would probably not go out and buy phonics workbooks for their preschool children or play phonological awareness game unless their children enjoyed these activities. There must be a basic interest in language and literacy for children to seek out these activities. This interest is sustained, however, by the ability to achieve high levels of success in these activities. If, for example, Alison struggled with the workbook activities or phonological awareness games, I doubt she would have kept doing them. My younger daughter, Franne, learned to read by age 6 1/2, about a year and a half later than Alison. On the surface, Franne appeared to show less interest than Alison in phonics activities, especially before she turned four. The difference, I think, was not so much in Franne's interest level, but in the difficulty she had doing the activities. As soon as Franne began to achieve some success with phonics activities, she pursued these activities with as much enthusiasm as Alison did. Today at age 11, she reads much more than Alison does. Interest and motivation are thus linked at least in part to ability level.

Learning about Print

As discussed in the previous section, joint book reading contributes to and facilitates the learning of letter names, shapes, and sounds. In homes where children are exposed to literacy artifacts and events (high-print homes), there are many other opportunities for young children to learn about print. For example, one of the first songs many children learn is the alphabet song. I have vivid memories of Alison, at age 2, entertaining several rows of passengers on a plane by reciting the alphabet song over and over again. After all of the letter names are mastered, children begin to learn the letter shapes. In high-print homes children are continually exposed to print through the multitude of literacy artifacts and toys that parents buy. Alison, like many of her friends, had a little desk with magnetic alphabet letters that she could place on the board. She began by learning all of the capital letters and once she mastered these, we bought her the magnetic lower case letters. She also had access to a keyboard with its slightly different orthography.

Adams (1990), in her seminal book on early reading, reviewed evidence showing that letter recognition accuracy and speed were critical determinants to reading proficiency. Letter recognition speed and accuracy are important for reading because the more time one spends identifying letters, the more difficult it will be to learn sound-letter correspondences and decode novel words. Learning sound-letter correspondences depends on solid knowledge of letters. Individuals who continue to have difficulty recognizing letters will inevitably have decoding problems, which, in turn, will lead to comprehension difficulties and frustration with the whole reading process.

The exposure to a variety of literacy artifacts, frequent joint book reading, and various experiences with letter names and sounds may lead preschoolers to the discovery of the alphabetic principle. The insight that letters stand for individual sounds in words requires knowing something about letters (e.g., their names, shapes, and sounds) and the awareness that words consist of discrete sounds. Phoneme awareness, or more generally, phonological awareness, has received considerable attention since the earlier version of this book.

Much has been written about the importance of phonological awareness for early reading (cf. Adams, 1990; Blachman, 1989, 1994; Torgeson, Wagner, & Rashotte, 1994). The important role phonological awareness plays in reading has led to an interest in how children become aware that words consist of discrete sounds. Children as young as 2 years old begin to show some appreciation of the sound system. This awareness is seen in children's spontaneous speech repairs, rhyming behaviors, and nonsense sound play. One of my favorite examples of early phonological awareness is when Alison, at around age 2, put a plastic letter *T* in a cup and said, "Look, Daddy, I'm pouring tea." This example indicates that Alison was able to make a correspondence between the word "tea" and the letter *T*. Her interest in how words sound was also seen in her interest in nursery rhymes and word games. Rhyming activities typically reflect awareness of syllabic and subsyllabic units, such as onsets and rimes (e.g., c-at, h-at, b-at).

Interest in rhyming and developing knowledge of rimes and onsets may lead some children to become interested in and aware of all the sounds in words. Children like Alison soon go beyond simple rhyming games to more challenging "letter and sound" games. One of Alison's favorite car games was to think of words beginning with a certain letter. When this game got too easy, we changed it to thinking of words ending with certain letters. Alison also enjoyed writing and doing worksheets from the workbooks my wife would buy her. The workbooks were filled with exercises that increased her knowledge of letters, sounds, and their correspondences. Although Alison may be an exception, she demonstrates that it is possible to acquire phoneme awareness without formal instruction. Most children, however, will need some formal instruction to direct their attention and become aware of phonemes. Because this instruction typically does not occur until kindergarten, many children may not develop phoneme awareness until sometime in the first grade (see Chapter 6).

So much attention has been devoted to the importance of joint book reading activities, letter recognition, and phonological awareness that the importance of general language and cognitive factors for reading sometimes get overlooked. Although language and cognitive abilities may not be highly correlated to early reading ability, they play an important role in reading comprehension (Hoover & Gough, 1990). Consider, for example, that during the emergent literacy period, children acquire considerable knowledge about language. This knowledge enables them to be fairly competent communicators by the time they enter school. By 5 years of age, children can express abstract conceptual notions involving temporal, spatial, and causal relations. These notions are often expressed in complex sentence structures that include multiple embeddings of subordinate, relative, and infinitive clauses. By five years of age, children also have considerable knowledge of familiar scripts and story structure. Children are also developing cognitively during the preschool years and their increasingly sophisticated reasoning and problem-solving abilities begin to be reflected in measures of reading comprehension during the middle elementary school years.

Summary

It should be apparent that young children learn a great deal about literacy during the emergent literacy period. It is not uncommon for children from high-print homes to enter kindergarten with the ability to recite the alphabet, recognize letters, use a typewriter or a computer, write their name and a few other words, and sight read a dozen or more written words. It is also not uncommon for a precocious child who enjoys literacy activities to enter school with fairly sophisticated decoding skills. Children who begin school with such extensive knowledge about literacy obviously have a considerable advantage over children who enter school without this knowledge and experience. Teachers need to be aware that children with limited literacy knowledge and experience are not slow learners or learning disabled. Children from low- and high-print homes may have comparable language, cognitive, and attentional abilities; however, in order for children with limited early literacy experiences to catch up to their more advantaged peers, they need focused and systematic instruction in phonological awareness and letter recognition in conjunction with enjoyable and interesting reading and writing activities. Much more will be said about phonological awareness training in Chapter 6. In the next section, we will consider how children become proficient in decoding print.

The Development of Word Recognition Skills

In considering how emergent readers become proficient readers, it is necessary to understand what it means to be a proficient reader. It is generally agreed that a proficient reader can recognize words accurately and with little effort. Accurate, effortless word recognition requires the use of visual decoding based on familiar letter sequences or orthographic patterns. Although phonetic decoding skills are necessary to develop proficient word recognition, these skills are rarely used by the mature fluent reader. With all the emphasis on phonological awareness and decoding/phonics approaches in recent years, we sometimes forget that proficient word recognition does not involve sounding words out. Proficient word recognition relies primarily on visual, orthographic information rather than phonological information. If you don't believe this, think about how you read the last sentence. Did you sound out the particular words in the sentence? Imagine sounding out a word like *proficient,* p-r-o-f-i-c-i-e-n-t. Sounding out words, letter by letter or even syllable by syllable, would make reading an incredibly tedious endeavor. Accurate, effortless word recognition requires the ability to use a direct visual route without phonological mediation to access semantic memory and word meaning.

Mature readers, of course, are still capable of sounding out words, but they rarely need to break down a word into its individual sounds in order to decode it. Even novel words usually have familiar syllable structures or orthographic sequences that can facilitate decoding. For example, most people would probably have little difficulty decoding an unfamiliar name like "Kafelnikov" because it contains familiar syllable structure and letter sequences. However, a name like "Kamhi" would be more likely to be sounded out and mispronounced because the syllable structure (e.g., stress) in unclear and there is no English word with the sequence "kamhi." One has to decide whether the "h" is aspirated or silent (silent) and also decide between the various pronunciations of the two vowels.

How children become automatic fluent readers has intrigued theorists for years. Stage models are a common way to capture the changes that occur in the acquisition of complex behaviors such as reading. Most reading specialists are probably familiar with Chall's (1983) stage theory of reading. Although stage theories have a number of shortcomings that will be discussed later, they provide a useful framework for understanding the basic developmental changes that occur as children learn to read.

Logographic Stage

Most stage theories of reading acknowledge an initial visual or logographic stage in learning to read (Ehri, 1991; Frith, 1985). Frith (1985), for example, has proposed a "logographic stage" to mark the end of the emergent literacy period and a transition to a phonetic or alphabetic stage of reading. In this stage, children construct associations between unanalyzed spoken words and one or more salient graphic features of the printed word or its surrounding context. During this stage, children do not use knowledge of letter names or sound-letter relationships to recognize words. Ehri (1991, p. 387) points out that if readers use letters as cues, they do so because their shapes are visually salient, not because the letters correspond to the sounds in the word. As a result, they cannot read new words and can be easily fooled by switching visual cues. For example, when the Coca Cola logo was pasted on a Rice Krispies box, more than half the preschoolers tested thought that it said "Rice Krispies" (Masonheimer, Drum, & Ehri, 1984). When one letter was changed in the Pepsi logo to read Xepsi, 74 percent of preschoolers read the label as Pepsi.

The role of logographic reading for the development of word recognition skills is controversial. Share and Stanovich (1995) suggest that it has no functional value because it ignores correspondences between print and sound at a sub-lexical level. If logographic reading had any functional value, one would expect to find positive correlations with reading ability. Share and Stanovich (1995) cite numerous studies that found no relationship between logographic reading and later reading ability, suggesting that from the standpoint of acquiring proficient word recognition skills, the logographic stage may best be regarded as pre-reading. Because logographic reading has no apparent developmental role in reading, children do not have to read logographically in order to begin to read phonetically. Most children from high-print homes probably go through a clearly defined period when they read logographically, but there would be no reason to teach children to read logographically if they entered school with limited literacy knowledge. The first "true" stage of word recognition would have to involve the use of at least some phonetic cues to recognize words.

Transition Phase

Stage theorists differ in the number of stages it takes to develop proficient word recognition skills (Chall, 1983; Ehri, 1991; Frith, 1985). Researchers agree that when children begin to read words by processing sound-letter correspondences, they move into the *alphabetic stage.* They differ, however, in whether there is a transition phase before the alphabetic stage. Ehri (1991), for example, believes that there is a transition phase in which children use partial phonetic cues to recognize words, typically the initial letter or the initial and final letters. The letters may be linked to sounds, such as /s/ and /i/ in *see* or letter names, such as the /be/ in *beat* or *beaver.* For example, children might recognize the word *beat* by the initial *b* and final *t,* but because they are not focusing on the vowels, they may confuse beat with *boot* or *boat.* Children in this phase are similar to logographic readers because they cannot read unfamiliar words, but differ from logographic readers because they are able to use sound-letter information to read familiar words.

Alphabetic Stage

Researchers such as Chall (1983) and Frith (1985) see no need for a transition phase involving the use of letter names. They believe that once children use the sounds of letters to read, they have entered the alphabetic stage. The disagreement about when the alphabetic stage begins is a relatively minor one because theorists agree that the alphabetic stage is characterized by the ability to use sound-letter correspondences to decode novel words. Most theories of reading development acknowledge that constructing associations between sounds and letters is the fundamental task facing the beginning reader. Importantly, productive learning of sound-letter correspondences involves more than just recognizing letters and coupling them with appropriate sounds. It is not enough to memorize the sounds that go with each letter. To make use of those sounds, the child must realize that they are the sounds that make up spoken language. The child needs to link the letters to the particular set of phonemic sounds that comprise spoken language (cf. Adams, 1990). This is the alphabetic insight that underlies the ability to phonetically decode words.

The alphabetic insight, like other insights, is a one-time occurrence. Having the insight does not make the task of learning all the sound-letter correspondences any easier. The sounds or phonemes that children must associate with letters are abstract linguistic concepts rather than physically real entities and, as such, do not always correspond to discrete and invariant sounds. As a result of coarticulation, the sound segments of speech blend together in running, conversational speech. Sounds that are less affected by coarticulation are thus inherently easier to associate with letters than sounds that are affected by coarticulation. This is why continuant sounds and letters (e.g., /s/, /f/, /m/) are often taught before stop sounds (/b/, /d/, /g/). In the word *see,* for example, it is easy to have the child listen for the /s/ sound (s-s-s-s-s) and separate it from the vowel (eeeee). For the word *bat,* however, it is not possible to separate the /b/ from its accompanying vowel. Without a vowel, the *b* in *bat* is nothing more than a burst of air that is more similar to a bird's chirp than the "buh" [bʌ] sound many people think a *b* makes. But if *b* was really a [bʌ] then the word *bat* would be pronounced "buh-at" not "bat."

There are many examples of the lack of correspondence between sounds and letters in English. This lack of correspondence makes learning to read a slow process and makes learning to spell even more difficult. Consider, for example, the words *writer* and *rider.* Most people think that the difference in these two words is in the medial consonant. *Writer* has a *t* whereas *rider* has a *d.* But if you say these two words to yourself and don't effect a British accent, the *t* and *d* in the two words are pronounced the same, as an alveolar flap /ɾ/. The two words sound different because the first vowel is longer in *rider* than it is in *writer.* Another frequently cited example is the *tr* in *truck.* It is difficult to say *tr* at a normal rate of speech without turning the /t/ into an affricate. Listen carefully and you will hear something resembling the "ch" sound. A common early spelling of *truck* is thus "ch-u-k." Children's invented spellings often reflect how words actually sound.

Learning sound-letter correspondences is further complicated by the allophonic variations of many English phonemes. In the *writer-rider* example above, the alveolar flap /ɾ/ is an allophonic variation of /t/ and /d/. Many teachers incorrectly assume, however, that phonemes have only one phonetic form. But many English phonemes have several phonetic variations depending on where they occur in words and the sounds around them. The phoneme /t/, for example, is produced with aspiration only before stressed vowels (e.g., *top, attack*). But as we saw with the word *writer,* an intervocalic /t/ is always flapped. A syllable final /t/ as in *pot* or *Kaitlin* may be unreleased. In s-clusters (e.g., *stop*), the /t/ actually sounds more like a /d/ than a /t/, and in words like *bottle,* the /t/ may become a glottal stop. These examples illustrate how phonemes can have several different phonetic variations. These phonetic variations make the task of learning what are actually phoneme-grapheme (rather than sound-letter) correspondences a difficult one.

Once one gets beyond the word level, there is even less correspondence between sounds and letters because the effects of coarticulation are greater in sentences and conversational speech. For example, in normal conversation, the phrase *did you know* is pronounced [dɪdʒəno]. A child who was told that the letter *y* corresponds to the "ya" sound would have difficulty constructing an association between this sound and letter because there is no "ya" sound in this sentence.

Another considerable obstacle facing young children is the irregularities of English spelling. Children must learn that many letters do not always sound like they should. There are 251 different spellings for the 44 sounds of English (Horn, 1926). Consider, for example, all of the different spellings of the vowel sound /i/—ie, e, ei, i, y, ea, ee—or the consonant /f/—f, ff, gh, ph. Children also have to learn that each grapheme (letter) may have a number of different forms. Most graphemes have different upper- and lowercase forms and a different script form. Some graphemes may also have a different typewritten form (e.g., lowercase a̲), meaning that a particular grapheme might have as many as four or five different letter forms.

Despite these obstacles, young children gradually begin to move beyond the inefficient strategy of sounding out every word. Whereas the alphabetic insight and learning of phoneme-grapheme relations mark the transition into the alphabetic stage and the true beginning of word recognition, orthographic knowledge is necessary to develop automatic, effortless word recognition skills. This stage is discussed in the next section.

Orthographic Stage and Automatic Word Recognition

The orthographic stage is characterized by the use of letter sequences and spelling patterns to recognize words visually without phonological conversion. The ability to use a direct visual route without phonological mediation to access semantic memory and word meaning is crucial for developing automatic word recognition skills. Although some theorists disagree about what to call this final stage of word recognition (e.g., orthographic or automatic), there is consensus that orthographic knowledge is necessary for automatic, effortless word recognition. Without orthographic knowledge, readers would continue to have to sound out long multisyllabic words and rely on the more inefficient and time-consuming indirect phonological route to access semantic memory.

According to Ehri (1991) and Frith (1985), the orthographic phase begins when children accumulate sufficient knowledge of spelling patterns so that they are able to recognize the words visually without phonological conversion. Orthographic knowledge accumulates as readers phonetically decode different words that share similar letter sequences, recognize these similarities, and store this information in memory. Phonetic decoding is thus necessary to become proficient at orthographic reading. If readers are not able to phonetically decode all the letters in a word, they will have difficulty learning to recognize letter patterns that occur in different words (Ehri, 1991).

What kinds of orthographic patterns do readers detect? It seems obvious that readers will most likely learn patterns that occur frequently. Morphemes (-*ing, -ed, -able, -ment, -ity*), with their consistent spelling and function, present an excellent starting point to focus on orthographic rather than phonological sequences. Ehri (1991, p. 405) cites a study by Becker, Dixon, and Anderson-Inman (1980) in which they analyzed 26,000 high-frequency English words into root words and morphemes. They found about 8,100 different root words and about 800 different morphemes that occurred in at least ten different words.

The other place to look for orthographic regularities is in words that share letter sequences. These words may be thought of as belonging to a particular word family or orthographic neighborhood. For example, *teach, reach, each,* and *preach* all have the common stem -*each,* whereas *cake, bake, take, make,* and *lake* all have the common stem -*ake.* In Chapter 6 of this book, Torgesen lists some common spelling patterns that are found at the end of single-syllable words: -*ack, -ight, -eat, -ay, -ash, -ip, -ore,* and -*ell.* As readers begin to focus on common spelling sequences, they begin to use an analogy strategy to read new words (Marsh, Friedman, Desberg, & Saterdahl, 1981). Rather than sounding out a new word sound-by-sound, mature readers compare the letter sequence of a new word to letter sequences of familiar words in semantic memory. Torgesen gives several examples of reading by analogy in his chapter. For example, the word *cart* might be read by noticing the word *car* and adding a /t/ sound at the end. A long word like *fountain* might initially be read by noticing its similarity to *mountain.*

As noted above, orthographic knowledge is crucial for the development of automatic word recognition skills because knowledge of letter sequences enables readers to set up access routes in memory to read words by sight. Although many theorists have characterized fluent word recognition as an automatic process, the concept of automaticity is not a simple one. Stanovich (1990, 1991) has discussed the difficulty involved in "unpacking" what automatic word recognition actually involves. He argues that the question of whether word recognition is automatic is not a good one because it confounds aspects of word recognition that can be differentiated such as speed, capacity usage, conscious control, obligatory execution, and influence of higher-level knowledge. Development of each of these factors does not coincide.

The concept of modularity provides a better way to characterize developing word recognition proficiency. A modular process is one that operates quickly and is not controlled or influenced by higher-level processes. Fodor (1983), who first proposed the concept of modularity, described modular systems as having functional autonomy and being cognitively impenetrable. Proficient word recognition fits the definition of a modular process because it is fast, requires little capacity and conscious attention, and is not affected by higher-level knowledge sources. In support of a modular view of word recognition, context effects have been shown to decrease as word recognition skills become more proficient (e.g., Gough, 1983). In other words, children rely less on higher-level knowledge sources as their word recognition skills become more modularized. Although most reading theorists and practitioners will probably continue to talk about automatization of word recognition, it may be useful to attempt to incorporate modular notions in characteristics of proficient word recognition skill.

Problems with Stage Theories of Word Recognition

Although the stages of word recognition described in the previous section accurately portray the kinds of knowledge and skills required to become a proficient reader, the actual stages do not seem to be supported by empirical evidence (Share & Stanovich, 1995). One consistent problem with stage theories is that the focus is primarily on what knowledge children need to become proficient readers rather than the mechanisms that underlie changes in reading proficiency. Another problem with stage theories is that each stage is associated with only one type of reading (logographic, alphabetic, orthographic), which implies that all words are read with the same approach at a particular stage. Although stage theorists often mention beginning and end points of stages, little attention is typically devoted to the actual development of the knowledge that characterizes these stages. For example, a common description of the alphabetic stage is that a child has little alphabetic knowledge at the beginning of the stage and is able to phonetically decode most words by the end of the stage. How a little knowledge becomes a lot of knowledge is often not addressed by most stage theorists (e.g., Spear-Swerling & Sternberg, 1996). Ehri (1991) is a notable exception. Another limitation of stage theories is that they tend to oversimplify development and obscure individual differences. Although there are certain things that all children must learn in order to become proficient readers, children may take different paths to becoming good readers.

The Self-Teaching Hypothesis

Share (1995) and Share and Stanovich (1995) have recently offered an alternative to stage-based theories. The key notion in what they refer to as the "self-teaching hypothesis" is that phonological decoding functions as a self-teaching mechanism that enables the learner to acquire the detailed orthographic representations necessary for fast and accurate visual word recognition and for proficient spelling. Although direct instruction and contextual guessing may play some role in developing orthographic knowledge, Share and Stanovich argue that only phonological decoding offers a viable means for the development of fast, efficient visual word recognition.

The problem with direct instruction is that children encounter too many unfamiliar words. The average fifth grader, for example, encounters around 10,000 new words per year (Nagy & Herman, 1987); there is no way teachers, parents, or peers can help children with all of these unfamiliar words. The problem with contextual guessing is that the primary purpose of text is to convey non-redundant information, not redundant information. Sentences like *We walked into the restaurant and sat down at a* ___" are rare because they violate a basic communicative convention of conveying new or non-redundant information. Gough (1983) has referred to context as a false friend because it helps you when you least need it. It works best for high-frequency function words, but not very well for content words.

To further support the inadequacy of contextual guessing, Share and Stanovich cite data from a study by Finn (1977/78) indicating that the average predictability of words when they were deleted was 29.5 percent. Guesses were thus twice as likely to be wrong than right. The inadequacy of contextual guessing is caused in part by the large number of synonyms or near-synonyms in English. But even if children are successful in guessing the correct word, this strategy is not a viable one to develop orthographic word recognition skills because children are not focusing on particular spelling patterns of the words.

Because of the inadequacy of direct instruction and contextual guessing for the development of efficient orthographic word recognition, Share and Stanovich (1995) contend that the ability to phonetically decode words and associate printed words with their spoken equivalents must play a pivotal role in the development of fluent word recognition. In their own words,

> According to the self-teaching hypothesis, each successful decoding encounter with an unfamiliar word provides an opportunity to acquire the word-specific orthographic information that is the foundation of skilled word recognition and spelling. In this way, phonological recoding acts as a self-teaching mechanism or built-in teacher enabling the child to independently develop knowledge of specific word spellings and more general knowledge of orthographic conventions. (p. 18)

The self-teaching hypothesis attempts to explain one of the long-standing puzzles of how children learn to read. I remember years ago wondering how my older daughter Alison seemed to change overnight from a slow plodding reader, asking about every other word, to a fluent reader. I read somewhere a long time ago that the transition to fluent, proficient decoding is like magic. I knew that helping Alison with unfamiliar words could not turn her into a fluent reader, so I just waited and assumed some day it would all come together. When the day finally came, I had no idea what the underlying factors were that led Alison (and other young children) to finally automatize the word recognition process.

The answer, and it is the only possible answer, is that children teach themselves to read fluently. This notion has apparently been around for a while, but Share was the first to articulate it (Share, 1995; Share & Stanovich, 1995). What makes learning to read seem magical is that parents and most professionals never could satisfactorily explain how children seemed to become fluent readers overnight. One reason that it has taken so long for a self-teaching theory of reading to be proposed and will take many more years to be accepted is that we have always assumed that teachers taught children to read. But as will become clear below, it is difficult to teach children all they need to know to become proficient readers.

There are four features of the self-teaching role of phonological decoding: (1) item- as opposed to stage-based role of decoding in development, (2) early onset, (3) progressive "lexicalization" of word recognition, and (4) the asymmetric relationship between primary phonological and secondary orthographic components in the self-teaching process. Each of these features is discussed in more detail below.

The stage theories reviewed in the previous section propose that all words are initially phonologically decoded with a later developmental shift to visual access using orthographic information. In reviewing the research that addresses the phonological-to-orthographic shift, Share and Stanovich (1995, p. 14) note that it is consistently inconsistent. Some studies find evidence of direct visual access in early grades with no indication of a transition from a phonological to a visual-orthographic stage (e.g., Barron & Baron, 1977). Other studies, in contrast, found evidence in support of the developmental phonological to visual-orthographic shift (e.g., Backman, Bruck, Hebert, & Seidenberg, 1984).

To resolve the conflicting findings, Share (1995) suggests that it is more appropriate to ask how children get meaning from *which* words. The process of word recognition depends on how often a child has been exposed to a particular word and the nature and success of decoding the particular word. Familiar high-frequency words are recognized visually with minimal phonetic decoding, whereas novel or low-frequency words for which the child has yet to develop orthographic representations will be more dependent on phonetic decoding. The frequency of phonetic decoding will thus vary according to children's familiarity with words in particular texts. If the reading is at the child's reading level or a little above, "a majority of the words will be recognized visually, while the smaller number of low-frequency unfamiliar words will provide opportunities for self-teaching with minimal disruption of ongoing comprehension processes" (Share, 1995, p. 155). Importantly, the self-teaching opportunities with these unfamiliar words represent the "cutting edge" of reading development not merely for the beginner, but for readers throughout the ability range (p. 156).

Evidence of self-teaching can be found at the very earliest stage of word recognition. In order for self-teaching to occur, children need to have at least some sound-letter knowledge, some phonological awareness, and the ability to use contextual information to determine exact word pronunciations based on partial decodings. The key point here is that children do not need to have accurate phonetic decoding skills in order to develop orthographic-based representations. These orthographic representations may, however, be somewhat incomplete or primitive, but the primitive nature of these representations does not prevent them from being used for direct (visual) access to meaning.

The lexicalization of phonological decoding is a central aspect of the self-teaching hypothesis. Early decoding skill is based on simple one-to-one correspondences between sounds and letters. There is little sensitivity to orthographic and morphemic context. Share and Stanovich (1995, p. 23) suggest that with print exposure, these early sound-letter correspondences become "lexicalized"; that is, they come to be associated with particular words. As the child becomes more attuned to spelling regularities beyond the level of simple one-to-one phoneme-grapheme correspondences, this orthographic information is used to modify the initial lexicalizations children develop. The outcome of this process of lexicalization, according to Share and Stanovich, "is a skilled reader whose knowledge of the relationships between print and sound has evolved to a degree that makes it indistinguishable from a purely whole-word mechanism that maintains no spelling-sound correspondence rules at the level of individual letters and digraphs" (pp. 23-24).

Share and Stanovich cite a number of studies in support of this view that the interested reader may wish to examine. These studies show that as children perform more detailed analyses of the internal structure of words, they develop more accurate orthographic representations. These more accurate representations lead, in turn, to more efficient word recognition because less attention needs to be focused on sound-letter correspondences or contextual cues that are needed to disambiguate homonyms.

The notion of lexicalization resolves one of the classic enigmas of decoding—that the rules required for proficient decoding are very different from the simplistic and sometimes incorrect rules (e.g., /b/ = "buh") taught to beginning readers. Basic knowledge of simple sound-letter correspondences are a logical starting point for the beginning reader, but it is impossible to become a proficient reader using these rules. These simple rules are used as a bootstrap or scaffold for developing the "complex lexically constrained knowledge of spelling-sound relationships that characterize the expert reader (Share & Stanovich, 1995, p. 25).

The final claim that the self-teaching hypothesis makes is that phonological skills are the primary self-teaching mechanism for the acquisition of fluent word recognition. The contribution of visual/orthographic factors is secondary and "largely parasitic upon the self-teaching opportunities provided by decoding and print exposure" (Share & Stanovich, 1995, p. 26). Phonetic decoding causes children to look at all the letters in a word, and this attention gradually leads to recognition of common letter sequences and other orthographic patterns. The evidence in support of this claim is found in studies documenting the strong relationship between pseudoword reading and word recognition (e.g., Stanovich & Siegel, 1994). Correlation coefficents typically exceed .70, indicating that a large part of the variance in word recognition is accounted for by the ability to phonetically decode. Although there is disagreement about how to evaluate the contribution of visual/orthographic factors, studies comparing pseudoword with exception word reading have consistently found that orthographic factors play less of a role in decoding than phonological factors (e.g., Baron & Treiman, 1980).

Further support for the primary role of phonetic decoding can be found in studies of disabled readers. As will be discussed in later chapters, poor readers almost always have deficits in phonetic decoding. On the other hand, poor readers, as a group, show comparable orthographic skills to children reading at the same overall reading level (Olson, Kliegl, Davidson, & Foltz, 1995; Stanovich & Siegel, 1994).

Considerable time in this section has been devoted to Share and Stanovich's self-teaching hypothesis. Unlike stage theories that focus on what children need to learn or do to become fluent readers, the self-teaching hypothesis attempts to explain how children become proficient at word recognition. The central claim of the theory is that phonological decoding functions as the primary self-teaching mechanism that enables the learner to acquire the detailed orthographic representations necessary for fast and accurate visual word recognition and for proficient spelling.

One possible point of confusion is that phonological decoding can occur on different size units of speech, such as phonemes, syllables, rimes/onsets, and morphemes. The most straightforward type of decoding involves identifying and blending together the individual sounds in words. Because simple one-to-one sound blending is a very inefficient way to decode long words and words with irregular spellings, children will try to find larger units to phonetically decode. For example, they may divide words into onsets and rimes. It is much easier to phonetically decode *fight* as f-ight and *bought* as b-ought than it is to sound out individual letters. As children begin to notice common morphemes in different words, they will use these language-based units to decode unfamiliar words. Once they get to this point, they should also be able to decode novel words by making analogies to other words that they already know (cf. the *mountain/fountain* example discussed earlier). As novel words become familiar, children will be able to visually recognize the whole word without having to phonetically decode any part of the word.

Share and Stanovich (1995) make it very clear that phonological decoding skill is no guarantee of self-teaching: "It only provides the opportunities for self-teaching. Other factors such as the quantity and quality of exposure to print together with the ability and/or inclination to attend to and remember orthographic detail will determine the extent to which these opportunities are exploited" (p. 25). In other words, there is a lot of room for individual differences in reading ability. At one end of the continuum, there will be cases of children with severe deficits in visual/orthographic memory. Even with good phonetic decoding skill, these children would have to tackle every word as if they were seeing it for the first time. At the other extreme are children who may recall word-specific letter patterns after only a single exposure. These children should become proficient readers at a relatively early age given adequate exposure to print.

Before moving on to discuss the development of comprehension, it is important to mention the role that writing may play in developing proficient word recognition skills. Adams, Treiman, and Pressley (1996) provide an excellent discussion of the impact of writing on learning to read. There is little doubt that writing provides an excellent medium for developing basic understanding of the sounds and spellings for words. Writing forces children to think about sound-letter correspondences, the relation of print to spoken language, and orthographic/spelling patterns. As such, writing may be an important part of the self-teaching mechanism that leads to fluent word recognition.

The Development of Reading Comprehension

In Chapter 1, the processes involved in reading comprehension were reviewed. In order to assign meaning to texts, readers rely on previously stored knowledge about language and the world as well as specific knowledge about different text structures and genres. Basic reasoning abilities, such as making analogies and inferences, as well as metacognitive abilities, also play an important role in text comprehension. A detailed discussion of how children develop conceptual knowledge, knowledge of text structure, reasoning, and metacognitive skills is beyond the scope of this chapter. It is important to consider, however, what such a discussion would need to entail.

An understanding of how text comprehension develops requires a consideration of the developmental changes that occur in listening and reading comprehension over the school years. For example, when children are first learning to read and their word recognition skills are inefficient, their ability to understand spoken discourse is necessarily much better than their ability to understand written texts. The development of proficient word recognition skills frees up attentional resources to focus on text comprehension and learning. Chall's stage theory of reading reflects this change in focus. In Chall's second stage of reading, children became unglued from print. In her third stage, which begins in about third grade and continues through middle school, children begin the long course of reading to learn. Chall noted that in traditional schools, children in the third/fourth grade begin to study the so-called subject areas, such as history, geography, and science. Content subjects such as these are purposely not introduced until children have presumably become relatively proficient readers (i.e., decoders). The reading in Stage 3, according to Chall, is primarily for facts, concepts, or how to do things. Chall divides Stage 3 into two phases. In the initial phase, children (age nine to eleven) can read serious material of adult length but cannot read most adult popular literature. During the second phase (junior-high level), preadolescents are able to read most popular magazines, popular adult fiction, *Reader's Digest,* and newspapers. Literary fiction and news magazines, such as *Newsweek* and *Time,* are still beyond the abilities of children at this stage.

Chall's "reading to learn" stage describes children's increasing ability to understand more sophisticated texts. As discussed in the previous section, stage theories typically do not address how processes become more proficient. In order to read more sophisticated texts, children need more than accurate, efficient word recognition. In addition to rapid lexical access, other aspects of linguistic processing, such as assigning syntactic/semantic roles, need to take place in a timely manner (Carlisle, 1991). Efficient linguistic processing plays an important role in one's ability to integrate ideas within and across sentences, paragraphs, and larger discourse units.

Children's facility for understanding texts increases as they become more familiar with the particular structure and function of different text genres. When children start school, their experience with different kinds of discourse genres is often fairly limited. As Carlisle (1991, p. 22) notes, they are most familiar with running commentaries of their playmates, explanations of events or simple phenomena, and narratives encountered in shared story reading with adults. In school, they gradually become exposed to different genres, such as biography, drama, poetry, and the various kinds of expository texts used in science and social studies. Comprehension of expository texts has been shown to lag behind comprehension of narrative until at least the third grade (Rasool & Royer, 1986). There is also evidence that developing awareness of text structures plays an important role in understanding and remembering texts (Richgels, McGee, Lomax, & Sheard, 1987).

As children develop more sophisticated reasoning skills, their comprehension of various texts necessarily increases. In our earlier book (Kamhi & Catts, 1989), we commented that Chall's final two stages of reading development are more appropriately viewed as stages of cognitive development. As adolescents become capable of more abstract levels of thought, the information they are able to learn from reading increases. The essential characteristic of Stage 4 (Multiple Viewpoints, 14–18) is that the reader can now deal with more than one point of view, whereas the essential characteristic of Stage 5 (Construction and Reconstruction, 18+) is that reading is viewed as constructive; that is, the reader constructs knowledge using basic reasoning processes, such as analysis, synthesis, and judgment. Not coincidentally, the ability to consider alternative solutions to problems, an aspect of hypothetical-deductive reasoning, is one of the hallmarks of the formal operational period that marks adolescent thought (Piaget, 1952). A true understanding of how individuals become more critical and thoughtful readers requires a comprehensive inquiry into cognitive development during the adolescent period.

It should be apparent that it is not possible to provide a straightforward simple developmental model of text comprehension. Even if one were able to accurately measure the various linguistic, conceptual, reasoning, metacognitive, and text-specific processes that contribute to reading comprehension, it would be difficult to relate these assessments to specific measures of text comprehension. Although standardized tests of reading comprehension lead one to believe that the development of comprehension follows a nice linear path during the school years, this view is more than a gross oversimplification; it is basically inaccurate because many of the factors that contribute to comprehension do not develop in discrete quantifiably measurable ways.

One factor that does seem to develop in a discrete quantifiable way is vocabulary. Measures of vocabulary are integral components of standardized measures of language and reading comprehension. In fact, vocabulary-oriented measures are central components of college and graduate aptitude tests (PSAT, ACT, SAT, GRE, and so forth). There is little doubt that receptive vocabulary knowledge is important for reading comprehension. But how important is it to know the meaning of words like *terpsichorean, cenotaph, nidificating,* and *importunity* in order to be a good reader? These words appear on the Form IIIA of the Peabody Picture Vocabulary Test-Third Edition. I think I'm a pretty good reader and I had no idea what these words meant until I looked them up a couple of months ago. I may have seen *importunity* before, but had never encountered the other three words. How could knowledge of these words possibly impact on reading comprehension if they occur so infrequently? Yet in order for vocabulary to be quantified in neat developmental increments across the school years, it is necessary to find increasingly obscure words that even very good readers will not know. One must be wary, then, of discrete quantifiable measures of reading comprehension because they may tap knowledge that has little bearing on actual reading ability.

If the development of comprehension abilities does not follow a nice linear path throughout the school years, how can educators determine what skills to teach children as they progress through school? In order to answer this question, it is necessary to consider what it means to understand a text. Does it mean understanding particular words, sentences, paragraphs, or chapters? Does it mean understanding plot, purpose, theme, character motives, or author's intent? Or does understanding involve the ability to evaluate the literary worth of a particular text? Standardized reading comprehension tests usually assess information reflected in the first two questions through multiple-choice or fill-in-the blank (cloze-type) questions.

One of the main problems with standardized measures of reading comprehension is their focus on informational types of answers. Because of their informational focus, these tests may be measuring something other than text-specific comprehension, such as the ability to eliminate options (i.e., test-taking strategy), familiarity with the topic of the text, or familiarity with the text structure and genre. More importantly, the ability to answer informational questions is a very different skill than the one required to answer questions about literary quality. To answer these questions one must be able to use interpretive and reasoning skills that go beyond the information in the text.

Another serious problem with standardized tests of reading comprehension is that they are based on the structuralist view of reading (cf. Kamhi, 1993) that meaning resides in the text, not in the transaction between the reader and the text. If meaning is in the text, then the task for readers is to figure out what the meaning is. Each text is viewed as having one correct or best interpretation. Students quickly learn that the teacher (or the workbook) will usually tell them the correct meaning or interpretation. They also learn that to perform well in class and on tests, they simply need to reconstruct or restate the meaning of the text as presented by the teacher or the workbook. Students who perform well on these assessments are thought to be good readers whereas students who perform poorly on these assessments are thought to be poor readers.

The way comprehension is measured does not change as students progress through the school years. Purves (1992), for example, has noted that students viewed English classes as part of a game that involved reading to take comprehension tests. They did not read for enjoyment or to enlarge their understanding; instead they focused on ways to get the information to pass tests. For example, students talked about how it was better to have English during second period so they could get the questions from first-period students.

It seems clear that another view of comprehension is needed. In a recent article (Kamhi, 1997), I presented two alternative views of comprehension, one that considered the multiple meanings available to readers and another that considered how texts can be processed at different levels of meaning. The first view has its roots in literary theory. Literary theorists (e.g., reader-response critics, new historicists, and so forth) are interested in how meaning is constructed from text during the process of reader-text interaction (see, for example, Brodkey, 1992; McLaren, 1992). Meaning is thought to reside not in the text, but in the transaction between reader and text. Some reader-response theorists (most notably, Stanley Fish, e.g., 1980) actually deny the existence of an independent text and view every aspect of a text as a product of an interpretive strategy initiated by a reader. Reader-response theorists (e.g., Iser, 1978; Langer, 1992) believe that a text is a series of changing understandings, interpretations, or envisionments. Because a text can never be grasped as a whole, a reader-response theorist would never ask "What is this story/book about?" The interpretation (meaning of the text) a reader constructs is influenced by a number of factors, including social and cultural attitudes, personality, and linguistic and conceptual skills. Some literary theorists also emphasize how meaning is influenced by the social-historical context of the author and the reader.

Although reader-response theories are concerned primarily with fiction, the notion of multiple meanings could apply to other genres as well. These theories reflect what Milosky (1992) has called "the indeterminacy of language," which is simply another way of saying that language is open to many different interpretations. How indeterminate a particular text is depends on a number of factors. Expository texts should be less indeterminate than fiction, poetry, and the other creative genres because ambiguity would detract from their overall purpose to inform or persuade.

Texts are not only open to many different interpretations, but also can be processed at several different levels. In a classic book first published almost sixty years ago, Adler and Van Doren (1940/1972) identified four levels of reading comprehension. The first or elementary level involved understanding the literal meaning of the words and sentences. This is the level typically assessed by standardized measures of reading comprehension. The second level was termed "inspectual reading" or "systematic skimming." When reading at this level, one has a set amount of time to complete an assigned amount of reading. The goal of inspectual reading is to get the most out of a book within a given time. Inspectual reading is not casual or random browsing; it is more accurately viewed as the art of skimming systematically (Adler & Van Doren, 1972, p. 18). For example, I remember in college being told that one way to get through large amounts of reading was to read the first and last sentences of paragraphs. After reading these sentences, I would decide whether to read the entire paragraph and if it needed to be read at a more analytic level.

In contrast to the previous two levels, analytic reading is thorough, complete reading—the best that you can do (Adler & Van Doren, 1972, p. 19). It is the best and most complete reading that is possible given unlimited time. The goal of analytic reading is more than simply understanding the main point or gist of the book; it requires a deeper more complete understanding of the contents of the book. In order to read analytically, it is necessary to consider the structure of the book, the author's intentions, characterization, plot, narrator, and so forth.

The fourth and final level is comparative reading. The comparative reader has read many books and is able to relate different books and topics to one another. Mere comparison of text is not enough, however, because the comparative reader must be able to generate a critical or novel interpretation of the text. In order to do this, the reader needs to use inspectual and analytic skills acquired previously. For example, in writing this chapter on reading development, I knew that there were hundreds, perhaps thousands, of articles that addressed this topic. If I had attempted to read each of these articles analytically, I would never have finished the chapter. To make the task manageable, I skimmed a number of articles and books to determine which ones I needed to read analytically. The act of writing the chapter pushed me to be a comparative reader because writing requires analysis, synthesis, and interpretation of different sources of information.

The notion that texts have different degrees of indeterminacy and can be processed at different levels has significant implications for how one views the development of text comprehension abilities. Consider, for example, if one's view of comprehension development was based on the way in which students responded to the following questions:

1. What made the book interesting?
2. Did you like the book? Why or why not?
3. Are there characters in the book who you would like to have as friends?
4. What other things would you like to see happen in the book?
5. If you were the main character, what would you have done differently in the story?
6. If you could meet the author of the book, what would you say?

7. What things would you change in the story?

8. Have you ever experienced some of the events or feelings that the characters in the book experienced?

Questions such as these require informational knowledge as well as interpretation and reasoning skills. Much has been written lately about how to use reader response in elementary classrooms to foster higher-level thinking skills. The National Council of Teachers of English has published a number of books in this area. A recent book edited by Karolides (1997) is filled with chapters about how elementary school teachers are encouraging student responses to literature in elementary classrooms.

Change is slow, however. Most students proceed through school thinking that meaning is in the text and getting good grades involves figuring out which answer the teacher wants. When my wife, who teaches first-year college literature classes, asks students if they liked the book they just read, they wonder if they are in the right class. After getting over the initial shock of being asked to offer a personal aesthetic judgment of the book, one of my wife's students might answer that they liked the book. My wife then asks the much more difficult question, "Why did you like the book?" The attempts by students to answer this question begins their initiation into the kind of reading expert readers do. With a good college English professor, students will learn the criteria literary theorists use to answer questions like, "What makes good literature?" "Why are some interpretations better than others?" "Why are doctoral students today still writing dissertations on Shakespeare?" The ability to explain, justify, and understand different aesthetic judgments requires interpretation and reasoning abilities that go way beyond the knowledge tapped by standardized reading comprehension measures. Importantly, it is not necessary to wait until college to assess and teach these skills. Elementary school children may not have the sophisticated reasoning skills of older students, but they can learn how to justify and defend their aesthetic judgments and appreciate the aesthetic judgments of others.

In addition to "reader-response" questions, such as those listed above, a number of other ways to assess comprehension have been developed by researchers. One of the most popular ways to evaluate comprehension is to have readers provide a running verbal commentary of their understanding and reaction to texts (e.g., Trabasso & Magliano, 1996). These commentaries are typically referred to as "think aloud" verbal protocols. After reading a sentence or paragraph, the experimenter might ask "Tell me more about that sentence/paragraph" or "Tell me in your own words what you just read." Think aloud protocols provide opportunities for students to relate text information to personal experiences and indicate where specific comprehension breakdowns may be occurring.

It should be clear from this discussion of alternative views of comprehension that simplistic views of reading comprehension lead to simplistic views of comprehension development. It is not possible to understand how children's comprehension abilities mature if one has a one-dimensional view of what comprehension is. The view of text comprehension that many teachers, students, and parents have is based on the way standardized reading tests measure comprehension. To begin to understand how children understand texts, it is necessary to consider how their interactions with texts become more complex and how they develop proficiency to read at different levels for different types of texts. This, of course, is in addition to considering the ways in which children's linguistic, reasoning, and metacognitive processes improve with age and how conceptual knowledge and specific knowledge of text structure and genre impact on comprehension.

Summary

In this chapter, I have attempted to provide a kind of road map for the development of proficient reading. The primary focus in the chapter has been on the development of proficient word recognition skills because one can restrict the discussion to how children acquire specific phonological and orthographic knowledge. Once one enters the realm of comprehension, it becomes necessary to talk about how good readers use higher-level analysis and reasoning skills to integrate information within and across texts. How children develop these skills was beyond the scope of this chapter on reading development because it requires a theory of higher-level cognitive development.

The developmental view presented in this chapter with its focus on word recognition has important implications for understanding reading disabilities. The importance of developmental models for notions of disability is a common theme in our field. Spear-Swerling and Sternberg (1996), for example, point out how an understanding of the factors that contribute to normal reading development can help differentiate the cognitive deficits that cause a reading problem from the cognitive deficits that may result from the reading problem. The factors that contribute to normal reading development also can provide a useful road map for considering the possible causes of reading problems and describing the specific problems children with reading disabilities experience. Chapters 4 and 5 cover these topics.

A theory of reading development can also influence how one defines and classifies children with reading disabilities. For example, in the next chapter, dyslexia is differentiated from a language-learning disability based on the extent to which the reading problem is restricted to problems with word recognition. And finally, knowledge of normal reading development can have significant educational and remedial implications, though as Spear-Swerling and Sternberg note, these implications are often not simple or straightforward. We may know from our developmental model, for example, that phonological awareness is important for learning sound-letter correspondences, but the developmental model does not prescribe how phonological awareness is best taught. Joe Torgesen will address this issue in Chapter 6.

References

Adams, M. (1990). *Beginning to read: Thinking and learning about print.* Cambridge, MA: MIT Press.

Adams, M., Treiman, R., & Pressley, M. (1996). Reading, writing, and literacy. In I. Sigel & A. Renninger (Eds.), *Mussen's handbook of child psychology, Volume 4: Child psychology in practice* (pp. 1–124). New York: Wiley.

Adler, M., & Van Doren, C. (1940/1972). *How to read a book.* New York: Simon & Schuster.

Backman, J., Bruck, M., Hebert, J., & Seidenberg, M. (1984). Acquisition and use of spelling-sound correspondences in reading. *Journal of Experimental Child Psychology, 38,* 114–133.

Baron, J., & Treiman, R. (1980). Use of orthography in

reading and learning to read. In J. Kavanagh & R. Venezky (Eds.), *Orthography, reading, and dyslexia* (pp. 171–189). Baltimore, MD: Park Press.

Barron, R., & Baron, J. (1977). How children get meaning from printed words. *Child Development, 48,* 587–594.

Becker, W., Dixon, R., & Anderson-Inman, L. (1980). *Morphographic and root word analysis of 26,000 high-frequency words.* Eugene, OR: University of Oregon College of Education.

Blachman, B. (1989). Phonological awareness and word recognition: Assessment and intervention. In A. Kamhi & H. Catts (Eds.), *Reading disabilities: A developmental language perspective* (pp. 133–158). Boston: Allyn & Bacon.

Blachman, B. (1994). What we have learned from longitudinal studies of phonological processing and reading, and some unanswered questions: A response to Torgesen, Wagner, and Rashotte. *Journal of Learning Disabilities, 27,* 287–291.

Brodkey, L. (1992). Articulating poststructural theory in research on literacy. In R. Beach, J. Green, M. Kamil, & T. Shanahan (Eds.), *Multidisciplinary perspectives on literacy research* (pp. 293–319). Urbana, IL: National Council of Teachers of English.

Bus, A., van IjzenDoorn, M., & Pellegrini, A. (1995). Joint book reading makes for success in learning to read: A meta-analysis on intergenerational transmission of literacy. *Review of Educational Research, 65,* 1–21.

Carlisle, J. (1991). Planning an assessment of listening and reading comprehension. *Topics in Language Disorders, 12*(1), 17–31.

Chall, J. (1983). *Stages of reading development.* New York: McGraw-Hill.

Commission on Reading (1985). *Becoming a nation of readers: The report of the Commission on Reading.* Washington, DC: The National Institute of Education.

Ehri, L. (1991). Development of the ability to read words. In R. Barr, M. Kamil, P. Mosenthal, & P. Pearson (Eds.), *Handbook of reading research* (Vol. 2, pp. 383–417). White Plains, NY: Longman.

Finn, P. (1977/78). Word frequency, information theory, and cloze performance: A transfer feature theory of processing in reading. *Reading Research Quarterly, 23,* 510–537.

Fish, S. (1980). *Is there a text in this class?* Cambridge MA: Harvard University Press.

Fodor, J. (1983). *The modularity of mind.* Cambridge, MA: MIT.

Frith, U. (1985). Beneath the surface of developmental dyslexia. In K. Patterson, J. Marshall, & M. Coltheart (Eds.), *Surface dyslexia* (pp. 301–330). London: Erlbaum.

Gibson, E., & Levine, H. (1975). *The psychology of reading.* Cambridge, MA: MIT Press.

Gough, P. (1983). Context, form, and interaction. In K. Rayner (Ed.), *Eye movements in reading* (pp. 203–211). New York: Academic Press.

Heath, S. (1982). What no bedtime story means: Narrative skills at home and at school. *Language in Society, 11,* 49–76.

Hoover, W., & Gough, P. (1990). The simple view of reading. *Reading and Writing: An Interdisciplinary Journal, 2,* 127–160.

Horn, E. (1926). *A basic writing vocabulary.* University of Iowa Monographs in Education, No. 4. Iowa City: University of Iowa Press.

Iser, W. (1978). *The act of reading: A theory of aesthetic response.* Baltimore: Johns Hopkins University Press.

Juel, C. (1991). Beginning reading. In R. Barr, M. Kamil, P. Mosenthal, & P. Pearson (Eds.), *Handbook of reading research* (Vol. 2, pp. 759–788). White Plains, NY: Longman.

Kamhi, A. (1993). Assessing complex behaviors: Problems with reification, quantification, and ranking. *Language, Speech, and Hearing Services in Schools, 24,* 110–113.

Kamhi, A. (1997). Three perspectives on comprehension: Implications for assessing and treating comprehension problems. *Topics in Language Disorders, 17*(3), 62–74.

Kamhi, A., & Catts, H. (1989). *Reading disabilities: A developmental language perspective.* Boston: Allyn & Bacon.

Karolides, N. (1997). *Reader response in elementary classrooms: Quest and discovery.* Mahwah, NJ: Erlbaum.

Langer, J. (1992). *Literature instruction: A focus on student response.* Urbana, IL: National Council of Teachers of English.

Marsh, G., Friedman, M., Desberg, P., & Saterdahl, K. (1981). Comparison of reading and spelling strategies in normal and reading-disabled children. In

M. Friedman, J. Das, & N. O'Connor (Eds.), *Intelligence and learning* (pp. 363–367). New York: Plenum.

Masonheimer, P., Drum, P., & Ehri, L. (1984). Does environmental print identification lead children into word reading? *Journal of Reading Behavior, 16,* 257–271.

McLaren, P. (1992). Literacy research on the postmodern turn: Cautions from the margins. In R. Beach, J. Green, M. Kamil, & T. Shanahan (Eds.), *Multidisciplinary perspectives on literacy research* (pp. 319–343). Urbana, IL:; National Council of Teachers of English.

Milosky, L. (1992). Children listening: The role of world knowledge in language comprehension. In R. Chapman (Ed.), *Processing in language acquisition and disorders* (pp. 20–44). St. Louis, MO: Mosby.

Nagy, W., & Herman, P. (1987). Breadth and depth of vocabulary knowledge: Implications for acquisition and instruction. In M. McKeown & M. Curtis (Eds.), *The nature of vocabulary acquisition* (pp. 19–35). Hillsdale, NJ: Erlbaum.

Olson, R.K., Kliegl, R., Davidson, B.J., & Foltz, G. (1985). Individual and developmental differences in reading disability. In C.E. MacKinnon & T. G. Waller (Eds.) *Reading Research: Advances in Theory and Practice: Vol 4.* New York: Academic Press.

Piaget, J. (1952). *The origins of intelligence in children.* New York: International Universities Press.

Purves, A. (1992). Testing literature. In J. Langer (Ed.), *Literature instruction: A focus on student response* (pp. 19–34). Urbana, IL: National Council of Teachers of English.

Rasool, J., & Royer, J. (1986). Assessment of reading comprehension using the sentence verification technique: Evidence from narrative and descriptive texts. *Journal of Educational Research, 79,* 180–184.

Richgels, D., McGee, L., Lomax, R., & Sheard, C. (1987). Awareness of four text structures: Effects on recall of expository texts. *Reading Research Quarterly, 22,* 177–196.

Royer, J. (1986). The sentence verification technique as a measure of comprehension: Validity, reliability, and practicality. Unpublished manuscript, University of Massachusetts.

Scarborough, H., & Dobrich, W. (1994). On the efficacy of reading to preschoolers. *Developmental Review, 14,* 245–302.

Share, D. (1995). Phonological recoding and self-teaching: *sine qua non* of reading acquisition. *Cognition, 55,* 151–218.

Share, D., & Stanovich, K. (1995). Cognitive processes in early reading development: Accommodating individual differences into a model of acquisition. *Issues in Education, 1,* 1–57.

Snow, C., & Goldfield, B. (1981). Building stories: The emergence of information structures from conversation. In D. Tannen (Ed.), *Analyzing discourse: Text and talk.* Washington, DC: Georgetown University Press.

Spear-Swerling, L., & Sternberg, R. (1996). *Off track: When poor readers become "learning disabled."* Boulder, CO: Westview Press.

Stanovich, K. (1990). Concepts in developmental theories of reading skill: Cognitive resources, automaticity, and modularity. *Developmental Review, 10,* 1–29.

Stanovich, K. (1991). Word recognition: Changing perspectives. In R. Barr, M. Kamil, P. Mosenthal, & P. Pearson (Eds.), *Handbook of reading research, Volume II* (pp. 418–452). White Plains, NY: Longman.

Stanovich, K., & Siegel, L. (1994). The phenotypic performance profile of reading-disabled children: A regression-based test of the phonological-core variable-difference model. *Journal of Educational Psychology, 86,* 24–53.

Stevenson, J., & Fredman, G. (1990). The social environmental correlates of reading ability. *Journal of Child Psychology and Psychiatry, 31,* 681–698.

Torgesen, J., Wagner, R., & Rashotte, C. (1994). Longitudinal studies of phonological processing and reading. *Journal of Learning Disabilities, 27,* 276–286.

Trabasso, T., & Magliano, J. (1996). Conscious understanding during comprehension. *Discourse Processes, 21,* 255–287.

van Kleeck, A. (1995). Emphasizing form and meaning separately in prereading and early reading instruction. *Topics in Language Disorders, 16*(1), 27–49.

van Kleeck, A., & Schuele, C. (1987). Precursors to literacy: Normal development. *Topics in Language Disorders, 7*(2), 13–31.

Wells, G. (1985). Preschool literacy-related activities and success in school. In D. Olson, N. Torrance, & A. Hildyard (Eds.), *Literacy, language, and learning: The nature and consequences of reading and writing* (pp. 229–255). New York: Cambridge University Press.

Wells, G. (1986). *The meaning makers.* Portsmouth, NH: Heinemann.

Chapter 3

Defining Reading Disabilities

HUGH W. CATTS   *ALAN G. KAMHI*

The development of reading is one of the major achievements of the early school years. For most children, learning to read is an enjoyable experience and one that comes without hardship. As noted in Chapter 2, some children enter school with a rich preschool history of literacy and in a few short months are well on their way to becoming skilled readers. Other children begin school with more limited literacy experiences, but with appropriate instruction, go on to become competent readers as well. Some children, on the other hand, experience significant difficulty learning to read and struggle for years with written language. These children with reading difficulties are the primary concern of this book. In this chapter, we begin by providing a historical perspective of reading disabilities that reflects our interest in the language basis of reading. After a brief discussion of the prevalence of reading disabilities, the remainder of the chapter focuses on terminology and definition issues associated with reading disabilities.

Historical Basis of Reading Disabilities

There is no such thing as an unbiased historical perspective. Historical reviews usually reflect the theoretical biases of the reviewer. One's biases influence not only the interpretation of the literature reviewed, but also what body of literature is reviewed. A few years ago, the second author (Kamhi, 1992) was asked to respond to Sylvia Richardson's historical perspective of dyslexia (Richardson, 1992). Richardson's medical orientation and background were clearly reflected in her review. She traced the roots of dyslexia to the medical literature of 100 years ago, wherein dyslexia was first viewed as a type of aphasia. She presented a brief history of aphasia, highlighting the work of Broca, Wernicke, and

Jackson, and then discussed the early accounts of dyslexia by other medical professionals such as Hinshelwood and Orton. Whereas Richardson's medical background influenced her historical perspective of dyslexia, our language background influences our historical perspective. The story we will tell about reading disabilities traces how reading problems have come to be viewed as a language-based disorder. There are, of course, other stories one could tell about reading disabilities. One could, for example, tell the story of the emergence of the field of learning disabilities and its relationship to reading disabilities (Lerner, 1985; Torgesen, 1991) or focus on perceptual-motor and visual correlates of reading disabilities (Benton, 1991).

In some respects, the different stories one can tell about reading disabilities should begin and end at the same place. It is hard to begin a story of reading disabilities without mention of Morgan and Hinshelwood, and it is hard to end the story without acknowledging the language bases of the disability. With these points in mind, here is our story of reading disabilities.

Early Reports

Reports of children with reading disabilities first began to appear in the late 1890s (Morgan, 1896). The identification of reading disabilities at that time was due, in part, to more widespread mandatory school attendance. As more and more children attended school on a regular basis, children who were experiencing difficulties learning to read despite adequate instruction became more apparent to educators. Some of these children were subsequently referred to physicians and other related professionals. Until the late 1800s, however, most physicians did not recognize the significance of these learning difficulties. Children with reading problems were generally thought to be poorly motivated or of low intelligence. Toward the end of the nineteenth century, however, reports began to be published that described patients who had lost spoken and/or written language abilities as the result of brain injury or illness (e.g., Berlin, 1887; Brodbent, 1872; Kussmaul, 1887). These accounts demonstrated that individuals could lose language abilities, but retain other aspects of intelligence. Physicians and other professionals soon began to recognize the similarities between acquired reading disabilities and the reading problems experienced by some children. This recognition led to the publication of scholarly reports of reading disabilities in children.

W. Pringle Morgan, an English physician, is generally given credit for the first published paper on developmental reading disabilities (Morgan, 1896). In this paper, he described the case of a bright 14-year-old boy who was "quick at games," but had great difficulty learning to read. Morgan reported that despite seven years of laborious and persistent instruction in reading, the boy could only read or spell the simplest of words. He described the boy's condition as *congenital word blindness*, a term coined by Hinshelwood (1895), a Scottish ophthalmologist, who had used *word blindness* to refer to the problems experienced by a school teacher with an acquired reading problem. Morgan found many similarities between the boy and the school teacher, but the boy's problems were not the result of an injury or illness. Because there was no obvious cause for the boy's reading problem, Morgan concluded that this problem must be congenital in nature.

Soon after Morgan's report, Hinshelwood (1900, 1917) published several accounts of congenital word blindness. He argued that the condition was the result of neurological deficits that impaired children's ability to remember visually presented letters and words. He also noted that the disorder ran in families and was probably hereditary. Hinshelwood also had some specific views on treatment and prognosis of the disorder. He believed strongly that all children with the disorder could learn to read and advocated for daily one-on-one instruction using the "old-fashioned" phonics method of teaching reading, rather than the look-and-say method that was commonly used at the time. He also recommended the use of multisensory input. Hinshelwood's views about treatment are remarkably consistent with current views on this subject (see Chapter 6).

Orton

One of the earliest accounts of developmental reading disabilities in the United States was by Samuel T. Orton. As the director of a mental health clinic in Iowa, Orton encountered a number of children whose primary problem was a difficulty learning to read. In 1925, he discussed these children's difficulties in a paper entitled "'Word Blindness' in School Children" (Orton, 1925). Following the publication of this paper, Orton began a comprehensive research program that included an investigation of speech and reading problems in children. In two years, he and his research team, employing a mobile clinic, examined more than a 1000 children across the state (J. Orton et al., 1975). This research and his subsequent work in private practice in New York laid the foundation for his seminal book, *Reading, Writing, and Speech Problems in Children* (Orton, 1937).

As a result of his extensive research, Orton recognized that reading disabilities were more common than generally thought. He believed that the prevalence rate was much higher than the 1/1000 estimate that had been reported by Hinshelwood and others. Orton's higher prevalence figure was due primarily to the way he defined the disability. Whereas others only recognized the most severe cases as instances of reading disabilities, he believed that reading disabilities were distributed along a graded continuum with no clear demarcation between the most and least severe cases. He maintained, as many do today, that the problems experienced by children with the most severe cases of reading disabilities are not qualitatively different from those found in the less severe cases.

Orton also attempted to explain the cause of reading disabilities. Rather than propose deficits in a specific area of the brain as Hinshelwood did, Orton argued that reading problems resulted from a failure to develop cerebral dominance for language in the left hemisphere. His theory is perhaps best known for its explanation of the reversal (e.g., *b/d*) and sequencing errors (e.g., *was/saw*) that had been observed in dyslexic individuals. Orton thought that insufficient cerebral dominance caused occasional confusion between the mirror images of words that he mistakenly believed were represented in each hemisphere. This confusion led to reversal or sequencing errors. While this account of reading errors is clearly inaccurate, many of Orton's other insights into the nature of reading disabilities are quite consistent with what we know today. In his 1937 book, he offered a classification system that included different types of spoken and written language disorders. He viewed reading disabilities as part of a larger set of developmental language disorders. He noted that many children who had problems reading also had difficulties in spoken language or had a history of spoken language difficulties. Orton's language-based view of reading disabilities was clearly way ahead of its time. In fact, it was so ahead of its time that it was ignored for decades.

Orton also developed a program of intervention for reading disabilities. Like Hinshelwood, he recommended a multisensory approach that involved explicit instruction in phoneme-grapheme associations. Children were first taught to link letters with their sounds and names. Once phoneme-grapheme correspondence was firmly established, children were taught to blend letter sounds together to form words. Orton believed all children with reading disabilities could learn to read using this approach. He later collaborated with Anna Gillingham to develop the Orton-Gillingham Approach. Currently, this program and ones like it are among the most popular methods of instruction for children with severe reading disabilities.

The important insights Orton and Hinshelwood made about the nature of reading disabilities had little impact on the prevailing views of reading disabilities held by most educators and other professionals of their time. In Orton's case this was probably because he was more known for his theory of cerebral dominance than for his language-based view of reading development. In any event, it would take about fifty years for researchers to begin to accumulate convincing evidence in support of a language-based view of reading. During these years, reading disabilities were attributed to an assortment of intellectual, perceptual, environmental, attitudinal, and/or educational problems (Critchley, 1970; Torgesen, 1991).

Johnson and Myklebust

Doris Johnson and Helmer Myklebust's contributions are of particular relevance to a language-based perspective of reading disabilities. Johnson and Myklebust were affiliated with the Institute for Language Disorders at Northwestern University. This institute was one of the first in which language specialists worked in conjunction with other professionals in the treatment of children with reading disabilities. Johnson and Myklebust's work at the Institute led to a seminal book on learning disabilities (Johnson & Myklebust, 1967). In this book, they offered a description and classification system for children with spoken and written language disorders. Among the problems described was auditory dyslexia, the term they used for a prominent form of reading disabilities. They reported that in addition to reading problems, children with auditory dyslexia had problems perceiving the similarities in the initial and final sounds in words. These children also had problems breaking words into syllables and phonemes, retrieving the names of letters and words, remembering verbal information, and pronouncing phonologically complex words in speech (e.g., pronouncing *enemy* as *emeny*). In providing this description of children with reading disabilities, Johnson and Mykelbust were the first to clearly delineate the extent of the phonological processing deficits experienced by these children. As will be discussed throughout this book, phonological processing deficits are now known to be strongly associated with developmental reading disabilities.

The Modern Era

The work of Orton and Johnson and Myklebust laid the foundation for the now widely accepted view that reading problems generally reflect limitations in language, rather than limitations in general cognitive abilities or visual perception. This view began to be espoused in the early 1970s by Mattingly (1972), Lerner (1972), and Shankweiler and Liberman (1972). Evidence in support of language-based theories of reading accumulated rapidly during the 1970s and 1980s. Lower-level phonological correlates of reading as well as higher-level syntactic and semantic correlates were studied in this work (Bradley & Bryant, 1983; Liberman & Shankweiler, 1985; Perfetti, 1985; Stanovich, 1988; Vellutino, 1979; Wagner & Torgesen, 1987). This research is discussed in several chapters of this book.

The change from visually based theories of reading disabilities to language-based theories opened the door for language specialists to become involved in reading problems. Speech-language pathologists with their knowledge and training in language and language disorders have become increasingly involved in the identification, assessment, and treatment of individuals with reading disabilities. The contribution a language specialist can make in serving individuals with reading disabilities is gradually becoming recognized by teachers, reading specialists, special educators, and psychologists. This recognition has led to an increase in the collaborative efforts between these professionals and language specialists.

Collaborative efforts have been encouraged and supported by writings and presentations from well-known language specialists. It is now more than twenty years since Norma Rees (1974) and Joel Stark (1975) began writing about the role of the speech-language pathologist in reading disabilities. It was another ten years before Wallach and Butler (1984) published their seminal book on language and learning disabilities. This book represented the first comprehensive attempt to integrate research on language development and disorders with research on learning and reading disabilities. Like the present book, contributors were language specialists. This book provided an important link for professionals involved in serving children and adolescents with language-based learning disorders. One of our goals in writing our first book on reading disabilities (Kamhi & Catts, 1989) was to make this link even stronger by focusing more closely on the language basis of reading disabilities.

It is always better to let others evaluate your contributions to history. Nevertheless, we would be remiss if we did not acknowledge the fortuitous timing of the publication of our book on reading disabilities in 1989. By the end of the 1980s, the so-called pragmatic revolution was well underway and many professionals were receptive to the consideration of language in multiple contexts. The American Speech-Language-Hearing Association (ASHA) was working closely with the National Joint Council on Learning Disabilities to develop a better definition of learning disabilities, ASHA committees were involved in developing position papers about serving children with language-learning disabilities, and prominent reading researchers were confirming the language basis of reading disabilities. In addition, researchers in speech-language pathology were presenting convincing evidence that many children with preschool language impairments developed reading problems when they entered school. Language specialists were thus primed to read about the language basis of reading disabilities and how they should be involved in the assessment and treatment of children with reading problems. During the ensuing ten years, language specialists have become increasingly involved in emergent literacy programs and in collaborative efforts with regular and special educators in elementary and secondary schools. With this increased scope of practice, language specialists and other educators need the most current information about reading disabilities. The present book attempts to address this need.

Terminology

Many different terms have been used to refer to individuals with reading disabilities (RD). As noted above, *congenital word blindness* was the first term to be employed. Other terms include *dyslexia, developmental dyslexia, specific reading disability*, and *reading disability*. The term *disability* is often used interchangeably with *disorder, impairment*, and in some cases, *retardation*. More general terms such as *learning disability* and *poor reader* are also used to characterize individuals with reading problems. The term *language-learning disability* has also been used by some to describe school-age children who have spoken and written language deficits (Gerber, 1993; Wallach & Butler, 1984, 1994). Occasionally, the word *developmental* is added in order to clarify that the disability is not an acquired problem, but rather one of initial learning.

Of all the terms used to refer to individuals with RD, the term *dyslexia* has been the most confusing and the most misunderstood. Etymologically, dyslexia means difficulty with words. Dyslexia was first used in the late nineteenth century to label reading problems associated with brain injury or illness (Berlin, 1887). The term was later applied to developmental reading disabilities where there was no evidence of brain damage. Dyslexia, however, eventually became a popular label for children who made reversal (*b/d*) or sequencing errors (*was/saw*). Most people outside the field of reading disabilities continue to think of dyslexia as reading or writing backwards. Although children with dyslexia do make reversal and sequencing errors, these errors represent only a small proportion of the total errors they make. More importantly, normally developing readers as well as nondyslexic poor readers also make these kinds of errors, so the occurrence of these errors has little diagnostic value (see Chapter 5 for more discussion of this issue). Despite the confusion surrounding the term dyslexia, it remains a popular label among researchers and clinicians who deal specifically with reading disabilities.

The standard educational term used to categorize children with reading disabilities in the United States is *learning disabled*. While the majority of children labeled learning disabled have received this designation on the basis of their poor reading skills, the term is also used for other learning problems (e.g., math difficulties). Because of the heterogeneity of children with learning disabilities, most investigators and clinicians agree that the term learning disability is too broad to be used to refer to reading disabilities. The term *language-learning disability* suffers from some of the same problems as the term learning disability. Use of this term is primarily restricted to speech-language pathologists, though some reading theorists have also embraced the term (Ceci & Baker, 1978). In the past, the term has not been well defined and has included a variety of problems beyond reading disabilities. In spite of these problems, by focusing attention on the language basis of many learning problems, the term language-learning disability has played an important role in getting language specialists involved in serving children with reading and other learning disabilities.

Throughout this book, we primarily use the term *reading disabilities*. This term is a common term used by researchers and practitioners to refer to a heterogeneous group of children who have difficulty learning to read. We also use the terms dyslexia and language-learning disabilities to refer to more specific types of reading problems. These latter terms are defined later in this chapter.

Prevalence

What is the prevalence of reading disabilities? For many years, it was thought that this question could be answered in a rather straightforward manner. Reading abilities were assumed to be distributed bimodally with normal readers constituting one group and children with RD the other. The reading achievement scores of the normal readers were thought to be distributed along a normal bell-shaped curve, whereas children with RD were thought to have reading scores that clustered together and formed a "hump" at the low end of the normal distribution. Children with RD could, therefore, be clearly distinguished from typically developing children, and the prevalence of reading disabilities could be easily determined.

Early support for the existence of a hump in the reading achievement distribution was provided by Rutter and Yule (1975) and Yule, Rutter, Berger, and Thompson (1974). In the 1960s, Rutter, Yule, and their colleagues conducted a large epidemiological study on the Isle of Wight in England. The study included the entire population of about 3,500 9- to 11-year-old children living on the island. One of the many goals of this investigation was to determine the prevalence of reading disabilities. A reading disability was operationally defined as performance on a reading achievement test (word recognition or reading comprehension) that was at least two standard deviations below normal. If scores were normally distributed without a hump in the low end, it would be predicted that 2.3 percent of the population of children should perform two standard deviations below the mean. Depending on how reading was measured (i.e., word recognition or reading comprehension) and the age of the children, the results indicated that between 3.1 and 4.4 percent of the subjects obtained reading scores more than two standard deviations below the mean. Yule and colleagues (1974) also reported that in a comparative group of children from London the prevalence rate was 6.3 to 9.3 percent. The researchers concluded that there was evidence of a hump at the low end of the reading achievement distribution and that this indicated the distinct nature of reading disabilities.

A number of investigators have questioned the validity of the prevalence data from the Isle of Wight study (Rodgers, 1983; Shaywitz, Escobar, Shaywitz, Fletcher, & Makuch, 1992; van der Wissel & Zegers, 1985). The primary criticism concerns the possible ceiling effects of the Neale Analysis of Reading Ability, the instrument used to measure reading achievement in this study. This reading test had an upper age limit of 12 years, which was exceeded by many of the subjects in the study. Van Wissel and Zegers (1995) argued that such a ceiling effect could result in an apparent hump in the low end of the reading distribution. To test this, they ran a computer simulation in which a ceiling effect was artificially imposed. This resulted in a hump at the low end of the distribution much like that reported by Rutter and Yule (1975) and Yule and colleagues (1974).

Recently, Shaywitz and co-workers (1992) attempted to replicate the results from the Isle of Wight study in their data from the Connecticut Longitudinal Study, an investigation involving approximately 400 Connecticut children who entered kindergarten in 1983. Their results indicated that regardless of the way in which reading disabilities were defined or the grade at which they were examined (first to sixth grade), there was no evidence of an excess of poor readers at the low end of the distribution. In other words, children with RD did not represent a distinct group. They were simply at the low end of the reading ability continuum (also see Rodgers, 1983; Share, McGee, McKenzie, Williams, & Silva, 1987).

If the above findings continue to be replicated in future studies, they will have important implications for the notion of the prevalence of reading disabilities. These results indicate that the distinction between normal children and those with RD is arbitrary. It depends on the specific cut-off score selected by the researcher or clinician. For example, if one standard deviation below the mean is selected as the sole criterion for defining a reading disability, then the prevalence of reading disabilities would be 16 percent. If two standard deviations is selected as the dividing line, then the prevalence of reading disabilities would decrease to 2.3 percent.

Just because the notion of prevalence is a relative one, it does not mean that reading disabilities are not a real phenomenon. This point has been made very clearly by Ellis (1985), who noted that a reading disability is like obesity. He stated that for any given age and height there is an uninterrupted continuum from painfully thin to inordinately fat. Where on the continuum obesity falls is entirely arbitrary, but the arbitrariness of the distinction between overweight and obese does not mean that obesity is not a real and worrysome condition, nor does it prevent research into the causes and cures of obesity from being both valuable and necessary (Ellis, 1985). Although the prevalence of reading disabilities, like obesity, depends on where one draws the line, reading disabilities are as real as obesity.

Gender Differences

It has been commonly assumed that the prevalence of reading disabilities is higher in boys than in girls (Critchley, 1970; Golderberg & Schiffman, 1972; Thomson, 1984). Most early studies of reading disabilities supported this assumption. For example, the boy-to-girl ratio of reading disabilities reported by Naidoo (1972) was 5:1 and by Rutter and colleagues (Rutter, Tizard, & Whitmore, 1970) was 3.3:1. More recent studies, however, have failed to find gender differences in the prevalence of reading disabilities (e.g., Prior, Sanson, Smart, & Oberlaid, 1995; Shaywitz, Shaywitz, Fletcher, & Escobar, 1990). Shaywitz and colleagues (1990) attributed the conflicting results in prevalence figures to whether the sample selected for study was identified by schools/clinics or by research. School and clinic samples typically showed a higher prevalence of boys with reading disabilities. Research-identified samples, they argued, were more likely to show no gender bias because objective criteria, based on achievement scores and/or IQ-achievement discrepancy, were used to identify the children with RD. The reason for the gender bias in schools or clinics is that factors other than reading performance have often been used for diagnostic or classification purposes. For example, children's attention, level of activity, or classroom behavior can influence identification. Shaywitz and colleagues noted that boys are more active, more inattentive, and more disruptive than girls. The prevalence of attention deficit disorders is also thought to be higher in boys than girls (Nass, 1993). Poor readers with behavior and attention problems are more likely to be identified as reading or learning disabled than poor readers without behavior and attention problems.

Shaywitz and colleagues (1990) tested this explanation in two samples of poor readers from the Connecticut Longitudinal Study. One sample included all children in the study whose reading achievement score was 1.5 standard deviations or more below their IQ (research-identified sample). The other sample consisted of all children who were classified by the school district as reading/learning disabled and who were receiving special services for their reading problems (school-identified sample). Consistent with their predictions, the researchers found a 4:1 ratio in favor of boys in the school-identified sample compared with a 1.3:1 ratio in a research-identified sample. These results indicate that a selection bias may account for the earlier findings of more boys than girls with reading disabilities. Until recently, most studies have employed samples of children with RD who have been identified by schools or clinics. However, it appears that if a low score on a reading achievement test (and/or a discrepancy between reading and IQ) is used as the primary criterion to identify a reading disability, then one should expect to find about as many girls with reading disabilities as boys.

Defining Reading Disability

It should be clear after the discussions of prevalence and gender that the way children with RD are defined has significant theoretical implications. Indeed, the validity of research on reading disabilities depends in large part on the operational definitions used to select participants for study. At least some of the inconsistencies in the literature can be attributed to the lack of uniformity in the criteria used to identify students with RD. As noted in the previous section, the reliance on school or clinic designations of reading/learning disabilities has led to the inclusion of children with behavior and attention problems in studies of children with RD. Research that has used such heterogeneous samples of poor readers has produced a host of questionable associations between reading disabilities and behavioral, cognitive, and environmental variables.

Definitions also affect the identification, assessment, and treatment of children with RD. Definitions are used to determine who is eligible for remedial services. Definitions of reading/learning disabilities vary from state to state and from school district to school district. This variability significantly influences whether a given child will receive remedial services. A particular child may qualify for special services in one state or school district, but not another. Definitions can also give direction for intervention. Specifying the nature of the problems associated with reading disabilities in a definition can lead professionals to areas of difficulty that should be considered in planning intervention. Clearly, definitions are not simply trivial matters for scholars to debate.

Defining reading disabilities has not proven to be an easy task, in part because several different disciplines are interested in reading disabilities. Reading problems have been the concern of special educators, reading specialists, physicians, optometrists, psychologists, and speech-language pathologists. These individuals have different orientations and theoretical biases that influence the way they define reading disabilities. As a result, different professionals may focus on different aspects of the problem. Despite these different orientations and theoretical biases, most professionals agree that the term reading disability should not be used to refer to all children who have problems in learning to read. For example, children who have had inadequate instruction are not considered reading disabled. In addition, children with severe visual impairment or mental retardation are seldom classified as reading disabled. Most professionals also agree that a group of children exist who have reading problems despite normal or above average levels of intelligence. The terms *specific reading disability* and *dyslexia* have typically been used to characterize this group of children.

In the sections that follow, we begin by considering the exclusionary criteria that have traditionally been used to define reading disabilities. The remaining sections consider the advantages of using inclusionary criteria to define reading disabilities and our attempt to differentiate between children with specific reading disabilities and those with more general language-learning problems. In these sections, we will use the term *dyslexia* to refer to children with a specific reading disability because much of the literature uses this label. This term also seems to be more appropriate for labeling a condition whose symptoms are seldom limited to reading problems.

Exclusionary Factors

Traditionally, definitions of dyslexia have focused heavily on exclusionary factors. For the most part, definitions have provided as much, if not more, information about what dyslexia is not than what it is. Consider, for example, an influential definition of dyslexia proposed by the World Federation of Neurology (Critchley, 1970):

> Dyslexia is a disorder manifested by difficulty learning to read despite conventional instruction, adequate intelligence, and socio-culture opportunity. It is dependent upon cognitive disabilities which are frequently of constitutional origin. (p. 11)

The World Federation definition excludes a number of causal factors from dyslexia. Although stated in a positive manner, inadequate instruction, lack of opportunity, and low intelligence are ruled out as potential causes of the reading problems found in dyslexia. Other definitions exclude sensory deficits such as impairments in hearing or visual acuity (Lyon, 1995; Miles, 1983). Emotional disturbances and brain damage are also sometimes ruled out in definitions of dyslexia (Heaton & Winterson, 1996).

Sensory/Emotional/Neurological Factors
Generally, hearing and visual acuity are assessed. For children to be labeled dyslexic, they must have sensory abilities within normal limits (this includes corrected vision). In some cases, children with sensory deficits can be diagnosed as dyslexic, provided their reading problems go beyond those predicted on the basis of the hearing or visual handicap. Identification of dyslexia also typically requires that emotional and behavioral problems be ruled out as the cause of the reading difficulties. Poor readers, for example, with autism, childhood schizophrenia, or significant behavioral problems, are not considered dyslexic. Finally, neurological impairments caused by injury or illness are excluded from the diagnosis of dyslexia.

Instructional Factors
To be identified as dyslexic, poor readers also must have had adequate literacy experience. Unlike the acquisition of spoken language, the development of reading requires explicit instruction. Therefore, an individual who has not had adequate opportunity and instruction should clearly not be labeled reading disabled. Operationalizing this exclusionary criterion, however, can be difficult. Practitioners and researchers have most often relied on enrollment in an age-appropriate grade as evidence of adequate literacy experience and instruction.

However, such a criterion is often not sufficient. In many inner-city schools, a large percentage of children in age-appropriate classrooms are reading well below national norms. Although these children clearly have reading problems, we do not consider them to be reading disabled.

Recent research suggests that the use of enrollment in an age-appropriate grade as an exclusionary criterion for reading disability may not even be sufficient for children attending middle-class schools. In a longitudinal study, Vellutino and colleagues (Vellutino, Scanlon, Sipay, Small, Chen, Pratt, & Denckla, 1996) sampled children from middle- and upper middle-class school districts in Albany, New York. From this sample, a group of poor readers was identified on the basis of first-grade reading achievement. The poor readers were subsequently provided with fifteen weeks of daily one-to-one tutoring (30 minutes per session). Following this intervention phase, the poor readers were divided into those who were hard to remediate and those who were easy to remediate. Vellutino and co-workers suggested that the former were truly reading disabled, whereas the latter simply lacked adequate literacy experience. The researchers further found that the so-called truly RD children (and not the readily remediated children), differed significantly from normal readers in cognitive abilities closely linked with reading development (namely, phonological processing). Vellutino and colleagues suggested that the diagnosis of dyslexia might be reserved for those children with phonological processing deficits who do not respond to short-term intervention efforts.

Some school districts have implemented procedures similar to those suggested by Vellutino and co-workers (1996). For example, public schools in Texas have begun to use a three-phase approach for the identification of dyslexia (Texas Education Agency, 1996). During Phase I, poor readers are identified and information is gathered from vision/hearing screening, teacher reports, and formal assessments. In Phase II, all poor readers are provided with remedial reading services in order to rule out environmental or instructional deficits. In Phase III, those students who continue to have reading problems after completion of remedial services may be diagnosed as dyslexic and receive special educational services for their problems.

Procedures such as these seem to better address exclusionary criteria related to instruction. However, many questions remain. For example, how intensive must remedial services be to rule out instructional deficits? What type of remedial instruction is most appropriate? Will children who respond favorably to remedial instruction continue to develop normally in reading, or will they again fall behind once services have been discontinued? If the latter is the case, should they now be labeled reading disabled? Finally, when it is not possible to provide short-term remedial services, what alternative procedures might be used to rule out instructional factors?

Intelligence

Among exclusionary factors, intelligence has been given the most attention by practitioners. To be diagnosed as dyslexic, an individual typically must demonstrate a significant difference between measured intelligence (IQ) and reading achievement. This is often referred to as an IQ-achievement discrepancy. Generally, this means that to be diagnosed as dyslexic, the individual must show poor reading achievement but normal or above normal intelligence.

Poor readers with low IQs and children who do not meet IQ-achievement criteria have been variously labeled backward readers (Jorm, Share, Maclean, & Matthews, 1986; Rutter & Yule, 1975), low achievers (Fletcher, Shaywitz, Shankweiler, Katz, Liberman, Stuebing, Francis, Fowler, & Shaywitz, 1994), or garden-variety poor readers (Gough & Tunmer, 1986; Stanovich, 1991). A common justification for the use of IQ-achievement discrepancy is that it differentiates children who have specific reading problems (i.e., dyslexics) and those who have more general learning difficulties.

Serious concerns have been raised about the use of IQ in definitions of dyslexia (Fletcher, Francis, Rourke, Shaywitz, & Shaywitz, 1992; Siegel, 1989; Stanovich, 1991, 1997). There are, for example, numerous methodological problems associated with selecting intelligence and achievement tests and comparing test performances. The tests used to measure IQ and achievement have been shown to significantly influence the magnitude of the discrepancy obtained. For example, Rudel (1985) found that a sample of fifty children referred for reading disabilities had a mean discrepancy of 23.9 months between mental age and reading age using the Gray Oral Reading Test, a timed test. In contrast, these same children had a mean discrepancy of only 8.6 months using the Wide Range Achievement Test, which tests the reading of single words and is timed. Another measurement issue concerns potential problems involving statistical regression. Because of regression toward the mean, the calculation of IQ-achievement discrepancy can result in the overidentification of dyslexia in students with high IQs and underidentification of those with low IQs (cf. Fletcher, 1992; Francis, Espy, Rourke, & Fletcher, 1987).

Another problem with the use of IQ in defining dyslexia is that IQ tests do not directly measure potential for reading achievement. Rather, they assess current cognitive abilities, some of which overlap with abilities important in reading. This is particularly true for verbal IQ tests that assess vocabulary and comprehension. Because of the overlap in the abilities measured by these tests and reading tests, many poor readers will have lower IQ levels than good readers. In addition, poor readers generally read less than good readers, and thus, may acquire less of the knowledge measured by verbal IQ tests. As a result, verbal IQ tests may underestimate the intelligence of poor readers and make it harder for them to show an IQ-achievement discrepancy (Siegel, 1989).

The problem with verbal IQ tests has led some investigators to argue for the use of nonverbal IQ measures to identify children with dyslexia. However, performance on nonverbal IQ tests has little direct relationship to reading achievement (Stanovich, 1991). Knowing how well a child matches block designs or perceives the missing parts of pictures tells us little about how he or she should read. Such an argument calls into question the practice of some language specialists who insist on using nonverbal IQ measures to estimate potential (or IQ-achievement discrepancy) of children with language-based reading disabilities.

Research has also challenged some of the basic assumptions associated with the use of IQ in defining dyslexia. Inherent to this approach is the belief that dyslexics have different profiles in reading and reading-related abilities than do poor readers with low IQs (Siegel, 1989; Stanovich, 1991; 1997). Contrary to this assumption, recent research has shown that dyslexics and low achievers typically have similar problems in learning to read (Felton & Wood, 1992; Fletcher et al., 1994; Francis, Fletcher, Shaywitz, Shaywitz, & Rourke, 1996; Share, 1997; Siegel, 1992; Stanovich & Siegel, 1994). Both groups of children have difficulty learning to use the phonetic route to decode words. Dyslexics and low achievers have also been shown to exhibit similar cognitive deficits, particularly in phonological processing (Das, Mensink, & Mishra, 1990; Das, Mishra, & Kirby, 1994; Hurford, Schauf, Bunce, Blaich, & Moore, 1994; Naglieri & Reardon, 1993; Taylor, Satz, & Friel, 1979; but see Eden, Stein, Wood, & Wood, 1995; Wolf & Obregon, 1989). Studies have also failed to find distinct differences between dyslexics and low achievers in terms of heritability of reading problems and the neurological basis of these problems (Olson, Rack, Conners, DeFries, & Fulker, 1991; Pennington, Gilger, Olson, & DeFries, 1992; Steveson, Graham, Fredman, & McLoughlin, 1987; but see Olson, Forsberg, Gayan, & Defries, in press).

A primary justification for the use of IQ in defining dyslexia has been its presumed prognostic value. It has been assumed that dyslexics, with their higher IQs, respond better to intervention than low achievers. Because of this assumption, dyslexics have often received special education while low achievers typically have not. This practice, unfortunately, has gone unchecked for years. Recently, however, researchers have begun to investigate intervention outcome in relation to IQ. In general, studies have failed to find an association between improvement in reading (primarily word recognition) and IQ (Kershner, 1990; Share et al., 1987; Torgesen, Wagner, & Rashotte, 1997). Torgesen, Wagner, and Rashotte (1997), for example, found that IQ was not a good predictor of outcome in children at risk for reading disabilities who were participating in a two-and-one-half-year intervention study.

It should be clear that there are a number of serious problems associated with the use of IQ in defining dyslexia. These problems have led some leading scholars to argue that IQ should not be used in defining or diagnosing dyslexia (Aaron, 1991; Siegel, 1989; Stanovich, 1991, 1997). The abandonment of IQ as an exclusionary factor, however, has been slow to gain acceptance, which is really not surprising, given that normal or above normal intelligence has always been a defining characteristic of dyslexia. In addition, IQ tests play a fundamental role in determining eligibility and placement for special education services. In most school systems, children cannot qualify for special education services for a reading disability without an IQ test. Because IQ is so entrenched in our definitions and practice involving reading disabilities, it is probably unrealistic to expect that researchers and practitioners would readily abandon its use. One way, however, to move beyond definitions based heavily on IQ-achievement discrepancy is to turn to definitions that specify inclusionary factors. By focusing on what dyslexia is and the inclusionary characteristics that define the disorder, we should be able to reduce the reliance on exclusionary factors such as IQ when identifying children with RD.

Inclusionary Factors

Most definitions of reading disabilities have provided only minimal information concerning inclusionary factors. For example, the World Federation definition of dyslexia simply states that dyslexia is a problem learning to read and that this problem is due to cognitive impairments that are presumed to be present from birth. In this definition, no information is provided about the nature of the reading problems or the specific cognitive deficits that underlie them. As recognition has grown about the importance of specifying the nature of reading and cognitive deficits found in dyslexia, inclusionary definitions have become more prominent. For example, the Research Committee of the International Dyslexia Association (formerly the Orton Dyslexia Society), a professional organization devoted to the study of dyslexia, has proposed the following working definition of dyslexia:

> Dyslexia is a specific language-based disorder of constitutional origin character-ized by difficulties in single word decoding, usually reflecting insufficient phono-logical processing. These difficulties in single word decoding are often unexpected in relationship to age and other cognitive and academic abilities; they are not the result of a generalized developmental disability or sensory impairment. Dyslexia is manifest by variable difficulty with different forms of language, often including, in addition to problems in learning to read, a conspicuous problem in acquiring proficiency in writing and spelling (cited in Lyon, 1995).

This definition not only includes the usual exclusionary criteria, but also provides some spe-cific information about what dyslexia is, namely, that dyslexia represents a problem in single word decoding. Such a statement is consistent with a large body of research that indicates that children with dyslexia have particular problems in word recognition (see Chapter 4). This work demonstrates that children with dyslexia have problems using the phonological route to decode words, which results in difficulty recognizing novel words and building a sight vocabulary (Share & Stanovich, 1995). The Dyslexia Association definition also acknowledges that dyslexia is often characterized by problems in writing and spelling. These problems are generally quite persistent, and even with intervention, often are present in adulthood (Clark & Uhry, 1995; Miles, 1983).

The International Dsylexia Association definition further states that dyslexia is a specific language-based disability of constitutional origin and that insufficient phonological pro-cessing underlies the difficulty dyslexics have in learning to read, write, and spell. Research now strongly documents the problems individuals with dyslexia have in storing and retriev-ing phonological memory codes and in the explicit awareness of these codes. These diffi-culties have been observed in speech perception (Brandt & Rosen, 1980; Godfrey, Lasky, Millag, & Knox, 1981; Werker & Tees, 1987), verbal short-term memory (Brady, Poggie, & Rapala, 1989; Cohen & Netley, 1981; Torgesen, 1985), retrieval of phonological informa-tion (Bowers & Swanson, 1991; Denckla & Rudel, 1976; Spring & Davis, 1988; Wolf, 1984), production of phonologically complex sequences (Catts, 1986; 1989b; Snowling, 1981; Taylor, Lean, & Schwartz, 1989), and phonological awareness (Bradley & Bryant, 1983; Mann & Liberman, 1984; Torgesen, Wagner, & Rashotte, 1994; Vellutino & Scanlon, 1987). The general consensus is that phonological processing deficiencies cause significant difficulties learning to decode and recognize words (Catts, 1989a; Liberman & Shankweiler, 1985; Stanovich, 1988).

Dyslexia as a Developmental Language Disorder

Our definition of dyslexia also emphasizes the language basis of the disorder. We define dyslexia in the following manner:

> Dyslexia is a developmental language disorder whose defining characteristic is difficulty in phonological processing. This disorder, which is often genetically

transmitted, is generally present at birth and persists throughout the lifespan. Phonological processing difficulties include problems storing, retrieving, and using phonological codes in memory as well as deficits in phonological awareness and speech production. A prominent characteristic of the disorder in school-age children is difficulties learning to decode and spell printed words. These difficulties, in turn, often lead to deficits in reading comprehension and writing.

Our definition is similar in many respects to the Dyslexia Association definition. We concur that dyslexia is a language-based disorder in which phonological processing difficulties disrupt word decoding and other aspects of written language. However, our definition places more emphasis on the developmental nature of the disorder. According to our definition, dyslexia is much more than a reading disability; it is a disorder in the development of spoken and written language. This language impairment begins early in life and continues throughout childhood into adolescence and adulthood. During the preschool years, the disorder manifests itself in problems with spoken language development (Badian, 1994; Catts, 1993; Scarborough, 1990). In some cases, problems will be seen in the development of vocabulary, morphology, and syntax (Catts, 1993; Scarborough, 1990). However, these problems will be limited. As will be discussed below, we use the term language-learning disability to refer to more widespread difficulties in language development. According to our definition, the primary language deficit experienced by preschool children with dyslexia is difficulty in phonological processing. Children with dyslexia generally have significant problems in phonological awareness. Many also have difficulties in other aspects of phonological processing, including phonological storage and retrieval, speech perception, and complex phonological production. These problems in phonological processing are generally biologically based and, at least in part, heritable (Olson et al., 1991).

Upon entering school, phonological processing problems make it difficult for children with dyslexia to learn to decode printed words. Decoding problems and the associated spelling difficulties that ensue are a prominent characteristic of dyslexia during the school years. Although many children with dyslexia will also experience problems in reading comprehension, decoding deficits are the major contributing factor to these problems. Many individuals with dyslexia go on to acquire some basic reading and writing skills. However, in adulthood, most still show problems in oral reading, writing, and spelling (Miles, 1983). Difficulties in phonological processing are also still frequently observed in spoken and written language (Blalock, 1982; Bruck, 1992; Felton, Naylor, & Wood, 1990).

Unlike many definitions of dyslexia, the severity of the reading disability is not a critical criterion of our definition. Granted, most individuals with dyslexia will demonstrate some reading difficulties during the school years. However, if these individuals have the developmental language impairment described above, they can be referred to as dyslexic before they have reading difficulties, as well as afterwards when they have acquired some reading skills. Traditionally, dyslexia has been tied closely to a reading disability. However, such an approach is problematic. Many factors can influence how well or poorly an individual reads, so reading performance by itself will not be able to differentiate dyslexia from other reading problems. By defining dyslexia as a developmental language disorder rather than a reading disability, we can better capture the language basis of the problem. This has the added advantage of allowing us to identify dyslexia early in development.

According to our definition, identification of dyslexia can be based on language deficits, particularly problems in phonological processing. Because such problems are present during the preschool years, dyslexia can be identified before children enter school and experience problems learning to read.

It is, of course, possible to have difficulties in the development of spoken language without being dyslexic. Some children have problems learning to talk and understand language during the preschool years, but demonstrate normal development in spoken and written language during the school years (Bishop & Adams, 1990; Catts, 1993). These children are not considered to be dyslexic. We also recognize that not all children with reading problems are dyslexic. Like others, we exclude sensory deficits and environmental factors from serving as the primary cause of dyslexia. Individuals with sensory impairments or environmental disadvantagement can be considered dyslexic if their developmental language disorder goes beyond problems caused by these factors. We also exclude most children with general intellectual impairments from dyslexia. If these children have low verbal IQs, they may be included in another language-based reading disability category that is discussed in the next section. Children with normal verbal IQs but below average nonverbal IQs may still be labeled dyslexic, provided they show the phonological processing and reading deficits associated with the disorder.

Finally, not all children with a specific reading disability necessarily have a developmental language disorder. A small percentage of children with specific reading disabilities (perhaps 10 to 15%) may have other primary cognitive-perceptual factors underlying their difficulties. Some have suggested that visual deficits may contribute to these reading problems, though the confirmatory evidence is still inconclusive at this time (see Chapter 5). If visual problems do turn out to be the principal cause of reading disabilities in some children, we suggest that these children not be considered dyslexic, but rather as having a "visual-based reading disability." Conversely, we may find that visual deficits co-occur with language deficits and reading disabilities, but are not causally related to them. As such, visual deficits might be considered correlated problems and possible symptoms of dyslexia. Others have suggested a similar status for factors such as right-left confusion (Miles, 1983) or motor and balance problems (Nicolson & Fawcett, 1995). As more converging evidence becomes available on these latter factors, they may also become part of the definition of dyslexia. Until then, however, dyslexia seems to best be defined on the basis of phonological processing deficits.

Language-Learning Disabilities

So far in this chapter, we have focused primarily on dyslexia. However, dyslexia is not the only type of language-based reading disability. Many poor readers have more widespread language impairments than are typically found in dyslexia. Catts, Fey, and Tomblin (1997) recently estimated that perhaps as many as 50 percent of poor readers have language deficits that go beyond phonological processing. These children may have limitations in vocabulary, morphology, syntax, and/or text-level processing (e.g., narrative comprehension). We will refer to this group of children as *language-learning disabled (LLD)*. Others have also used this term to describe school-age children with problems in language development (Gerber, 1993; Wallach & Butler, 1984, 1994). Like dyslexia, signs of a more widespread language-learning impairment first appear during the preschool years. At this time, children with LLD show deficits in vocabulary and grammar. Most of these children also have problems in phonological processing similar to those found in children with dyslexia (Kamhi & Catts, 1986; Kamhi, Catts, Mauer, Apel, & Gentry, 1988). Many children with LLD are seen by speech-language pathologists in the preschool years. At school age, children with LLD demonstrate difficulty in listening comprehension, discourse, and narrative production (Gerber, 1993; Wallach & Butler, 1994). Children with LLD will also have significant problems learning to read, including difficulties in word recognition and reading comprehension. However, unlike children with dyslexia, children with LLD have broad-based problems in comprehension. This distinction will be discussed in more detail in the next chapter.

For some children with LLD, language difficulties are their primary cognitive deficits. These children have been called *specific language impaired* by language specialists (Johnston, 1988; Leonard, 1989). Considerable research attention has been focused on this group of children (Bishop, 1992). A portion of this research clearly demonstrates the problems these children have in learning to read (Bishop & Adams, 1990; Catts, 1993; Menyuk, Chesnick, Liebergott, Korngold, D'Agostino, Belanger, 1993). While some children with LLD have problems specific to language, others have more extensive cognitive impairments including deficits in both verbal and nonverbal abilities. These children are sometimes referred to as *nonspecific language impaired* (Tomblin, Records, Buckwalter, Zhang, Smith, & O'Brian, 1997). In our definition of language-learning disabilities, we make no distinction between children with specific and nonspecific language impairments. Both groups of children have language deficits, and it is these impairments, not nonverbal cognitive deficits, that should be most directly related to reading development. Only recently has research begun to compare the reading and reading-related cognitive abilities of specific and nonspecific language impaired children (Catts & Fey, 1995). As this and other work is completed, we will be better able to evaluate the need for a distinction between these groups of children.

When more traditional diagnostic approaches are used, some children with LLD will be classified as dyslexic, especially if their impairments in vocabulary, morphology, syntax, and text-level processing are relatively mild. However, the more severe the language impairment is, the less likely children with LLD will demonstrate the IQ-achievement discrepancy needed to be considered dyslexic. This is because children with significant language impairments will perform poorly on the verbal scales of IQ tests, thus lowering overall IQ. The lower overall IQ will make it more difficult to meet the discrepancy criteria for dyslexia. As noted above, these children have been referred to as low achievers or garden-variety poor readers (Fletcher et al., 1994; Gough & Tunmer, 1986). We prefer to call these children language-learning disabled because this term focuses attention on the central role that language-learning difficulties play in these children's reading, writing, and other learning problems.

We recommend that rather than relying on IQ tests to distinguish between dyslexic and LLD children, that more direct measures of language development be used. These measures might include tests of semantic, syntactic, and text-level processing (sometimes referred to as higher-level language processing). Some have suggested the use of tests of listening comprehension that provide an overall measure of higher-level language processing. Children with RD who perform within normal age limits on these higher-level language tests would be classified as dyslexic, whereas children who perform below age limits would be referred to as language-learning disabled. Measures of higher-level language processing would also need to be used in conjunction with measures of phonological processing and reading. Differentiating children based on their higher-level language abilities should lead to more appropriate intervention programs for both groups of children. Children with dyslexia need intervention directed primarily at phonological processing and word recognition, while those with language-learning disabilities will require intervention that targets language comprehension abilities in addition to phonological processing and word recognition abilities.[1]

The use of higher-level language tests to distinguish dyslexia from language-learning disabilities does not mean we are advocating that language tests simply replace IQ measures in discrepancy approaches used for practice or research. We see no clinical or theoretical basis for using discrepancy formulas at all. Traditionally, these formulas have resulted in the provision of special services to dyslexic children. Children with LLD have had to meet additional criteria in order to qualify for special services for reading. As discussed above, this practice is based, in part, on the assumption that dyslexics benefit more from reading intervention than do children with LLD. This assumption, however, has not been adequately tested. Very few investigations have compared the intervention outcomes of dyslexic and LLD children. Related research suggests that in some ways these groups of children might be expected to have similar outcomes (Torgesen, Wagner, & Rashotte, 1997). Children with dyslexia and LLD have comparable deficits in word decoding and in phonological processing. Because of these similarities, intervention directed at phonological processing and word recognition might be expected to have similar results across these subgroups of poor readers. As discussed above, children with LLD have problems in language and reading that go beyond those of dyslexics. Therefore, they will need intervention in reading comprehension in addition to word recognition. However, there is no reason to believe that such intervention cannot be successful. Studies have shown that the higher-level language deficits that underlie reading comprehension problems can be effectively addressed (e.g., Dollaghan & Kaston, 1986; Ellis-Weismer & Hesketh, 1993).

Using measures of higher-level language abilities to distinguish between dyslexia and language-learning disabilities should help both subgroups to receive the kind of reading and language services they need. It is important to recognize, however, that the higher-level language abilities that distinguish these groups of RD children vary in a continuous rather than a categorical manner. Thus, there is no clear dividing line between children with dyslexia and children with LLD. This does not mean that the distinction is not useful. What it does mean is that clinicians and educators need to perform comprehensive assessments of children's reading, language, and phonological processing abilities in order to develop the most appropriate intervention programs.

---

[1]A diagnostic system that considers language comprehension deficits in addition to reading problems has the potential of identifying a third subgroup of children with language-based reading disabilities. These children, sometimes referred to as *hyperlexic,* are poor readers who have problems in listening comprehension but few difficulties in phonological processing and word recognition. Because much less is known about this subgroup of poor readers, we have chosen to delay consideration of them until we discuss classification issues in Chapter 4.

Summary

It has been recognized now, for over a century, that some children have difficulties learning to read despite adequate opportunity and experience. Almost from the beginning, researchers and practitioners have suspected the importance of language deficits in reading problems. Over the last several decades, considerable evidence has emerged in support of the language basis of reading disabilities. Research clearly demonstrates that phonological processing deficits, which are present early in life, are closely associated with many reading problems in school-age children. This research has led us to define dyslexia as a developmental language disorder. Investigations also indicate that in addition to phonological processing deficits, higher-level language problems contribute to reading disabilities in some children. We have referred to these children as language-learning disabled and discussed ways to differentiate these children from those with dyslexia. The use of language abilities to differentiate children with RD has several advantages over distinguishing children based on the nature or severity of the reading problem. Some of the advantages for planning treatment were briefly discussed in this chapter. In the chapters that follow, we will attempt to show how a language focus allows us to better understand the nature and causes of reading disabilities which, in turn, should lead to more efficient and effective assessment and treatment procedures.

References

Aaron, P.G. (1991). Can reading disabilities be diagnosed without using intelligence tests? *Journal of Learning Disabilities, 24,* 178–186.

Badian, N.A. (1994). Preschool prediction: Orthographic and phonological skills and reading. *Annals of Dyslexia, 44,* 3–25.

Benton, A. (1991). Dyslexia and visual dyslexia. In J. Stein (Ed.), *Vision and visual dysfunction: Vol. 13. Visual dyslexia.* London: Macmillan Press.

Berlin, R. (1887). *Eine besondere art der wortblindheit: Dyslexia [A special type of wordblindness: Dyslexia].* Wiesbaden: J.F. Bergmann.

Bishop, D.V.M. (1992). The underlying nature of specific language impairment. *Journal of Child Psychology and Psychiatry, 33,* 3–66.

Bishop, D.V.M., & Adams, C. (1990). A prospective study of the relationship between specific language impairment, phonological disorders and reading retardation. *Journal of Child Psychology and Psychiatry, 31,* 1027–1050.

Blalock, J.W. (1982). Persistent auditory language deficits in adults with learning disabilities. *Journal of Learning Disabilities, 15,* 604–609.

Bowers, P.G., & Swanson, L.B. (1991). Naming speed deficits in reading disability: Multiple measures of a singular process. *Journal of Experimental Child Psychology, 51,* 195–219.

Bradley, L., & Bryant, P. (1983). Categorizing sounds and learning to read: A causal connection. *Nature, 301,* 419–421.

Brady, S., Poggie, E., & Rapala, M.M. (1989). Speech repetition abilities in children who differ in reading skill. *Language and Speech, 32,* 109–122.

Brandt, J., & Rosen, J.J. (1980). Auditory phonemic perception in dyslexia: Categorical identification and discrimination of stop consonants. *Brain and Language, 9,* 324–337.

Brodbent, W.H. (1872). On the cerebral mechanism of speech and thought. *Transactions of the Royal Medical and Chirurgical Society, 15,* 330–357.

Bruck, M. (1992). Persistence of dyslexics' phonoloical awareness deficits. *Developmental Psychology, 28,* 874–886.

Catts, H.W. (1986). Speech production/phonological deficits in reading-disordered children. *Journal of Learning Disabilities, 19,* 504–508.

Catts, H.W. (1989a). Defining dyslexia as a developmental language disorder. *Annals of Dyslexia, 39,* 50–64.

Catts, H.W. (1989b). Speech production deficits in developmental dyslexia. *Journal of Speech and Hearing Disorders, 54,* 422–428.

Catts, H.W. (1993). The relationship between speech-language impairments and reading disabilities. *Journal of Speech and Hearing Research, 36,* 948–958.

Catts, H.W., & Fey, M. (1995). Written language outcomes of children with language impairments. Grant proposal funded by The National Institute of Deafness and Other Communicative Disorders. Bethesda, MD.

Catts, H.W., Fey, M., & Tomblin, B. (1997). *Language basis of reading disabilities.* Paper presented at the Society for the Scientific Study of Reading, Chicago, IL.

Ceci, S., & Baker, S. (1978). Commentary: How should we conceptualize the language problems of learning disabled children? In S. Ceci (Ed.), *Handbook of cognitive, social, and neuropsychological aspects of learning disabilities* (pp. 102–115). Hillsdale, NJ: Erlbaum.

Clark, D.B., & Uhry, J.K. (1995). *Dyslexia: Theory and practice of remedial instruction.* Baltimore, MD: York Press.

Cohen, R.L., & Netley, C. (1981). Short-term memory deficits in reading disabled children, in the absence of opportunity for rehearsal strategies. *Intelligence, 5,* 69–76.

Critchley, M. (1970). *The dyslexic child.* Springfield, IL: Charles C. Thomas.

Das, J., Mensink, D., & Mishra, R. (1990). Cognitive processes separating good and poor readers when IQ is covaried. *Learning and Individual Differences, 2,* 423–436.

Das, J.P., Mishra, R.K., & Kirby, J.R. (1994). Cognitive patterns of children with dyslexia: A comparison between groups with high and average nonverbal intelligence. *Journal of Learning Disabilities, 27,* 235–242, 253.

Denckla, M.B., & Rudel, R.G. (1976). Rapid automatized naming (RAN): Dyslexia differentiated from other learning disabilities. *Neuropsychologia, 14,* 471–479.

Dollaghan, C., & Kaston, N. (1986). A comprehension monitoring program for language-impaired children. *Journal of Speech and Hearing Disorders, 51,* 264–271.

Eden, G.F., Stein, J.F., Wood, M.H., & Wood, F.B. (1995). Verbal and visual problems in reading disability. *Journal of Learning Disabilities, 28,* 272–290.

Ellis, A.W. (1985). The cognitive neuropsychology of developmental (and acquired) dyslexia: A critical survey. *Cognitive Neuropsychology, 2,* 196–205.

Ellis-Weismer, S., & Hesketh, L. (1993). The influence of prosodic and gestural cues on novel word acquisition by children with specific language impairment. *Journal of Speech and Hearing Research, 36,* 1013–1025.

Felton, R.H., Naylor, C.E., & Wood, F.B. (1990). Neuropsychological profile of adult dyslexics. *Brain and Language, 39,* 485–497.

Felton, R.H., & Wood, F.B. (1992). A reading level match study of nonword reading skills in poor readers with varying IQ. *Journal of Learning Disabilities, 25,* 318–326.

Fletcher, J.M. (1992). The validity of distinguishing children with language and learning disabilities according to discrepancies with IQ: Introduction to the special series. *Journal of Learning Disabilities, 25,* 546–548.

Fletcher, J.M., Francis, D.J., Rourke, B.P., Shaywitz, S.E., & Shaywitz, B.A. (1992). The validity of discrepancy-based definitions of reading disabilities. *Journal of Learning Disabilities, 25,* 555–561, 573.

Fletcher, J.M., Shaywitz, S.E., Shankweiler, D.P., Katz, L., Liberman, I.Y., Stuebing, K.K., Francis, D.J., Fowler, A.E., & Shaywitz, B.A. (1994). Cognitive profiles of reading disability: Comparisons of discrepancy and low achievement definitions. *Journal of Educational Psychology, 86,* 6–23.

Francis, D.J., Espy, K.A., Rourke, B.P., & Fletcher, J.M. (1987). Validity of intelligence test scores in the definition of learning disability: A critical analysis. In B.P. Rourke (Ed.), *Neuropsychological validation of learning disability subtypes* (pp. 15–44). New York: Guilford Press.

Francis, D.J., Fletcher, J.M., Shaywitz, B.A., Shaywitz, S.E., & Rourke, B. (1996). Defining learning and language abilities: Conceptual and psychometric issues with the use of IQ tests. *Language, Speech, and Hearing Services in Schools, 27,* 132–143.

Gerber, A. (1993). *Language-related learning disabilities: Their nature and treatment.* Baltimore: Paul H. Brooks.

Godfrey, J.J., Lasky, A.K., Millag, K.K., & Knox, C.M. (1981). Performance of dyslexic children on speech perception tests. *Journal of Experimental Child Psychology, 32,* 401–424.

Golderberg, H., & Schiffman, G. (1972). *Dyslexia: problems of reading disabilities.* New York: Grune & Stratton.

Gough, P.B., & Tunmer, W.E. (1986). Decoding, reading, and reading disability. *Remedial and Special Education, 7,* 6–10.

Heaton, P., & Winterson, P. (1996). *Dealing with dyslexia.* San Diego, CA: Singular.

Hinshelwood, J. (1895). Letter-word- and mind-blindness. *Lancet, December 21.*

Hinshelwood, J. (1900). Congenital word-blindness. *Lancet, 1,* 1506–1508.

Hinshelwood, J. (1917). *Congenital word blindness.* London: H.K. Lewis.

Hurford, D.P., Schauf, J.D., Bunce, L., Blaich, T., & Moore, K. (1994). Early identification of children at risk for reading disabilities. *Journal of Learning Disabilities, 27,* 371–382.

Johnson, D., & Myklebust, H. (1967). *Learning disabilities: Educational principles and practice.* New York: Grune & Stratton.

Johnston, J.R. (1988). Specific language disorders in the child. In N. Lass, J. Northern, L. McReynolds, & D. Yoder (Eds.), *Handbook of speech-language pathology and audiology.* Philadelphia: B.C. Decker.

Jorm, A.F., Share, D.L., Maclean, R., & Matthews, R. (1986). Cognitive factors at school entry predictive of specific reading retardation and general reading backwardness: A research note. *Journal of Child Psychology and Psychiatry, 27,* 45–54.

Kamhi, A., Catts, H., Mauer, D., Apel, K., & Gentry, B. (1988). Phonological and spatial processing abilities in language and reading impaired children. *Journal of Hearing and Speech Disorders, 53,* 316–327.

Kamhi, A.G. (1992). Response to historical perspective: A developmental language perspective. *Journal of Learning Disabilities, 25,* 48–52.

Kamhi, A.G., & Catts, H.W. (1986). Toward an understanding of developmental language and reading disorders. *Journal of Speech and Hearing Disorders, 51,* 337–347.

Kamhi, A.G., & Catts, H.W. (1989). *Reading disabilities: A developmental language perspective.* Boston: Allyn & Bacon.

Kershner, J.R. (1990). Self-concept and IQ as predictors of remedial success in children with learning disabilities. *Journal of Learning Disabilities, 23,* 368–374.

Kussmaul, A. (1887). Disturbances of speech. In H. von Ziemssen (Ed.), *Cycolpedia of the practice of medicine.* New York: William Wood.

Leonard, L.B. (1989). Language learnability and specific language impairment in children. *Applied Psycholinguistics, 10,* 179–202.

Lerner, J. (1985). *Learning disabilities: Theories, diagnosis, and teaching strategies.* Boston: Houghton Mifflin Co.

Lerner, J.W. (1972). Reading disability as a language disorder. *Acta Symbolica, 3,* 39–45.

Liberman, I.Y., & Shankweiler, D. (1985). Phonology and the problems of learning to read and write. *Remedial and Special Education, 6,* 8–17.

Lyon, G.R. (1995). Toward a definition of dyslexia. *Annals of Dyslexia, 4,* 3–30.

Mann, V.A., & Liberman, I.Y. (1984). Phonological awareness and verbal short-term memory. *Journal of Learning Disabilities, 17,* 592–599.

Mattingly, I. (1972). Reading the linguistic process, and linguistic awareness. In J. Kavanaugh & I. Mattingly (Eds.), *Language by ear and by eye* (pp. 133–147). Cambridge, MA: MIT Press.

Menyuk, P., Chesnick, M., Liebergott, J., Korngold, B., D'Agostino, R., & Belanger, A. (1993). Predicting reading problems in at-risk children. *Journal of Speech and Hearing Research, 34,* 893–903.

Miles, T. (1983). *Dyslexia: The pattern of difficulties.* Springfield, IL: Charles C. Thomas.

Morgan, W. (1896). A case of congenital word-blindness. *British Medical Journal, 2,* 1,378.

Naglieri, J.A., & Reardon, S.M. (1993). Traditional IQ is irrelevant to learning disabilities—intelligence is not. *Journal of Learning Disabilities, 26,* 127–133.

Naidoo, S. (1972). *Specific dyslexia.* London: Pitman.

Nass, R.D. (1993). Sex differences in learning abilities and disabilities. *Annals of Dyslexia, 43,* 61–77.

Nicolson, R.I., & Fawcett, A. (1995). Dyslexia is more than phonological disability. *Dyslexia: An International Journal of Research and Practice, 1,* 19–36.

Olson, R.K., Forsberg, H., Gayan, J. & DeFries, J.C. (in press). A behavioral-genetic analysis of reading disabilities and component processes. In R.M.

Klein & P.A. MacMullen (Eds.), *Converging methods for understanding reading and dyslexia.* Cambridge, MA: MIT Press.

Olson, R.K., Rack, J., Conners, F., DeFries, J., & Fulker, D. (1991). Genetic etiology of individual differences in reading disability. In L. Feagans, E. Short, & L. Meltzer (Eds.), *Subtypes of learning disabilities.* Hillsdale, NJ: Erlbaum.

Orton, J.L., Thompson, L.J., Buncy, P.C., Bender, L., Robinson, M.H., & Rome, P.D. (1975). Samuel T. Orton, Who was he: Part 1. Biographical sketch and personal memories. *Bulletin of Orton Society, 25,* 145–155.

Orton, S. (1925). Word-blindness in school children. *Archives of Neurology and Psychiatry, 14,* 581–615.

Orton, S. (1937). *Reading, writing and speech problems in children.* London, UK: Chapman Hall.

Pennington, B.F., Gilger, J.W., Olson, R.K., & DeFries, J.C. (1992). The external validity of age- versus IQ-discrepancy definitions of reading disability: Lessons from a twin study. *Journal of Learning Disabilities, 25,* 562–573.

Perfetti, C. (12985). *Reading ability.* New York: Oxford University Press.

Prior, M., Sanson, A., Smart, D., & Oberklaid, F. (1995). Reading disability in an Australian community sample. *Australian Journal of Psychology, 47,* 32–37.

Rees, N.S. (1974). The speech pathologist and the reading process. *ASHA, 16,* 255–258.

Richardson, S.O. (1992). Historical perspectives on dyslexia. *Journal of Learning Disabilities, 25,* 40–47.

Rodgers, B. (1983). The identification and prevalence of specific reading retardation. *British Journal of Educational Psychology, 3,* 369–373.

Rudel, R. (1985). The definition of dyslexia: Language and motor deficits. In F.H. Duffy & N. Geschwind (Eds.), *Dyslexia: A neuroscientific approach to clinical evaluation* (pp. 33–53). Boston: Little, Brown and Company.

Rutter, M., Tizard, J., & Whitmore, K. (1970). *Education, health and behaviour.* London: Longman.

Rutter, M., & Yule, W. (1975). The concept of specific reading retardation. *Journal of Child Psychology and Psychiatry, 16,* 181–197.

Scarborough, H.S. (1990). Very early language deficits in dyslexic children. *Child Development, 61,* 1728–1743.

Shankweiler, D., & Liberman, I. (1972). Misreading: A search for causes. In J. Kavanaugh & I. Mattingly (Eds.), *Language by ear and by eye* (pp. 293–317). Cambridge, MA: MIT Press.

Share, D. (1997). Word recognition and spelling processes in specific reading disabled and garden-variety poor readers. *Dyslexia: An International Journal of Theory and Practice, 2,* 167–174.

Share, D.L., McGee, R., McKenzie, D., Williams, S., & Silva, P. (1987). Further evidence relating to the distinction between specific reading retardation and general reading backwardness. *British Journal of Developmental Psychology, 5,* 35–44.

Share, D.L., & Stanovich, K.E. (1995). Cognitive processes in early reading development: Accommodating individual differences into a model of acquisition. *Issues in Education, 1,* 1–57.

Shaywitz, S.E., Escobar, M.D., Shaywitz, B.A., Fletcher, J.M., & Makuch, R. (1992). Evidence that dyslexia may represent the lower tail of a normal distribution of reading ability. *The New England Journal of Medicine, 326,* 145–193.

Shaywitz, S.E., Shaywitz, B.A., Fletcher, J.M., & Escobar, M.D. (1990). Prevalence of reading disability in boys and girls. *Journal of the American Medical Association, 264,* 998–1002.

Siegel, L.S. (1989). IQ is irrelevant to the definition of learning disabilities. *Journal of Learning Disabilities, 22,* 469–478.

Siegel, L.S. (1992). An evaluation of the discrepancy definition of dyslexia. *Journal of Learning Disabilities, 25,* 618–629.

Snowling, M. (1981). Phonemic deficits in developmental dyslexia. *Psychological Research, 43,* 219–234.

Spring, C., & Davis, J.M. (1988). Relations of digit naming speed with three components of reading. *Applied Psycholinguistics, 9,* 315–334.

Stanovich, K.E. (1988). The right and wrong places to look for the cognitive locus of reading disability. *Annals of Dyslexia, 38,* 154–177.

Stanovich, K.E. (1991). Discrepancy definitions of reading disability: Has intelligence led us astray? *Reading Research Quarterly, 26,* 7–29.

Stanovich, K.E. (1997). Toward a more inclusive definition of dyslexia. *Dyslexia: An International Journal of Theory and Practice, 2,* 154–166.

Stanovich, K.E., & Siegel, L.S. (1994). The phenotypic performance profile of reading-disabled children: A regression-based test of the phonological-core variable-difference model. *Journal of Educational Psychology, 86,* 24–53.

Stark, J. (1975). Reading failure: A language-based problem. *ASHA, 17,* 832–834.

Steveson, J., Graham, P., Fredman, G., & McLoughlin, V. (1987). A twin study of genetic influences on reading and spelling ability and disability. *Journal of Child Psychology and Psychiatry, 28,* 229–247.

Taylor, H.G., Lean, D., & Schwartz, S. (1989). Pseudo-word repetition ability in learning-disabled children. *Applied Psycholinguistics, 10,* 203–219.

Taylor, H.G., Satz, P., & Friel, J. (1979). Developmental dyslexia in relation to other childhood reading disorders: Significance and clinical utility. *Reading Research Quarterly, 15,* 84–101.

Texas Education Agency (1996). Dyslexia and related disorders: An overview of state and federal requirements. Austin, TX: Author.

Thomson, M. (1984). *Developmental dyslexia: Its nature, assessment and remediation.* London: Edward Arnold.

Tomblin, J.B., Records, N.L., Buckwalter, P., Zhang, X., Smith, E., & O'Brian, M. (1997). The prevalence of specific language impairments in kindergarten children. *Journal of Speech, Language, and Hearing Research, 40,* 1245–1260.

Torgesen, J.K. (1985). Memory processes in reading disabled children. *Journal of Learning Disabilities, 18,* 350–357.

Torgesen, J.K. (1991). Learning disabilities: Historical and conceptual issues. In B. Wong (Ed.), *Learning about learning disabilities.* Orlando, FL: Academic Press.

Torgesen, J.K., Wagner, R.K., & Rashotte, C.A. (1994). Longitudinal studies of phonological processing and reading. *Journal of Learning Disabilities, 27,* 276–286.

Torgesen, J.K., Wagner, R.K., & Rashotte, C.A. (1997). *Preventing reading disabilities: Results from 2 1/2 years of intervention.* Paper presented at the Society for the Scientific Study of Reading, Chicago.

van der Wissel, A., & Zegers, F.E. (1985). Reading retardation revisited. *British Journal of Developmental Psychology, 3,* 3–9.

Vellutino, F. (1979). *Dyslexia: Theory and research.* Cambridge, MA: MIT Press.

Vellutino, F.R., & Scanlon, D. (1987). Phonological coding, phonological awareness, and reading ability: Evidence from a longitudinal and experimental study. *Merrill-Palmer Quarterly, 33*(87), 321–363.

Vellutino, F.R., Scanlon, D.M., Sipay, E.R., Small, S.G., Chen, R., Pratt, A., & Denckla, M.B. (1996). Cognitive profiles of difficult-to-remediate and readily remediated poor readers: Early intervention as a vehicle for distinguishing between cognitive and experiential deficits as basic causes of specific reading disabilities. *Journal of Educational Psychology, 88,* 601–638.

Wagner, R.K., & Torgesen, J.K. (1987). The nature of phonological processing and its causal role in the acquisition of reading skills. *Psychological Bulletin, 101,* 1–21.

Wallach, G.P., & Butler, K.G. (Eds.). (1984). *Language learning disabilities in school-age children.* Baltimore: Williams & Wilkins.

Wallach, G.P., & Butler, K.G. (Eds.). (1994). *Language-learning disabilities in school-age children and adolescents.* New York: Merrill.

Werker, J.F., & Tees, R.C. (1987). Speech perception in severely disabled and average reading children. *Canadian Journal of Psychology, 41,* 48–61.

Wolf, M. (1984). Naming, reading, and the dyslexias: A longitudinal overview. *Annals of Dyslexia, 34,* 87–136.

Wolf, M., & Obregon, M. (1989). *88 children in search of a name: A 5-year investigation of rate, word-retrieval, and vocabulary in reading development and dyslexia.* Paper presented at the Society for Research in Child Development, Kansas City, MO.

Yule, W., Rutter, M., Berger, M., & Thompson, J. (1974). Over and under achievement in reading: Distribution in the general population. *British Journal of Educational Psychology, 44,* 1–12.

Chapter 4

Classification of Reading Disabilities

HUGH W. CATTS   *ALAN G. KAMHI*

Practitioners and researchers have long recognized that children with RD are a heterogeneous group. Poor readers show variability in the nature of their reading problems and in the factors associated with these problems. This has frequently led to classification systems that have divided children with RD into subgroups or subtypes based on their similarities and differences (see Feagan & McKinney, 1991; Hooper & Willis, 1989; Newby & Lyon, 1991 for reviews). Some of these attempts have proven useful and continue to provide insights into the nature and treatment of reading disabilities. For example, in the previous chapter, we proposed that many reading disabilities are developmental language disorders and suggested that language abilities should be used to differentiate subtypes of reading problems. We obviously think that it is useful to classify children with RD into at least two primary subtypes, dyslexia and language-learning disability. In the first part of this chapter, we expand on this classification system and, in doing so, add a third subgroup of children (i.e., hyperlexia) to the system.

Subtypes based on the nature of deficits in word recognition may also be helpful in understanding and treating reading disabilities (e.g., Lovett, 1987; Murphy & Pollatsek, 1994; Stanovich, Siegel, & Gottardo, 1997). Poor readers have been shown to vary in their abilities in phonetic decoding and sight-word reading, as well as in word recognition accuracy versus rate. In the second part of the chapter, we consider how word recognition strengths and weaknesses can be used to differentiate children with RD. We believe that a good subtyping system should lead to more efficient and effective assessment and treatment. Assessment and treatment implications thus become an important criterion for evaluating the usefulness of a classification system of reading disabilities. In the final section of the chapter, we consider some of the clinical/educational implications of subtyping systems.

Before discussing other classification systems, we should briefly mention two popular approaches that have not proven to be that useful, one based on IQ-achievement discrepancy and the other on neuropsychological profiles. As discussed in the last chapter, a prominent approach to subgrouping poor readers is one based on IQ-achievement discrepancy. This approach, however, has not stood up well to empirical investigation. Research has generally failed to find important reading (primarily word recognition) and reading-related differences between subgroups based on IQ-achievement discrepancy (Fletcher, Shaywitz, Shankweiler, Katz, Liberman, Stuebing, Francis, Fowler, & Shaywitz, 1994; Siegel, 1989; Stanovich & Siegel, 1994). IQ-based subtypes have also failed to show expected differences in response to intervention (Kershner, 1990; Share, McGee, McKenzie, Williams, & Silva, 1987; Torgesen, Wagner, & Rashotte, 1997). For these and other reasons, many have argued against the use of classification systems based on IQ (e.g., Aaron, 1991; Catts, 1996; Siegel, 1989; Stanovich, 1991, 1997).

In another common subtyping approach, researchers have used large neuropsychological test batteries and complex statistical procedures to subgroup poor readers (Lyon, 1983; Morris, Satz, & Blashfield, 1981; Petrauskas & Rourke, 1979). This approach, however, has not proven to be very enlightening. Although this research uncovered cognitive processes that were related to various subtypes of reading disabilities (predominantly language processes), there was so much diversity in the measures and techniques employed that it has been difficult to draw generalizations. In addition, this work, for the most part, was not theory driven and consequently failed to explain how the specific cognitive processes associated with various subtypes impact reading development.

Subtypes Based on Comprehension versus Word Recognition Problems

Because of the problems in these approaches, researchers and practitioners have turned to classification systems that focus more directly on reading itself and on the individual differences children display in learning to read. In the previous chapter, we introduced a system that divided poor readers into subtypes based on reading and language differences. This system involved a distinction between those poor readers who have deficits in word recognition and those who have deficits in both word recognition and language comprehension. This distinction is based, to a large extent, on a theory of reading proposed by Gough and his colleagues (Gough & Tunmer, 1986; Hoover & Gough, 1990). According to this theory, called the *Simple View of Reading,* reading comprehension can be thought of as word recognition plus listening comprehension. It is argued that if one wants to know how well individuals understand what they read, one needs simply to measure how well they recognize words and how well they understand those words (and sentences) when read to them. Hoover and Gough (1990) tested the simple view of reading in a longitudinal study of English-Spanish bilingual children in first through fourth grades. As predicted, they found that word recognition and listening comprehension accounted for independent variance in reading comprehension. Their results showed that a linear combination of these variables explained between 72 and 85 percent of the variance in reading comprehension. In grades 1 and 2, word recognition accounted for most of the variance, whereas by grades 3 and 4 listening comprehension explained more sizable amounts of variance. In a more recent study, Hoover (1994) replicated these various findings using data from 900 children who were administered the Iowa Test of Basic Skills. Other studies have also provided support for the role of both word recognition and listening comprehension in reading (Aaron, 1991; Carver, 1993; Curtis, 1980; Jackson & McClelland, 1979; Palmer, MacLeod, Hunt, & Davidson, 1985; Singer & Crouse, 1981).

The simple view of reading suggests that children with RD can be divided into different subgroups on the basis of word recognition and listening comprehension abilities (see Table 4-1). One subgroup, traditionally referred to as *dyslexic*, has poor word recognition abilities, but good listening comprehension. Another subgroup has poor word recognition abilities and poor listening comprehension abilities. We have called this subgroup of children *language-learning disabled*. The simple view also suggests the possibility of a third subgroup of poor readers. This subgroup, referred to as *hyperlexic*, has good word recognition abilities but poor listening comprehension. All three of these subgroups have reading comprehension problems, but for different reasons. Children with dyslexia show poor reading comprehension because of their inaccurate and/or slow decoding skills. Children with hyperlexia have poor reading comprehension because of their language and cognitive deficits. Finally, children with language-learning disabilities (LLD) have poor reading comprehension because of deficits in both word recognition and listening comprehension. The extent of the reading comprehension deficits in each group depends on the severity of the deficit in word recognition and listening comprehension.

There is growing support for a subtyping system based on comprehension and/or word recognition deficits (Aaron, 1991; Catts, 1996; Padget, 1998). Most researchers, however, have examined these subgroups individually. Considerable attention has been devoted to poor readers whose primary problems are in word recognition (Carver, 1993; Clark & Uhry, 1995; Critchley, 1970; Stanovich, 1985; Thomson, 1984; Vellutino, 1979). As noted

TABLE 4-1   Subtypes Based on Word Recognition and Listening Comprehension

	Word Recognition	
	Poor	Good
Listening Comprehension — Good	Dyslexia	Other
Listening Comprehension — Poor	Language-Learning Disability	Hyperlexia

above, these poor readers have traditionally been referred to as dyslexic. The problems dyslexics have in word recognition are well documented (Bruck, 1988; Olson, Kliegl, David-son, & Foltz, 1985; Rack, Snowling, & Olson, 1992; Snowling, 1981; Stanovich & Siegel, 1994). From the beginning, children with dyslexia have difficulties learning to phoneti-cally decode words and to develop a sight-word vocabulary. As we discussed in the previ-ous chapter, most recent definitions of dyslexia, including ours, specifies word recognition deficits (and associated phonological processing deficits) as a primary symptom of the dis-order. Most definitions also state that children with dyslexia have at least normal intelli-gence. Because intelligence is generally measured by verbally loaded tests, most children meeting the latter criterion would be expected to have normal listening comprehension abilities. Indeed, research confirms that, as a group, children defined as dyslexic have lis-tening comprehension abilities that are within the normal range (Aaron, 1989; Ellis, McDougall, & Monk, 1996; Fletcher et al., 1994; Shankweiler, Crain, Katz, Fowler, Liberman, Brady, Thornton, Ludquist, Dreyer, Fletcher, Stuebing, Shaywitz, & Shaywitz, 1995). Bruck (1990) has further reported that in some cases, individuals with dyslexia may have exceptional listening comprehension abilities that allow them to compensate for their poor decoding skills. Consequently, these individuals' reading difficulties are often missed when using untimed tests of reading comprehension.

Children who have problems in both word recognition and listening comprehension have also been the focus of research investigations. These children generally comprise groups of poor readers who fail to meet IQ-achievement discrepancy criterion for dyslexia. As noted above, they have been referred to as backward readers (Jorm, Share, Maclean, & Matthews, 1986; Rutter & Yule, 1975), low achievers (Fletcher et al., 1994), or garden-variety poor readers (Gough & Tunmer, 1986; Stanovich, Nathan, & Zolman, 1988). We pre-fer to call them children with LLD, because this term focuses attention on the central role that language-learning difficulties play in these children's reading problems.

Studies have compared the reading and reading-related problems of children with dyslexia and LLD. These studies indicate that children with LLD have similar difficulties in word recognition to children with dyslexia (Ellis, McDougall, & Monk, 1996; Felton & Wood, 1992; Jorm et al., 1986; Stanovich & Siegel, 1994). Research also indicates that phonological processing deficits underlie many of the problems children with LLD have in recognizing printed words (Fletcher et al., 1994; Hurford, Schauf, Bunce, Blaich, & Moore, 1994; Shaywitz, Fletcher, Holahan, & Shaywitz, 1992). Unlike children with dyslexia, children with LLD have been shown to have significant deficits in listening comprehension (Aaron, Joshi, & Williams, 1995; Ellis et al., 1996; Fletcher et al., 1994; Stanovich & Siegel, 1994). These problems are sometimes associated with more global cognitive deficits. In such cases, children have problems in both verbal and nonverbal processing. In other cases, however, LLD children's difficulties are specific to language processing. These chil-dren may show deficits in vocabulary, morphosyntax, and text-level processing, but have normal nonverbal abilities (Catts, 1993; Catts, Fey, & Tomblin, 1997).

A third subgroup in this system is comprised of children with problems in listening comprehension, but with normal or above normal word recognition abilities. This reading/ language profile has sometimes been referred to as *hyperlexia* (Aaron, Frantz, & Manges, 1990; Aram & Healy, 1988; Elliott & Needleman, 1976; Silberberg & Silberberg, 1967).

Hyperlexia, as it was originally conceived, was used to refer to children with exceptional word decoding skills. Children with hyperlexia were observed to be quite precocious and learn "to read" before they entered school. Despite their exceptional word recognition abilities, hyperlexic children have been found to demonstrate significant problems in comprehension. Huttenlocher and Huttenlocher (1973) described the case of M.K. who by the age of four years, six months had learned to read with minimal parental help. At four years, ten months he could read a third-grade passage fluently. M.K. enjoyed reading and, in fact, was quite compulsive about it. He would read any written material in sight. His comprehension of what he read, however, was severely impaired.

Aram (1997) recently reviewed research concerning hyperlexia. She reported that children with hyperlexia generally have exceptional phonetic decoding skills. These children also have good sight-word reading abilities. These abilities, however, may not be at the same level as those in phonetic decoding. Aram further noted that children with hyperlexia typically have impairments in spoken language. Of particular significance are their deficits in listening comprehension. Children with hyperlexia have been shown to perform poorly on tests of semantic and syntactic processing (Aram, Ekelman, & Healy, 1984; Siegel, 1984). Hyperlexia, in its extreme case, has also been found to be associated with one or more developmental disabilities such as mental retardation, autism, and schizophrenia (see Aram & Healy, 1988). In some cases, it co-occurs with other "splinter skills" such as exceptional music talent or memory for names and dates.

Not all poor readers who demonstrate primarily listening comprehension deficits fit this description of hyperlexia. For example, Stothard and Hulme (1992) identified a group of poor readers who had better word recognition than reading comprehension. These children did not demonstrate precocious or exceptional decoding ability or a history of autism or mental retardation. They did, however, have significant problems in listening comprehension and adequate or better word recognition abilities. Other studies have also described children with this profile (Oakhill, 1982, 1984). These children may be among those that have reading problems only after they have reached the fourth or fifth grade. Presumably, these children's word recognition skills have been sufficient enough to master the reading curriculum of the primary grades. However, as curricular demands increase and more emphasis is placed on comprehension, these children begin to have trouble and are identified as poor readers. While these latter children do not fit the clinical profile of hyperlexia as it was originally conceived (e.g., precocious word recognition, autism), the term hyperlexia still seems to be an appropriate one to characterize these children.

Classification Studies

Currently, only a few studies have attempted to classify groups of children with RD on the basis of word recognition and listening comprehension abilities. In a recent study, Aaron, and colleagues (1995) examined the reading comprehension abilities of 139 children in third, fourth, and sixth grades and identified 16 children who were performing at least one standard deviation (SD) below the mean. They found that 13 of the 16 children with RD could be classified into subtypes on the basis of word recognition and/or listening comprehension deficits. Results showed that 6 of the children had problems in word recognition, but not listening comprehension (i.e., dyslexic). Four children were observed to have deficits in listening comprehension, but had normal word recognition abilities (i.e., hyperlexic). Additionally, three children performed poorly in both word recognition and listening comprehension (i.e., language-learning disabled). Aaron, Joshi, and Williams also noted that two of the unclassified children had deficits primarily in reading rate. Consequently, they suggested that reading rate problems, particularly in older children, might qualify as another subgroup of poor readers. Such a suggestion is consistent with the word recognition subtypes that will be discussed later in the chapter.

Data from an ongoing longitudinal study conducted by the first author and his colleagues (Catts, Fey, Zhang, & Tomblin, 1998) can also be used to classify children with RD according to word recognition and/or listening comprehension deficits. In this project, we identified 180 second-grade children who performed one or more SDs below the mean of a normative sample on a composite measure of reading comprehension. These poor readers were subsequently divided into subgroups on the basis of whether they had word recognition and/or listening comprehension deficits (defined as performance of at least one SD below the mean of the normative group). Our results showed that approximately 85 percent of the poor readers fall into one of the three poor reading subgroups. We found that 34.5 percent of the poor readers had deficits primarily in word recognition and could be classified as dyslexic. Results showed that 14.4 percent of the poor readers had problems in listening comprehension, but not word recognition, and could be classified as hyperlexic. Finally, we observed that 36.8 percent of the poor readers demonstrated a language-learning disabled profile and had deficits in both listening comprehension and word recognition. Further observation indicated that there were no definitive cutoff points for identifying subgroup membership. However, using various cutoff points to identify poor readers and subgroups, we continued to observe three subgroups, each with a somewhat comparable prevalence to that reported above. Our preliminary analyses have also indicated that some of the subgroups can be differentiated from others on the basis of performance on measures of listening comprehension and letter identification in kindergarten. We are following these children into the fourth grade and plan to evaluate the stability of these poor reader subgroups over time.

These studies thus provide some initial support for a classification system based on word recognition versus comprehension deficits. More in-depth investigations will be necessary to fully evaluate the usefulness of this subtyping approach. This work will need to compare subtypes of poor readers on a variety of reading and reading-related measures to better understand the similarities and differences between subtypes. Reading-level matched control group designs like that described in a later section (Stanovich, et al., 1997) could also prove insightful. It will also be important to conduct longitudinal investigations of this classification system. Recall that word recognition and listening comprehension vary in their relative contribution to reading comprehension depending on the grade level considered (Hoover & Gough, 1990). This could influence the size and nature of subtypes across grades.

Perhaps of more significance is the possible interaction between word recognition and listening comprehension across grades. Initially, word recognition and listening comprehension are largely independent, each comprised of a distinct set of cognitive processes. Over time, however, deficits in one area may influence abilities in the other. Specifically, prolonged deficits in word recognition could adversely influence children's listening comprehension abilities. Listening comprehension depends in part on children's language competence and world knowledge. Language competence and world knowledge are influenced to some degree by reading experience. Reading provides opportunities to learn new vocabulary, grammatical structures, and knowledge of a variety of topics. Because children with poor word recognition skills typically do not read as much as those with good word recognition skills, they will acquire less language and world knowledge. In turn, these children may perform more poorly on measures of listening comprehension than good decoders.

Unfortunately, there is little data concerning how word recognition abilities may interact with listening comprehension abilities over time. As more longitudinal studies consider this relationship, we will better understand the implications that this association has for subtyping children with RD. It seems likely, however, that the confounding effects of word recognition on listening comprehension will be most significant in the later school grades when the cumulative effects of lack of reading experience are the greatest. However, in the early grades, word recognition and listening comprehension abilities should be independent enough to allow for the identification of distinct subgroups. Even in the later grades, a classification system based on word recognition and listening comprehension still can have clinical/educational significance. Regardless of whether listening comprehension deficits stem from intrinsic problems with language or from environmental factors involving reading experience, children with these problems will need intervention directed at their comprehension deficits.

Subtypes Based on Nature of Word Recognition Deficits

Another body of research suggests that individual differences in word recognition abilities may be a useful way to classify poor readers. Recall that in Chapter 1, we noted that there are two routes for word recognition. One is the visual route in which words are recognized directly on the basis of their spelling or orthographic patterns. The other route is the phonological route in which words are recognized indirectly by using sound-letter correspondence rules to decode the word. Much attention has been devoted to possible individual differences in children's abilities to use these word recognition routes.

Reading Styles

A popular view in "folk psychology" and education is that children can be divided into two distinct subgroups based on whether they learn to read more easily by the visual route or phonological route (Carbo, 1987, 1992; Dunn, 1990). Carbo (1992), for example, divides children into global learners and analytic learners. Global learners or readers are argued to learn to recognize words best through a sight-word approach that makes use of the visual route. Analytic readers, on the other hand, learn to read best by a phonics method that takes advantage of the phonological route. Many in early education also refer to these groups as visual and auditory learners and believe that teachers should identify a child's learning style and teach to that style.

Despite the widespread appeal of reading/learning styles, the evidence is not very compelling that children can be divided into homogeneous subgroups on the basis of their reading strengths (or preferences), or that teaching to these strengths is an effective strategy for improving reading ability (Kavale, Forness, & Bender, 1987; Stahl, 1988; Stahl & Kuhn, 1995; Turner & Dawson, 1978). Relatively few studies have actually addressed this issue. Those studies that have offered some support for reading style subgroups and instruction (Holt & O'Tuel, 1990; Thomasson, 1990) have typically been reported outside the peer-review process. As a result, this work has not had the level of scrutiny and evaluation that is needed in order to effectively guide educational practice. This view is also contrary to most current theories of reading development. As discussed in Chapter 2, most research suggests the importance of both the visual and the phonological routes in learning to read (Share, 1995; Share & Stanovich, 1995). Children need to have good phonetic decoding skills to break the alphabetic code (i.e., self-teach) as well as good orthographic skills to develop accurate and automatic word recognition.

Dysphonetic, Dyseidetic, and Alexic Subgroups

While evidence supporting the existence of word recognition subgroups in the population as a whole is not strong, there is converging research that indicates that such a classification system may be of value for subgrouping poor readers. There is a long history of poor readers being classified on the basis of individual differences in reading by the phonological versus the visual route (Boder, 1971, 1973; Ingram, 1964). Ingram (1964), for example, grouped poor readers into audio-phonetic dyslexics and visuo-spatial dyslexics. The audio-phonetic dyslexics were argued to have problems in sound discrimination and blending and to be poor in phonetic decoding. The visuo-spatial dyslexics, on the other hand, were proposed to have difficulties in visual discrimination and spatial skills and problems reading by the sight-word route.

Elena Boder (1971, 1973) developed a classification system that recognized three subgroups of poor readers based on misreadings and/or misspellings: the *dysphonetic, dyseidetic*, and *alexic*. The dysphonetic subgroup has a primary deficit in auditory analytic skills. Children in this subgroup have great difficulty learning and using the phonological route. These children display misreadings and misspellings that are phonetically inaccurate. For example, the dysphonetic reader might pronounce *block* as *book* or spell *scramble* as *sleber*. Dyseidetic readers, on the other hand, have a deficit in the visual route. Consequently, they have particular problems with exception words (e.g., have, colonel). These words are misspelled or misread as phonetic renditions; for example, reading *talc* for *talk* or spelling *laugh* as *laf*. Finally, the alexic subgroup have a deficit in both phonetic and visual reading/spelling skills. This subgroup is the most handicapped of the three groups.

The primary evidence for the validity of these subgroups comes from a study of 107 dyslexic children (Boder, 1973). Using an in-depth analysis of reading and spelling abilities, 100 of these children were divided into one of the three subgroups. Boder reported that 67 of the dyslexic children were dysphonetic, 10 were dyseidetic, and 23 were alexic. Boder and a colleague (Boder & Jarrico, 1982) later developed a diagnostic screening test for subtyping dyslexia. Researchers, utilizing this test, have provided some evidence of behavioral and electrophysiological differences between subtypes of dyslexics (Dalby & Gibson,

1981; Flynn & Deering, 1989). Flynn and Deering (1989), for example, found that dyseidetic children demonstrated greater EEG activity in the left temporal-parietal region during reading than did dysphonetic children. They suggested that this was evidence of different processing capabilities between these subgroups. Others, however, have failed to uncover reading-related differences between these subgroups of poor readers (Godfrey, Lasky, Millag, & Knox, 1981; van den Bos, 1982). Godfrey and colleagues (1981), for example, failed to find an advantage in speech perception abilities among dyseidetic dyslexics as compared to dysphonetic dyslexics. Such a difference would be expected if dysphonetic dyslexics had a phonetic processing problem.

Deep, Phonological, and Surface Dyslexia

Cognitive neuropsychologists have also considered subgroups similar to those proposed by Boder (Coltheart, Patterson, & Marshall, 1980; Marshall & Newcombe, 1973). This work, however, has used terminology and procedures borrowed from the study of acquired dyslexia. *Acquired dyslexia* is a reading disability in previously literate individuals following neurological damage. Three syndromes are often identified: *deep, phonological,* and *surface dyslexia.* Individuals with deep and phonological dyslexia have considerable difficulty in phonetic decoding. They are identified primarily on the basis of their problems pronouncing nonwords such as *zun* or *vope.* Such words cannot be recognized by the visual route and must be sounded out using sound-letter correspondence rules. Individuals with deep dyslexia, unlike those with phonological dyslexia, also make semantic errors in reading. For example, when asked to read a word like "tulip" they might say "crocus" or they might read "sun" for "moon." Other symptoms include visual errors (confusing words like "wife" and "life"), morphological errors (misreading prefixes or suffixes), and greater facility recognizing content words as opposed to function words (Thomson, 1984). Finally, individuals with surface dyslexia have problems with the visual route. They are identified on the basis of their misreading of exception words. Whereas the terms phonological and surface dyslexia roughly correspond to dysphonetic and dyseidetic readers, the former terms have become more popular in recent years.

Using primarily case studies, cognitive neuropsychologists have subtyped individuals with developmental reading disabilities as phonological or surface dyslexics (Coltheart, Materson, Byng, Prior, & Riddoch, 1983; Holmes, 1978; Marshall, 1984; Temple & Marshall, 1983; see Rayner & Pollatsek, 1989 for review). For example, Temple and Marshall (1983) described a case of developmental phonological dyslexia. This student, a 17-year-old girl, had considerable difficulty reading nonwords compared to real words. Her responses to nonwords were typically real words that were visually similar to the target words. Marshall (1984) noted that this developmental case was very similar to the case of acquired phonological dyslexia reported by Patterson (1982). Coltheart and colleagues (1983) and Holmes (1978), on the other hand, identified a number of cases of developmental surface dyslexia. Holmes reported on four boys, between 9 and 13 years of age, who had great difficulty reading exception words. They often made phonetic errors, regularizing words like "bread" as "breed." Coltheart and colleagues (1983) identified a 15-year-old dyslexic girl who had many problems with homophones. For example, she was noted to read "pane" correctly, but to define it as "something that hurts."

Heterogeneity without Clusters

The classification system proposed by cognitive neuropsychologists may lead to the impression that poor readers can be divided into distinct and homogeneous subgroups based on word recognition deficits. Ellis (1985), however, has argued that while there may be heterogeneity among poor readers in terms of word recognition strengths and weaknesses, poor readers do not form distinct subgroups. He proposed that word recognition abilities can be viewed according to two dimensions: one dimension corresponding to reading by the visual route and the other dimension representing reading by the phonological route. He maintained that readers' abilities are distributed continuously along each of these dimensions. Readers may show similar abilities in these dimensions or have abilities in one dimension that are significantly better than those in the other.

Operationally, these abilities can be displayed on a scatterplot in which performance on exception word reading represents one axis and scores on nonword reading constitutes the other. Ellis noted that when plotted like this, the distinct subtype view of cognitive neuropsychologists assumes that there will be "galaxies" of dyslexics within the scatterplot. That is, phonological dyslexics would be expected to represent a cluster of poor readers who are separated from other readers by their distinct pattern of poor phonetic decoding skills and good exception word reading skills. The surface dyslexics, on the other hand, would be predicted to cluster together in this two-dimensional space as a result of their poor exception word reading skills and good phonetic decoding skills. Ellis, however, argued that a more valid conceptualization of heterogeneity is one without clusters or galaxies. He suggested that poor readers are more likely to be distributed continuously in this multidimensional space, such that "there will be a complete and unbroken gradation of intermediate dyslexics linking the extreme cases" (Ellis, 1985, p. 192). In proposing this model, Ellis does not deny individual differences, only the homogeneity of subgroups. In other words, he argues that children with RD do not fall into distinct categories in terms of their word recognition skills. While some children can be characterized as surface or phonological dyslexics, these children will differ by degree of impairment and not type of impairment.

Recently, Ellis and his colleagues (Ellis et al., 1996) tested this view of the heterogeneity of word recognition by examining a group of thirteen children with RD. These children, who were 9 to 11 years old, had normal or above normal IQs and a reading age eighteen or more months behind their chronological age. Three control groups, each consisting of thirteen children and matched for reading level to the dyslexic group, were also included. One group consisted of poor readers of the same age as the children with RD, but with lower IQ scores. Another group contained younger children who were reading at a level predicted for their age. The final group was an even younger group of precocious readers, children who were reading well above their age. All children read a list of nonwords and real words (half of which were exception words). A scatterplot of nonword reading abilities versus sight-word reading abilities showed considerable variability among the dyslexic children. However, there was no evidence of clustering among the dyslexic readers. Instead, the dyslexic children were distributed continuously throughout the scatterplot. Ellis and his colleagues also found similar heterogeneity in the three control groups.

Murphy and Pollatsek (1994) also examined the heterogeneity of word recognition abilities, but in a much larger sample of children with RD. Sixty-five children with RD, 10 to

13 years of age, were administered a variety of measures designed to test children's ability to read by the visual or phonological routes. These included timed and untimed reading of regular, exception, and nonwords; a lexical decision task; and a homophone definition task. Participants' phonological awareness and word retrieval abilities were also assessed.

Despite finding much hetergeneity between poor readers in word recognition abilities, they too failed to uncover distinct clusters of poor readers. Poor readers differed primarily in terms of the severity of deficits, and not in the kind of deficits. Most children with RD were poor at reading by both a visual and phonological route. In addition, a moderate correlation was found between nonword and exception word reading. If discrete subgroups had been present, such a correlation would have been negative, or at least absent. Nevertheless, there were some children with RD who did show a dissociation between phonetic decoding and sight-word reading. These children, however, were still part of the same continuum and did not cluster together into discrete subgroups.

Murphy and Pollatsek (1994) further speculated on the reasons for the dissociation in some children with RD. They noted that children fitting the profile of phonological dyslexics performed less well on a phonological awareness task and better on a phonological retrieval task than did children who displayed a surface dyslexia profile. They also speculated that instructional factors may have contributed to individual differences. Several of the surface dyslexics had been enrolled in intensive phonics programs that taught them to read nonwords and real words, but few exception words. Such instruction could have led to the error pattern of a surface dyslexic.

The results of these studies strongly suggest that poor readers cannot be divided into homogeneous subgroups based on their word recognition abilities. Some poor readers do, however, display a dissociation in their ability to use the phonological as opposed to the visual route. This dissociation may be related to differences in cognitive processing or reading instruction/experience (Murphy & Pollatsek, 1994). The fact that poor readers do display a dissociation despite the absence of distinct and homogeneous clusters suggests that the classification of poor readers on the basis of word recognition abilities might have some clinical/educational validity.

Hard versus Soft Subtypes

For a classification system based on word recognition to be of use, it is necessary to have a reliable procedure to differentiate children with phonological and surface dyslexia. Recall, that cognitive neuropsychologists have used the comparison of nonword and exception reading abilities (e.g., Coltheart et al., 1983; Holmes, 1978). Nonword reading relies primarily on phonological decoding, while exception word reading is dependent on sight-word reading abilities. The case reports presented by cognitive neuropsychologists give the impression that phonological dyslexics had poor nonword reading, but *normal* exception word reading, while surface dyslexics had poor exception word reading, but *normal* nonword reading. Such "purity" of subtype was seldom the case. Most reports concerned individuals with *relative* differences in nonword and exception word reading accuracy. For example, the surface dyslexic described by Coltheart and colleagues had problems reading both nonwords and exception words, but her problem was more pronounced for exception words.

Recently, Castles and Coltheart (1993) investigated different ways of identifying word recognition subtypes. They administered measures of exception word and nonword reading to 53 dyslexics and 56 normal children matched for chronological age. Initially, they divided the poor readers into what can be called "hard" subtypes (Stanovich, et al., 1997). According to this approach, dyslexics who performed poorly in exception word reading, as compared to same age peers, but normally in nonword reading were defined as surface dyslexics. Phonological dyslexics were defined as those students who showed poor nonword reading, but normal exception word reading. Castles and Coltheart found that these procedures led to the identification of only 8 phonological dyslexics and 10 surface dyslexics. These numbers were smaller than were expected on the basis of previous reports. Castles and Coltheart noted, however, that many of the poor readers showed a relative difference between nonword and exception word reading. Accordingly, the researchers proposed a statistical procedure that would identify children who showed relative differences, but not necessarily deficits, in one or the other area of reading. These can be called "soft subtypes." This technique involved the use of regression analyses to subgroup children with RD into those with better nonword reading than would be predicted on the basis of exception word reading (i.e., surface dyslexic), or those with better exception word reading than would be predicted on the basis of nonword reading (i.e., phonological dyslexic). In each case, predictions and confidence intervals were based on data from the chronological age-matched control group. Using this approach, Castles and Coltheart identified 16 surface and 29 phonological dyslexics. Thus, most of their poor readers (45 out of 53) showed a relative dissociation between nonword and exception word reading. The researchers argued that although these poor readers, for the most part, did not represent hard cases of surface or phonological dyslexia, the apparent dissociation in word recognition profiles could have important implications for understanding and treating reading disabilities.

Whereas the identification of soft subtypes seems profitable, some have questioned how to best evaluate poor readers' relative strengths in nonword and exception word reading. Recall, Castles and Coltheart (1993) used a chronological-age matched control group to estimate the relationship between nonword and exception word reading. In other words, they used same age peers to determine how many nonwords poor readers should read correctly, given their exception word reading score and vice versa. Stanovich and colleagues (1997) maintained that age-related data may not be appropriate for evaluating the relative strengths of poor readers who are reading at a level well below that of chronological age-matched children. The relationship between nonword and exception word reading at different reading levels may not be the same. Less skilled readers may, for example, be expected to read fewer exception words for a given nonword reading score than more skilled readers. Stanovich and colleagues (1997) suggested that the more appropriate comparison for poor readers is a younger group of normal children reading at the same overall level as the poor readers.

To evaluate this claim, Stanovich and colleagues (1997) used regression analyses based on both chronological age (CA) and reading level (RL) matched control groups to divide 68 third-grade children with RD into phonological and surface dyslexic subtypes. When using regression-based predictions from CA-matched children, the researchers found that approximately half of the children with RD (53%) were poor in reading both exception words and nonwords. However, some children with RD showed relative strengths on one or the other set of words. Specifically, 22 percent of the sample performed better on nonwords than exception words (i.e., surface dyslexics), while 25 percent scored better on exception words than nonwords (i.e., phonological dyslexics). When using predictions based on RL-matched controls, again 25 percent of the children with RD could be classified as phonological dyslexics. However, using these data, only one child was identified as a surface dyslexic. That is, compared to RL-matched children, surface dyslexia essentially disappeared. A similar finding was also reported by Manis, Seidenberg, Doi, McBride-Chang, & Petersen (1996).

The findings from this study provide some insights into the nature of the reading problems of phonological and surface dyslexics. Children identified as surface dyslexics, when compared to CA controls, may best be characterized as showing a developmental lag. These children did not display deviant reading abilities; rather, their nonword and exception word reading was like that of younger normal children. These children appear to be taking longer than same age peers to learn to read. Stanovich and colleagues suggested that these children may have a mild form of a phonological processing deficit. They further speculated that this deficit when combined with exceptionally inadequate reading experience could result in a surface dyslexic profile. In contrast to surface dyslexia, phonological dyslexia may constitute a true developmental disorder. Phonological dyslexics continued to show a distinctly different pattern of performance when compared to younger normal children. Furthermore, the phonological dyslexics, in contrast to the surface dyslexics, performed less well than the RL-matched children on tests of phonological awareness, working memory, and syntactic processing.

The results of Stanovich and colleagues (1997) are consistent with those of Murphy and Pollatsek (1994) who found that phonological dyslexics had deficits in phonological awareness. Murphy and Pollatsek also suggested that instructional factors contributed to the reading profiles of some of their cases of surface dyslexia. A recent investigation by Vellutino and colleagues (Vellutino, Scanlon, Sipay, Small, Chen, Pratt, & Denckla, 1996) also provides some converging evidence. As will be discussed in more detail in the next chapter, Vellutino and his colleagues found that some children with RD could be "readily remediated" with short-term intervention. These children, who Vellutino and colleagues believed to have instructional or experiential deficits (and may have also had mild phonological processing deficits), may overlap with the surface dyslexics identified by Stanovich and his colleagues. In contrast, Vellutino and colleagues also identified a group of "hard to remediate" poor readers who seem to fit the profile of phonological dyslexics in that these children had deficits in phonetic decoding and phonological processing.

In summary, it may seem that we have taken a circuitous and bumpy path in our attempt to understand the often conflicting research on word recognition subgroups. It is important to recognize that although poor readers do not cluster into homogeneous subgroups, they do show dissociations in their ability to use the phonological or visual route. It is these dissociations that may prove to have some utility for understanding and treating word recognition problems found in dyslexia (and language-learning disabilities). We will elaborate on possible clinical implications later in this chapter. Before doing so, however, we need to consider one further subtyping system related to word recognition abilities.

Rate-Disabled versus Accuracy-Disabled Readers

Recall that Aaron, Joshi, and Williams (1995) indicated that slow but accurate word recognition might be characteristic of a subgroup of poor readers. Others have also suggested a distinction between rate-disabled and accuracy-disabled poor readers. Specifically, Lovett and her colleagues (Lovett, 1984a, 1984b, 1987; Lovett, Ransby, & Barron, 1988; Lovett, Ransby, Hardwick, & Johns, 1989) proposed two subtypes of reading disabilities. One subtype, *accuracy-disabled* children, was defined as those with significant problems in decoding accuracy, while the other, *rate-disabled* children, were those with a marked deficit in reading rate despite grade-appropriate decoding ability. To be classified as accuracy-disabled, a child had to score at least one and a half years below grade level expectations on at least four of five different measures of word recognition. To be classified as rate-disabled, a child had to perform close to, at, or above grade level on four or more measures of word recognition and at least one and half years below grade-level on four of five measures of reading speed.

In an attempt to validate the above subgroups, Lovett (1987) administered a battery of oral and written language tests to 32 accuracy-disabled, 32 rate-disabled, and 32 normal children. The children were matched for chronological age, sex, and IQ. The oral language tests measured lexical, morphological, and syntactic knowledge. The written language battery included standardized and experimental measures of single word recognition, decoding in context, reading rate, reading comprehension, sound-letter processing, and related academic skills. The results confirmed the distinctiveness of the three groups. The accuracy-disabled children produced more errors, read more slowly, and showed poorer comprehension than the rate-disabled and normal children. The errors the accuracy-disabled children made in reading nonwords indicated that they still had not acquired basic knowledge of sound-letter correspondence rules. With respect to oral language abilities, the accuracy-disabled children demonstrated deficits in morphological and syntactic knowledge. They also were significantly slower than rate-disabled children in naming serial-letter arrays and analyzing individual speech sounds. Lovett concluded that, "these data suggest that accuracy-disabled children suffer a multidimensional language impairment coupled with specific sound analysis difficulties and a seemingly inability to automatize or consolidate single letter identities and/or names." (Lovett, 1987, p. 257)

The reading abilities of the rate-disabled sample were more selectively impaired. There were no differences between these children and the normal readers in their identification of regular and exception words, suggesting that the groups were equally adept at phonetic decoding and sight-word reading. Although these groups were equivalent in accuracy, the rate-disabled subjects exhibited significant impairments in word recognition speed. This was particularly the case in connected text, where these children appear to become functionally overloaded by the demands of processing large units of text. With respect to oral language abilities, the rate-disabled and normal readers were similar with one exception. The rate-disabled children were significantly slower on tasks measuring rapid automatic naming.

Lovett's research thus indicates the existence of another subgroup of poor readers based on word recognition deficits. These children, rate-disabled readers, are accurate in word recognition, but are slow in reading rate. It is unclear from the current research, however, exactly how these children fit into a developmental model of reading. For example, do these children have accuracy problems that later turn into rate problems? It has been our experience that at least some rate-disabled readers do not have a pronounced history of difficulties with accuracy of word recognition. These children appear to develop normally through the primary grades, but then experience significant difficulties in reading more advanced material.

What underlies these children's problems is unclear at present. Some may not have had an adequate amount of reading experience. Because automaticity of word recognition increases with practice, they may lag behind their normal peers in speed of word recognition. Many rate-disabled readers, however, continue to have problems with reading rate despite considerable literacy experience. As noted above, reading rate problems may also be related to phonological retrieval deficits. Lovett's results seem to confirm the problems these children have in the rapid retrieval of verbal labels.

Finally, Lovett's more recent work (Lovett, Benson, & Olds, 1990) is consistent with issues concerning the heterogeneity of clustering. Rather than treat accuracy-disabled and rate-disabled poor readers as distinct subgroups, she and her colleagues have begun to consider the dimensions that underlie these subgroups as continuous variables. For example, they investigated how the continuous variables of reading rate and accuracy are related to intervention outcome.

Combining Subtypes in Research and Practice

In the previous sections, we have described several classification systems for subtyping children with RD. Although presented separately, these systems overlap quite a bit. As seen in Table 4-2, poor readers can be divided into three primary subtypes: children with dyslexia, LLD, and hyperlexia. Children with LLD and those with hyperlexia share deficits in listening comprehension, while children with dyslexia and LLD share problems in word recognition (and associated phonological processing deficits). Because children with LLD and dyslexia both have deficits in word recognition, they can further be divided into word recognition subgroups. These subgroups include children displaying problems in accuracy, either phonological or surface profiles, or those with difficulties in rate. The latter word recognition subtypes, of course, do not apply to children with hyperlexia, because these children have average or above average word recognition abilities.

Whereas this combined classification system has some research support, further empirical validation is necessary. More comprehensive studies are needed to classify and compare subgroups of poor readers. We need to know, for example, if children with LLD show the same profiles in word recognition abilities and phonological processing as children with dyslexia. Some studies (Ellis, McDougall, & Monk, 1996; Felton & Wood, 1992; Stanovich & Siegel, 1994) have shown similarities between these subgroups in these areas, but further investigation is needed. We could find, for example, that because of their language deficits, children with LLD might show particular difficulties using context to develop a sight-word vocabulary. As a result, these children may be more likely to demonstrate a surface dyslexia profile. Lovett's (1987) results further suggest that children with dyslexia may be more likely to show rate problems than children with LLD. We also need to compare

TABLE 4-2   Subtypes of Reading Disabilities

Subtype	Listening Comprehension	Word Recognition
Dyslexia	Good	Phonological
		Surface
		Rate Disabled
Language-Learning Disability	Poor	Phonological
		Surface
		Rate Disabled
Hyperlexia	Poor	Good

children with hyperlexia and LLD. Do these children show similar deficits in listening comprehension? Are there other subgroups within language-learning disabilities and hyperlexia? Listening comprehension is a complex process that consists of linguistic, conceptual, and metacognitive processes. It may be the case that poor readers can be differentiated according to their strengths and weaknesses in these various processes.

Whereas comparative investigations can further our understanding of reading disabilities, theoretical advancements may better be made by treating variables of interest in a continuous rather than categorical fashion. As we noted, poor readers do not cluster together in terms of their word recognition abilities, but rather fall continuously along several dimensions. We would expect the same to be true for listening comprehension and the factors that underlie it. Research designs and statistical analyses that examine the continuous relationships between reading ability, word recognition, listening comprehension, and related factors (cognitive and environmental variables) could provide us with a better understanding of reading disabilities.

Clinical Implications

Despite the lack of homogeneous subgroups, the classification system presented here has some important clinical and educational implications. By considering children's strengths and weaknesses in listening comprehension and accuracy/rate of word recognition, practitioners may be better able to describe reading problems, plan intervention, monitor progress, and determine prognosis (Aaron, 1991). Our classification system suggests that all children with RD need an assessment that includes measures of word recognition, listening comprehension, and related cognitive processes. Word recognition abilities can be evaluated by standardized tests such as the Woodcock Reading Mastery Tests-Revised (Woodcock, 1991). This battery of tests provides an assessment of children's abilities to read real and nonsense words. These tests can be supplemented by lists of exception words in order to more directly evaluate reading by the visual route (see Manis et al., 1996). These measures should allow practitioners to uncover discrepancies between nonword and exception word reading, however, local normative data must be gathered to fully appreciate the meaning of these discrepancies (Stanovich et al., 1997). Rate and fluency of word recognition will also need to be considered. In Chapter 6, Torgesen discusses various ways to measure this aspect of word recognition. He also provides other suggestions for the assessment of word recognition and related language processes (e.g., phonological awareness).

Our classification system further suggests that assessment for reading disabilities should include an evaluation of children's listening comprehension abilities. This may involve the use of measures traditionally employed to assess receptive vocabulary and grammatical knowledge (Bishop, 1989; Carrow-Woolfolk, 1985; DiSimoni, 1978; Dunn & Dunn, 1981), as well as measures of the comprehension of extended spoken texts. Although standardized measures involving extended spoken texts are currently available (Newcomer, 1990; Wechsler, 1991; Wiig, Semel, & Second, 1995; Woodcock, 1991), practitioners may also consider the use of alternate forms of a reading comprehension test administered in a spoken form to assess listening comprehension (Aaron, 1991; Fletcher et al., 1994; Jackson & McClelland, 1979). For example, Aaron (1991) used Form G of the Passage Comprehension subtest of the Woodcock Reading Mastery Tests (Woodcock, 1987) to measure reading comprehension and Form H to assess listening comprehension. Because of the significance of language assessment in the evaluation of reading disabilities, speech-language pathologists can play an important role in the evaluation process.

The proposed classification system should also help clinicians plan intervention programs. This system suggests that children with dyslexia and LLD share the need for intervention directed at word recognition abilities. The nature of this intervention may vary, however, depending on the specific problems a poor reader has in word recognition. For those poor readers who are primarily rate-disabled, intervention will need to provide opportunities to increase the automaticity of word recognition. Automaticity of word recognition comes mainly from practice and repetition in reading. Repeated readings of the same passage can be helpful in this regard (Rashotte & Torgesen, 1985; Samuels, 1977). Paired reading, in which the student alternates turns reading the same passage, reading with audio support, in which the student reads along with an audiorecording of the passage, and imitative reading, in which the teacher reads a passage aloud followed by the student rereading the passage, have also been found to improve reading rate and fluency (Clark & Uhry, 1995; Rashotte & Torgesen, 1985; Samuels, 1977). These activities may also give the poor reader a sense of success and appreciation for fluent reading.

Many children with dyslexia and LLD have problems with word recognition accuracy. Most of these children will have deficits in both phonetic decoding and sight-word reading. Some will show a phonological dyslexic profile, while others will display a surface dyslexic profile. Unfortunately, current research only provides limited direction for differential treatment of these subgroups. As more intervention studies consider the interaction between word recognition subtypes and treatment outcomes, we will be better able to design appropriate intervention programs. While awaiting these results, some insights may be taken from current research. This work suggests that children with phonological dyslexia can benefit from direct and explicit instruction in the use of the phonological route. Rather than "teaching to strengths" as some have maintained, research indicates that children with phonological processing deficits may learn to read most effectively by receiving multisensory training in phonological awareness and phonetic decoding. In Chapter 6, Torgesen describes an intervention program that has been effective in improving the nonword reading abilities of poor readers (also see Lovett, Bordon, DeLuca, Lacerenza, Benson, & Brackstone, 1994).

Children with surface dyslexia have been hypothesized to have a developmental lag (Stanovich et al., 1997). If this turns out to be the case, these poor readers may be able to catch up with their peers with more instruction and practice in reading. They may also benefit from intervention directed at mild phonological processing problems. Vellutino and colleagues (1996) showed that poor readers with less severe phonological deficits responded well to short-term intensive remedial instruction that provided training in phonological processing and reading experience. It is important not to assume that because surface dyslexics are like younger normal children, that they will catch up on their own. They have significant reading problems and, without intervention, they may fall further behind their peers.

Intervention for children with LLD will need to focus on comprehension skills as well as word recognition abilities. In Chapter 7, Westby provides detailed suggestions for assessing and facilitating comprehension. These suggestions include activities to improve vocabulary, schema knowledge, grammatical understanding, and the use of text structure and metacognitive strategies to aid comprehension. In Chapter 9, Westby also offers intervention suggestions for improving the writing abilities of children with LLD. Finally, less is known about effective instruction for children with hyperlexia. However, because of their weakness in listening comprehension, these children should also benefit from intervention directed to comprehension and writing skills.

References

Aaron, P.G. (1989). Qualitative and quantitative differences among dyslexic, normal, and nondyslexic poor readers. *Reading and Writing: An Interdisciplinary Journal, 1,* 291–308.

Aaron, P.G. (1991). Can reading disabilities be diagnosed without using intelligence tests? *Journal of Learning Disabilities, 24,* 178–186.

Aaron, P.G., Frantz, S.S., & Manges, A.R. (1990). Dissociation between comprehension and pronunciation in dyslexic and hyperlexic children. *Reading*

and Writing: An Interdisciplinary Journal, 2, 243–264.

Aaron, P.G., Joshi, R.M., & Williams, K. (1995). *Not all reading disabilities are alike.* Unpublished manuscript.

Aram, D. (1997). Hyperlexia: Reading without meaning in young children. *Topics in Language Disorders, 17,* 1–13.

Aram, D.M., Ekelman, B.L., & Healy, J.M. (1984). *Reading profiles of hyperlexic children.* Paper presented at the International Neuropsychology Society, Aachen, Germany.

Aram, D.M., & Healy, J.M. (Eds.). (1988). *Hyperlexia: A review of extraordinary word recognition.* New York: Guilford Press.

Bishop, D. (1989). *Test of Reception of Grammar* (2nd ed.). University of Manchester, Department of Psychology.

Boder, E. (1971). Developmental dyslexia: Prevailing diagnostic concepts and a new diagnostic approach. In H.R. Myklebust (Ed.), *Progress in learning disabilities* (Vol. 2, pp. 293–321). New York: Grune & Stratton.

Boder, E. (1973). Developmental dyslexia: A diagnostic approach based on three atypical reading-spelling patterns. *Developmental Medicine and Child Neurology, 15,* 663–687.

Boder, E., & Jarrico, S. (1982). *The Boder Test of Reading-Spelling Patterns: A diagnostic screening test for subtypes of reading disability.* New York: Grune & Stratton.

Bruck, M. (1988). The word recognition and spelling of dyslexic children. *Reading Research Quarterly, 23,* 51–69.

Bruck, M. (1990). Word recognition skills of adults with a childhood diagnosis of dyslexia. *Developmental Psychology, 26,* 439–454.

Carbo, M. (1987). Reading styles research: "What words" isn't always phonics. *Phi Delta Kappan, 68,* 431–445.

Carbo, M. (1992). Giving unequal learners an equal chance: A reply to a biased critique of learning styles. *Remedial and Special Education, 13,* 19–29.

Carrow-Woolfolk, E. (1985). *Test for Auditory Comprehension of Language-Revised.* Allen, TX: DLM Teaching Resources.

Carver, R. (1993). Merging the simple view of reading with reading theory. *Journal of Reading Behavior, 25,* 439–455.

Castles, A., & Coltheart, M. (1993). Varieties of developmental dyslexia. *Cognition, 47,* 149–180.

Catts, H.W. (1996). Defining dyslexia as a developmental language disorder: An expanded view. *Topics in Language Disorders, 16,* 14–29.

Catts, H.W. (1993). The relationship between speech-language impairments and reading disabilities. *Journal of Speech and Hearing Research, 36,* 948–958.

Catts, H.W., & Fey, M.E. (1995). Written language outcomes of children with language impairments. Grant proposal funded by The National Institute of Deafness and Other Communicative Disorders, Bethesda, MD.

Catts, H.W. (1989a). Defining dyslexia as a developmental language disorder. *Annals of Dyslexia, 39,* 50–64.

Catts, H.W. (1989b). Speech production deficits in developmental dyslexia. *Journal of Speech and Hearing Disorders, 54,* 422–428.

Catts, H.W., Fey, M., & Tomblin, B. (1997). *Language basis of reading disabilities.* Paper presented at the Society for the Scientific Study of Reading, Chicago.

Catts, H.W., Fey, M., Zhang, X., Tomblin, B. (1998). *Subtypes of reading disabilities.* Paper presented at the Conference for the Society for the Scientific Study of Reading, San Diego.

Clark, D.B., & Uhry, J.K. (1995). *Dyslexia: Theory and practice of remedial instruction.* Baltimore, MD: York Press.

Coltheart, M., Materson, J., Byng, S., Prior, M., & Riddoch, J. (1983). Surface dyslexia. *Quarterly Journal of Experimental Psychology, 35A,* 469–496.

Coltheart, M., Patterson, K., & Marshall, J. (Eds.). (1980). *Deep dyslexia.* London: Routledge and Kegan Paul.

Critchley, M. (1970). *The dyslexic child.* Springfield, IL: Thomas.

Curtis, M. (1980). Development of the components of reading skill. *Journal of Educational Psychology, 72,* 656–669.

Dalby, J.T., & Gibson, D. (1981). Functional cerebral lateralization in subtypes of disabled readers. *Brain and Language, 14,* 34–48.

DiSimoni, F. (1978). *The Token Test for Children.* Boston: Teaching Resources Corporation.

Dunn, L., & Dunn, L. (1981). *Peabody Picture Vocabulary Test-Revised.* Circle Pines, MN: American Guidance.

Dunn, R. (1990). Teaching young children to read: Matching methods to learning style perceptual processing strengths, Part 1. *International Education, 17,* 5–7.

Elliott, D.E., & Needleman, R.M. (1976). The syndrome of hyperlexia. *Brain and Language, 3,* 339–349.

Ellis, A.W. (1985). The cognitive neuropsychology of developmental (and acquired) dyslexia: A critical survey. *Cognitive Neuropsychology, 2,* 196–205.

Ellis, A.W., McDougall, S., & Monk, A.F. (1996). Are dyslexics different? II. A comparison between dyslexics, reading age controls, poor readers, and precocious readers. *Dyslexia: An International Journal of Practice and Research, 2,* 59–68.

Feagan, L.V., & McKinney, J.D. (1991). Subtypes of learning disabilities: A review. In L.V. Feagan, E.J. Short, & E.J. Meltzer (Eds.), *Subtypes of learning disabilities* (pp. 3–32). Hillsdale, NJ: Lawrence Erlbaum.

Felton, R.H., & Wood, F.B. (1992). A reading level match study of nonword reading skills in poor readers with varying IQ. *Journal of Learning Disabilities, 25,* 318–326.

Fletcher, J.M., Shaywitz, S.E., Shankweiler, D.P., Katz, L., Liberman, I.Y., Stuebing, K.K. Francis, D.J., Fowler, A.E., & Shaywitz, B.A. (1994). Cognitive profiles of reading disability: Comparisons of discrepancy and low achievement definitions. *Journal of Educational Psychology, 86,* 6–23.

Flynn, J.M., & Deering, W.M. (1989). Subtypes of dyslexia: Investigation of Boder's system using quantative neurophysiology. *Developmental Medicine and Child Neurology, 31,* 215–223.

Godfrey, J.J., Lasky, A.K., Millag, K.K., & Knox, C.M. (1981). Performance of dyslexic children on speech perception tests. *Journal of Experimental Child Psychology, 32,* 401–424.

Gough, P.B., & Tunmer, W.E. (1986). Decoding, reading, and reading disability. *Remedial and Special Education, 7,* 6–10.

Holmes, J. (1978). Regression and reading breakdown. In C.A. & E. Zurif (Eds.), *Language acquisition and language breakdown.* Baltimore, MD: Johns Hopkins University Press.

Holt, S.B., & O'Tuel, F. (1990). *Reading styles program evaluation.* Lake City, SC: Florence County School District.

Hooper, S.R., & Willis, W.G. (1989). *Learning disability subtyping: Neuropsychological foundations, conceptual models, and issues in clinical differentiation.* New York: Springer-Verlag.

Hoover, W.A. (1994). *The simple view of reading: Analyses based on a monolingual sample.* Paper presented at the NATO Advanced Study Institute: Cognitive and Linguistic Bases of Reading, Writing, and Spelling, Alvor-Algarve, Portugal.

Hoover, W.A., & Gough, P.B. (1990). The simple view of reading. *Reading and Writing: An Interdisciplinary Journal, 2,* 127–160.

Hurford, D.P., Schauf, J.D., Bunce, L., Blaich, T., & Moore, K. (1994). Early identification of children at risk for reading disabilities. *Journal of Learning Disabilities, 27,* 371–382.

Huttenlocher, P.R., & Huttenlocher, J. (1973). A study of children with hyperlexia. *Neurology, 23,* 1107–1116.

Ingram, T.T.S. (1964). The nature of dyslexia. In F.A. Young & D.B. Lindsley (Eds.), *Early experience and visual information processing in perceptual and reading disorders.* Washington, DC: National Academy of Sciences.

Jackson, M.D., & McClelland, J.L. (1979). Processing determinants of reading speed. *Journal of Experimental Psychology: Human Perception and Performance, 108,* 151–181.

Jorm, A.F., Share, D.L., Maclean, R., & Matthews, R. (1986). Cognitive factors at school entry predictive of specific reading retardation and general reading backwardness: A research note. *Journal of Child Psychology and Psychiatry, 27,* 45–54.

Kavale, K.A., Forness, S.R., & Bender, M. (Eds.). (1987). *Handbook of learning disabilities: Dimensions and diagnosis* (Vol. 1). Boston: Little, Brown, and Company.

Kershner, J.R. (1990). Self-concept and IQ as predictors of remedial success in children with learning disabilities. *Journal of Learning Disabilities, 23,* 368–374.

Lovett, M.W. (1984a). A developmental perspective on reading dysfunction: Accuracy and rate criteria in the subtyping of dyslexic children. *Brain and Language, 22,* 67–91.

Lovett, M.W. (1984b). The search for subtypes of specific reading disability: Reflections from a cognitive perspective. *Annals of Dyslexia, 34,* 155–178.

Lovett, M.W. (1987). A developmental approach to reading disability: Accuracy and speed criteria of normal and deficient reading skill. *Child Development, 58,* 234–260.

Lovett, M.W., Benson, N.J., & Olds, J. (1990). Individual difference predictors of treatment outcome in remediation of specific reading disability. *Learning and Individual Differences, 2,* 287–314.

Lovett, M.W., Bordon, S.L., DeLuca, T., Lacerenza, L., Benson, N.J., & Brackstone, D. (1994). Treating the core deficits of developmental dyslexia: Evidence of transfer-of-learning following phonologically and strategy-based reading training programs. *Developmental Psychology, 30,* 805–822.

Lovett, M.W., Ransby, M.J., & Barron, R.W. (1988). Treatment, subtype, and word type effects in dyslexic children's response to remediation. *Brain & Language, 34,* 328–349.

Lovett, M.W., Ransby, M.J., Hardwick, N., & Johns, M.S. (1989). Can dyslexia be treated? Treatment-specific and generalized treatment effects in dyslexic children's response to remediation. *Brain & Language, 37,* 90–121.

Lyon, R. (1983). Learning-disabled readers: Identification of subgroups. In H. Myklebust (Ed.), *Progress in learning disabilities* (Vol. 5, pp. 103–134). New York: Grune & Stratton.

Manis, F.R., Seidenberg, M.S., Doi, L.M., McBride-Chang, C., & Petersen, A. (1996). On the basis of two subtypes of developmental dyslexia. *Cognition, 58,* 157–195.

Marshall, J. (1984). Toward a rational taxonomy of developmental dylexias. In R. Malatesha & H. Whitaker (Eds.), *Dyslexia: A global issue.* The Hague: Martinus Nighoff.

Marshall, J., & Newcombe, F. (1973). Patterns of paralexia: A psycholinguistic approach. *Journal of Psycholinguistic Research, 2,* 175–200.

Morris, R., Satz, P., & Blashfield, R. (1981). Neuropsychology and cluster analysis: Potentials and problems. *Journal of Clinical Neuropsychology, 3,* 77–79.

Murphy, L., & Pollatsek, A. (1994). Developmental dyslexia: Heterogeneity without discrete subgroups. *Annals of Dyslexia, 44,* 120–146.

Newby, R., & Lyon, G.R. (1991). Neuropsychological subtypes of learning disabilities. In J.E. Obrzut & G.W. Hynd (Eds.), *Neuropsychological foundations of learning disabilities: A handbook of issues, methods, and practice* (pp. 355–386). San Diego: Academic Press.

Newcomer, P. (1990). *Diagnostic Achievement Battery.* Austin, TX: Pro-Ed.

Oakhill, J. (1982). Constructive processes in skilled and less-skilled comprehender's memory for sentences. *British Journal of Psychology, 73,* 13–20.

Oakhill, J. (1984). Inferential and memory skills in children's comprehension of stories. *British Journal of Educational Psychology, 54,* 31–39.

Padget, Y. (1998). Lessons from research on dyslexia: Implications for a classification system for learning disabilities. *Learning Disability Quarterly, 21,* 167.

Palmer, J., MacLeod, C., Hunt, E., & Davidson, J. (1985). Information processing correlates of reading. *Journal of Memory and Language, 24,* 59–88.

Patterson, K. (1982). The relationship between reading and phonological coding: Further neuropsychological observations. In A. Ellis (Ed.), *Normality and pathology in cognitive functions.* London: Academic Press.

Petrauskas, R.J., & Rourke, B.P. (1979). Identification of subtypes of retarded readers: A neuropsychological, multivariate approach. *Journal of Clinical Neuropsychology, 1,* 17–37.

Rack, J.P., Snowling, M.J., & Olson, R.K. (1992). The nonword reading deficit in developmental dyslexia: A review. *Reading Research Quarterly, 27,* 28–53.

Rashotte, C.A., & Torgesen, J.K. (1985). Repeated reading and reading fluency in reading disabled children. *Reading Research Quarterly, 20,* 180–188.

Rayner, K., & Pollatsek, A. (1989). *The psychology of reading.* Englewood Cliffs, NJ: Prentice Hall.

Rutter, M., & Yule, W. (1975). The concept of specific reading retardation. *Journal of Child Psychology and Psychiatry, 16,* 181–197.

Samuels, S.J. (1977). The method of reacted reading. *The Reading Teacher, 32,* 403–408.

Shankweiler, D., Crain, S., Katz, L., Fowler, A.E., Liberman, A.M., Brady, S.A., Thornton, R., Lundquist, E., Dreyer, L., Fletcher, J.M., Stuebing, K.K., Shaywitz, S.E., & Shaywitz, B.A. (1995). Cognitive profiles of reading-disabled children: Comparison of language skills in phonology, morphology, and syntax. *Psychological Science, 6,* 149–156.

Share, D. (1995). Phonological recoding and self-teaching: Sine qua non of reading acquisition. *Cognition, 55,* 151–218.

Share, D.L., McGee, R., McKenzie, D., Williams, S., & Silva, P. (1987). Further evidence relating to the distinction between specific reading retardation and general reading backwardness. *British Journal of Developmental Psychology, 5,* 35–44.

Share, D.L., & Stanovich, K.E. (1995). Cognitive processes in early reading development: Accommodating individual differences into a model of acquisition. *Issues in Education, 1,* 1–57.

Shaywitz, B.A., Fletcher, J.M., Holahan, J.M., & Shaywitz, S.E. (1992). Discrepancy compared to low achievement definitions of reading disability: Results from the Connecticut Longitudinal Study. *Journal of Learning Disabilities, 25,* 639–648.

Siegel, L.S. (1984). A longitudinal study of a hyperlexic child: Hyperlexia as a language disorder. *Neuropsychologia, 22,* 577–585.

Siegel, L.S. (1989). IQ is irrelevant to the definition of learning disabilities. *Journal of Learning Disabilities, 22,* 469–478.

Silberberg, N.E., & Silberberg, M.C. (1967). Hyperlexia: Specific word recognition skills in young children. *Exceptional Children, 34,* 41–42.

Singer, M., & Crouse, J. (1981). The relationship of context-use skills to reading: A case for an alternative experimental logic. *Child Development, 52,* 1326–1329.

Snowling, M. (1981). Phonemic deficits in developmental dyslexia. *Psychological Research, 43,* 219–234.

Stahl, S.A. (1988). Is there evidence to support matching reading styles and initial reading methods? *Phi Delta Kappan,* 317–322.

Stahl, S.A., & Kuhn, M.R. (1995). Does whole language or instruction matched to learning styles help children learn to read? *School Psychology Review, 24,* 393–404.

Stanovich, K.E. (1985). Explaining the variance in reading ability in terms of psychological processes: What have we learned? *Annals of Dyslexia, 85,* 67–96.

Stanovich, K.E. (1991). Discrepancy definitions of reading disability: Has intelligence led us astray? *Reading Research Quarterly, 26,* 7–29.

Stanovich, K.E. (1997). Toward a more inclusive definition of dyslexia. *Dyslexia: An International Journal of Research and Practice, 2,* 154–166.

Stanovich, K.E., Nathan, R.G., & Zolman, J.E. (1988). The developmental lag hypothesis in reading: Longitudinal and matched reading-level comparisons. *Child Development, 59,* 71–86.

Stanovich, K.E., & Siegel, L.S. (1994). The phenotypic performance profile of reading-disabled children: A regression-based test of the phonological-core variable-difference model. *Journal of Educational Psychology, 86,* 24–53.

Stanovich, K.E., Siegel, L.S., & Gottardo, A. (1997). Converging evidence for phonological and surface subtypes of reading disability. *Journal of Educational Psychology, 89,* 114–127.

Stothard, S., & Hulme, C. (1992). Reading comprehension difficulties in children: The role of language comprehension and working memory skills. *Reading and Writing: An Interdisciplinary Journal, 4,* 245–256.

Temple, C.M., & Marshall, J.C. (1983). A case study of developmental phonological dyslexia. *British Journal of Psychology, 74,* 517–533.

Thomasson, R. (1990). *Reading style teaching districtwide.* Pine Bluff, AZ: Pine Bluff School District.

Thomson, M. (1984). *Developmental dyslexia: Its nature, assessment and remediation.* London: Edward Arnold.

Torgesen, J.K., Wagner, R.K., Rashotte, C.A. (1997). *Preventing reading disabilities: Results from 2 1/2 years of intervention.* Paper presented at the Society for the Scientific Study of Reading, Chicago, IL.

Turner, S., & Dawson, M. (1978). The teaching of reading: A review. *Journal of Learning Disabilities, 11,* 17–27.

van den Bos, K.P. (1982). *Letter span, scanning, and code matching in dyslexic subgroups.* Paper presented at the Orton Dyslexia Society, Baltimore, MD.

Vellutino, F. (1979). *Dyslexia: Theory and research.* Cambridge, MA: MIT Press.

Vellutino, F.R., Scanlon, D.M., Sipay, E.R., Small, S.G., Chen, R., Pratt, A., & Denckla, M.B. (1996). Cognitive profiles of difficult-to-remediate and readily remediated poor readers: Early intervention as a vehicle for distinguishing between cognitive and experiential deficits as basic causes of specific reading disabilities. *Journal of Educational Psychology, 88,* 601–638.

Wechsler, D. (1991). *Wechsler Individual Achievement Test.* San Antonio, TX: The Psychological Corporation.

Wiig, E., Semel, E., & Second, W. (1995). *Clinical Evaluation of Language Fundamentals–III.* San Antonio, TX: The Psychological Corporation.

Woodcock, R.W. (1987). *Woodcock Reading Mastery Tests-Revised.* Circle Pines, MN: American Guidance Service.

Woodcock, R. (1991). *Woodcock Language Proficiency Battery-Revised.* Chicago, IL: Riverside.

Chapter 5

Causes of Reading Disabilities

HUGH W. CATTS   *ALAN G. KAMHI*

When a parent or teacher learns that a child has a reading disability, he or she inevitably wants to know what has caused the disability. Providing answers about the causes of reading disabilities can be a difficult task. Reading is a complex ability and breakdowns in the acquisition of this ability can be difficult to understand. Recent research, however, has begun to provide some answers concerning the causes of reading disabilities. This work indicates that reading disabilities are the result of an interplay of intrinsic and extrinsic factors. Intrinsic factors refer to internal or child-based processes, while extrinsic factors concern environmental variables. As discussed in Chapter 3, intrinsic factors have long been thought to play a major role in most cases of reading disabilities (Critchley, 1970; Hinshelwood, 1917; Orton, 1937). Definitions have emphasized the intrinsic or constitutional nature of reading disabilities and the majority of the research has been driven by the quest to find the intrinsic cause of reading problems. As a result, there is now a large body of evidence that indicates the significance of biological factors in reading development and disorders.

Extrinsic factors also appear to play a role in reading disabilities. Although definitions generally exclude factors such as a lack of literacy experience or inadequate instruction from being a cause of reading disabilities, many children diagnosed with reading disabilities have experiential or instructional deficits. These deficits may be the initial cause of reading problems or they may occur secondary to intrinsic factors.

In this chapter, we will discuss the intrinsic and extrinsic causes of reading disabilities. Much of the research we will review has focused on dyslexia. Only a few studies have examined the causes of language-learning disabilities. However, from what is known, there is considerable overlap in the causal basis of these disorders. Therefore, in this chapter, we will not make a distinction between dyslexia and language-learning disabilities, but will consider the causal factors that underlie these reading disabilities.

Extrinsic Causes of Reading Disabilities

In order to learn to read, children need exposure to print, explicit instruction in how print works, and opportunity to practice their reading skills (Adams, 1990). Without opportunity and instruction, children will not learn to be skilled readers. Although literacy experience is critical for reading acquisition, it generally has been neglected in causal explanations of reading disabilities. As noted in the previous chapter, most definitions exclude extrinsic factors such as lack of opportunity or inadequate instruction as causes of reading disabilities. However, in most cases practitioners and researchers have paid only limited attention to whether poor readers have met this exclusionary criterion. Generally, if children are in age-appropriate grades, attend school regularly, and do not come from improvished homes, they are considered to have had adequate opportunity and instruction to learn to read. In evaluating children for reading disabilities, seldom do professionals closely consider the nature of the literacy experiences poor readers have had. As a result, variability in literacy experience often goes unnoticed and can potentially influence reading disabilities.

Unfortunately, the full extent of the contribution of limited literacy experiences to reading disabilities is not known. Because environmental factors have been excluded from definitions of reading disabilities, most researchers in the field have not examined literacy experience in relationship to reading disabilities. Spear-Swerling and Sternberg (1996) have noted that, for the most part, the study of the influence of environmental factors on reading disabilities has come from outside of the field of reading disabilities. One body of research that is relevant to the role of literacy experience in reading disabilities concerns the impact of early joint book reading on subsequent reading development.

Early Literacy Experience

In Chapter 2, we noted that it was quite common in many homes to find parents reading to their children from an early age. Whereas such practice occurs frequently in mainstream homes, some children enter school without this experience. It seems reasonable to ask about the possible causal role a lack of early joint book reading might play in later reading problems. Although there are many anecdotal claims of children with limited exposure to print having difficulty learning to read (e.g., Spear-Swerling & Sternberg, 1996), few studies have actually examined the influence of a lack of early literacy experience on reading disabilities. As discussed in Chapter 2, research has focused primarily on the relationship between joint book reading and reading development in the general population. Overall, this research has shown only a weak association between early joint book reading and subsequent reading development. Several recent meta-analyses of this literature (Bus, van Ijzendoorn, & Pellegrini, 1995; Scarborough & Dobrich, 1994) have indicated that on the average joint book reading accounted for only about 8 percent of the variance in reading outcome measures. Furthermore, this effect appeared to decrease with age, suggesting that school instruction in reading may compensate for a lack of home literacy experience.

Although an absence of joint book reading during the preschool years does not seem to be a primary cause of reading disabilities, it may still play some role in reading problems. For example, a lack of early literacy experience may be particularly detrimental to children with other risk factors. Children from low socioeconomic status backgrounds and/or those with language impairments may be at increased risk for reading disabilities if they have not had home literacy experiences.

Reading Instruction

Because reading is a skill that, for the most part, must be taught, differences in the quality and/or quantity of instruction clearly affect reading development. However, the role instructional factors play in reading disabilities is not well understood. Traditionally, it has been thought that instructional factors have little causal impact on reading disabilities. By definition, children with reading disabilities (RD) do not have instructional deficits. However, as noted above, this exclusionary criterion is seldom carefully assessed. Typically, if poor readers are in a grade that is appropriate for their age and attend school regularly, they are assumed to have had the necessary instruction to learn to read. These procedures, however, allow for considerable variability in the quality and quantity of instruction that poor readers may have received. It is likely that this variability has some impact on reading disabilities. Until recently, though, instructional variables have not been examined in children with RD.

Vellutino and his colleagues (Scanlon & Vellutino, 1996, 1997; Vellutino, Scanlon, Sipay, Small, Chen, Pratt, & Denckla, 1996), in a large longitudinal investigation, examined the role of instructional deficits in reading disabilities. From a total sample of 1,400 kindergarten children attending middle- to upper middle-class schools, they identified 151 children who were at risk for reading disabilities based on poor performance on a letter identification test (Scanlon & Vellutino, 1996, 1997). These children also met exclusionary criteria that included no sensory or intellectual handicaps. Researchers conducted classroom observations in which they evaluated the nature of reading/literacy instruction these children were receiving. They noted, for example, the materials being used (e.g., books, letters, spoken language), the activities in which the children were engaged (e.g., reading text, phoneme awareness, letter naming), and the expected responses of the children (e.g., reading, writing, looking). The participants were subsequently followed into first grade and were divided into those who were good, average, or poor readers based on teacher ratings and tests of reading achievement. Comparisons between outcome groups indicated that the at-risk children who became good readers received more instruction in analyzing the structural (sound and spelling) aspects of spoken and written language than did the other outcome groups. Reader groups did not differ, however, on variables such as time spent reading connected text or in discussions of word meanings. The researchers concluded that differences in instruction do make a difference in whether or not at-risk children become reading disabled.

More direct evidence of the role instructional variables play in reading disabilities comes from another component of this longitudinal investigation (Vellutino et al., 1996). As part of their study, Vellutino and his colleagues provided remedial instruction to those children in their sample who had significant reading problems at mid-first grade. These children performed at or below the 15th percentile on tests of reading achievement and met typical exclusionary criteria for reading disabilities. During the second semester of first grade, the children received daily one-to-one tutoring (30 minutes per session) for a minimum of fifteen weeks (typically 70 to 80 sessions). It was thought that this remedial instruction might be sufficient to eliminate reading problems in those children who suffered from instructional or experiential deficits, rather than intrinsic problems. Vellutino and his colleagues found that after remedial instruction, 67 percent of the poor readers scored in the average or above average range on tests of reading achievement. They concluded that among children meeting typical exclusionary criteria for reading disabilities, there will be many who have no intrinsic problems, but who have had inadequate instruction or opportunity to learn to read.

Although the above study points to the significance of extrinsic factors in reading disabilities, strong conclusions would be premature. Specifically, data showing that instruction can improve reading does not necessarily mean that instructional deficits were the cause of the reading problem in the first place. Children with phonological processing deficits or other intrinsic deficiencies may also benefit from instruction. In support of their conclusions, Vellutino and co-workers (1996) did show that the "readily remediated" poor readers had fewer problems in phonological processing than poor readers who were difficult to remediate. However, some of the former poor readers could have had mild phonological processing deficits or other intrinsic problems that were amenable to instruction. Clearly, more research is needed to understand the role of instructional variables in reading disabilities.

Matthew Effects

Although studies have not yet clearly shown that extrinsic factors play a primary role in recognized cases of reading disabilities, there is little doubt that these factors function to maintain, and in some instances, increase the severity of reading problems. In fact, some have argued that merely considering children to be reading disabled can set into motion a host of negative consequences that can influence reading development (Cole, 1987; Spear-Swerling & Stenberg, 1996). Spear-Swerling and Sternberg (1996) maintain that placing children in low ability or remedial reading groups or in special education classes can itself bring on further reading problems. Children in low ability or special reading groups often have low expectations placed on them by their teachers and parents. Their low ability peers offer them little support, and their teachers provide them with little challenge. These children become less motivated to read and may have other attentional or behavior problems. Spear-Swerling and Sternberg argue that these factors can actually lead to children receiving less instruction and practice in reading. In turn, these children may fall farther and farther behind their peers.

Stanovich (1986, 1988) has used the term Matthew effects to describe the negative consequences associated with failure in reading. The term comes from a biblical passage in the book of Matthew that comments on how the rich get richer and the poor get poorer. Stanovich argues that because of factors such as low expectations, limited practice, and poor motivation, those who get off to a slow start in reading often get caught in a downward spiral of failure. Spear-Swerling and Sternberg (1994) describe these factors as a kind of swamp. They state that "once children have entered the 'swamp' of negative expectations, lowered motivation, and limited practice, it may be very difficult for them to get back on the right road" (p. 99). Thus, it seems clear that even if extrinsic factors do no.. initial role in reading disabilities, they soon become an integral part of the disorder.

One particularly relevant consequence of Matthew effects is language problems. Because reading is a key source for new vocabulary and advanced grammatical and discourse knowledge, children who do not read much will often begin to fall behind their peers in language development (e.g., Stothard, Snowling, & Bishop 1996). Thus, as a result of their limited reading experience, poor readers who do not necessarily have a developmental language disorder will soon develop language problems.

Intrinsic Causes of Reading Disabilities

Factors intrinsic to the child have traditionally played a prominent role in causal explanations of reading disabilities. Consequently, considerable research attention has been devoted to the study of these factors. This research has examined the genetic and neurological bases of reading disabilities, as well as the cognitive-perceptual deficits that are believed to result from these bases.

Genetic Basis

From the earliest reports, it was recognized that reading disabilities often ran in families (Hallgren, 1950; Hinshelwood, 1917; Stephenson, 1907). For example, Hinshelwood (1917) noted that reading disabilities were often found in siblings and/or multiple generations of a family. More recently, investigations have confirmed the familial basis of reading disabilities (Finucci, Gutherie, Childs, Abbey, & Childs, 1976; Gilger, Pennington, & DeFries, 1991; Vogler, DeFries, & Decker, 1985). Taken together, these studies have shown that a brother or sister of a RD child has an approximately 40 percent chance of having a reading disability, while a parent of a RD child has a 30 to 40 percent likelihood of having a history of a reading disability.

Although reading disabilities are clearly familial, this does not mean that they are necessarily heritable. Bad table manners and cake recipes are among the common examples of things that run in families, but are not genetically transmitted. In order to determine the heritability of a complex behavior such as reading disability, researchers often examined identical and fraternal twins (DeFries, Fulker, & LaBuda, 1987; Light & DeFries, 1995). Identical or monozygotic twins share all the same genes, while fraternal or dizygotic twins only share half their genes on average. If a reading disability is heritable, it should co-occur in identical twins more often than it does in fraternal twins. This is essentially what researchers have found. In a representative study, Light and DeFries (1995) reported that in 68 percent of identical twins, when one twin had a reading disability, the other twin also had a reading problem. The corresponding rate in fraternal twins was 40 percent. Although these results support the heritability of reading disabilities, they also indicate that genes do not act alone. The co-occurence of reading problems in identical twins is far from 100 percent, suggesting that factors other than genetics also contribute to reading development. Thus, just because an individual has the gene(s) for reading disabilities, does not mean he or she will develop reading problems; rather, it indicates that the likelihood of having the disorder is much higher.

Researchers have also examined data from family studies to determine if reading disabilities are the result of a single gene or a combination of multiple genes (Pennington, Gilger, Pauls, Smith, Smith, & DeFries, 1991). Current thinking is that a limited number of genes work together in an additive manner to influence reading ability (Pennington & Gilger, 1996). However, these genes vary in their relative strength, with a major gene or genes having primary influence. In this view, referred to as the *quantitative trait locus model,* the major genes of concern are thought to influence reading ability in general, not just reading disability. Individuals with favorable forms of these genes are believed to have a biological advantage for learning to read, while those with unfavorable forms of these genes are at risk for reading disabilities.

Finally, studies have sought to determine which chromosome(s) contains the major gene(s) associated with reading ability/disability (Bisgaard, Eiberg, Moller, Neihbar, & Mohr, 1987; Cardon & Fulker, 1994; Grigorenko, Wood, Meyer, Hart, Speed, Shuster, & Pauls, 1997; Smith, Kimberling, & Pennington, 1991; Smith, Kimberling, Pennington, & Lubs, 1983). While this work is only in its early stages, researchers have already pinpointed regions on chromosomes 6 and 15 as likely locations for major gene(s) associated with reading ability. In the coming years, researchers should be able to locate the specific genes that influence reading. This knowledge should prove to be quite useful in the early identification of reading disabilities.

Neurological Basis

Considerable attention has been devoted to the study of the brain and its role in reading disabilities. Early accounts suggested that children with RD lacked cerebral dominance for language (Orton, 1937). In most individuals, the left cortical hemisphere plays a more dominant role in language processing than does the right. Orton (1937) and other early investigators proposed that in children with RD, the right hemisphere shared language dominance with the left (i.e., mixed dominance) or was the dominant hemisphere for language. To test this proposal, researchers initially had to rely on behavioral data, such as handedness. Because left-handedness is sometimes associated with mixed or right dominance, the study of handedness was seen as a way to examine brain laterality in individuals with RD. This work, however, has found no consistent association between handedness and reading disabilities (see Bishop, 1990; Bryden, 1982).

Other behavioral techniques have also been used to study laterality differences in reading disabilities. These have included dichotic listening (Obrzat, 1979; Satz & Sparrow, 1970; Thomson, 1976), visual split-field (Keefe & Swinney, 1979; Marcel, Katz, & Smith, 1974; Olson, 1973), and time-sharing studies (Obrzat, 1979; Stellern, Collins, & Bayne, 1987). This research has been fraught with mixed results and methodological shortcomings (Obrzat, Hynd, & Boliek, 1986; Satz, 1977). However, most reviews of this work (e.g., Bryden, 1982; Gerber, 1993) have concluded that the evidence seems to support the view that individuals with RD, as a group, show less left dominance for language than normal readers.

More recently, researchers have directly examined the brains of individuals with RD for evidence of abnormalities. Specifically, Galaburda and his colleagues have conducted postmortem examinations of the brains of a small number of individuals who had previously been diagnosed as dyslexic (Galaburda, 1988; Galaburda, Corsiglia, Rosen, & Sherman, 1987; Galaburda, Sherman, Rosen, Aboitiz, & Geschwind, 1985). One noteworthy observation concerned the planum temporale, a structure in the temporal lobe thought to be involved in language processing (Foundas, Leonard, Gilmore, et al., 1994). In nondisabled individuals the planum is generally larger in the left hemisphere than in the right. The researchers observed, however, that in the dyslexic brains the temporal plana were symmetrical. This symmetry was accounted for, not by a smaller than normal left planum, but rather a larger than expected right planum.

Galaburda and his team also identified microscopic anomalies in the dyslexic brains. These involved focal dysplasia that are nests of neurons in areas of the cortex where they are seldom found. Galaburda (1991) suggested that in dyslexics, neuronal pruning necessary to refine neuron networks and correct developmental errors may be disrupted. This disruption could account for the larger than normal right planum as well as the focal dysplasias.

Recent advancements in technology have provided additional ways to examine the brain structure and function of individuals with RD. This work has involved the use of magnetic resonance imaging, cortical blood flow measurement, and electrophysiological recordings. *Magnetic resonace imaging* (MRI) is an noninvasive technique that uses a strong magnetic field and high-frequency radio waves to produce precise two- or three-dimensional images of the brain. These images are much superior to those available by traditional x-ray technology. A number of studies have employed MRI techniques to examine the brains of individuals with RD. These studies have uncovered some structural differences between RD and normal individuals in the planum temporale (Hynd, Semrud-Clikeman, Lorys, Novey, & Eliopulos, 1990; Larsen, Hoien, & Odegaard, 1992) and other regions of the temporal lobe (Hynd et al., 1990; Jernigan, Hesselink, Sowell, & Tallal, 1991). Group differences have also been found in the corpus callosum (Duara et al., 1991; Hynd, Hall, Novey, Eliopules, Black, Gonzalez, Edmonds, Riccio, & Cohen, 1995; Lubs, Duara, Levin, Jallard, Lubs, Rabin, Kushch, & Gross-Glenn, 1991) and in the inferior parietal lobe (Lubs et al., 1991). Despite the observed group differences, there are some inconsistencies across studies, suggesting that one must be cautious about drawing conclusions concerning structural anomalies in individuals with reading disabilities (cf. Filipek, 1995).

Functional aspects of the brain have also been examined in individuals with RD. As part of this work, cortical blood flow techniques have been employed (Flowers, Wood, & Naylor, 1991; Paulesu, Frith, Snowling, Gallagher, Morton, Frackowiak, & Frith, 1992; Rumsey, Andreason, Zametkin, Aquino, King, Hamburger, Pikus, Rapoport, & Cohen, 1992; Rumsey, Nace, Donohue, Wise, Maisog, & Andreason, 1997). These techniques measure contrast in blood flow across various regions of the brain as an indication of the level of activity of these areas during specific tasks. In one such technique, called *positron emission tomography* (PET), regional blood flow is monitored by recording the distribution of cerebral radioactivity following the intravenous injection of a radioactive isotope. Using PET scan technology, Rumsey and her colleagues (Rumsey et al., 1997) found dyslexics showed less activation than controls in the mid- to posterior temporal cortex bilaterally and in the left inferior parietal cortex during several reading tasks. These regions have been linked with phonological processing (Paulesu, Connelly, Frith, Friston, Heather, & Myers, 1995; Paulesu, Frith, & Frackowiak, 1993). Paulesu and colleagues (1996) have further reported that dyslexics had less widespread blood flow across language areas while performing rhyming and phonological memory tasks.

Functional MRI (fMRI) techniques have also been employed to study brain activity in individuals with RD. Because differences in blood oxygenation correspond to differences in magnetic resonance, fMRI can provide a noninvasive measure of blood flow and regional brain activity. Using fMRI, Eden and colleagues (Eden, VanMeter, Rumsey, Maisog, Woods, & Zeffro, 1996) reported that adult dyslexics differed from controls in task-related functional activation of a specific region of the visual cortex. This region is the magnocellar layers of the lateral geniculate nucleus located at the junction of the occipital and temporal lobes. This brain area appears to be responsive to visual motion and has been implicated in behavioral studies of dyslexia (see below).

Electrophysiological measurements such as *electroencephalography, evoked potential, magnetoencephalogy* have further been used to examine brain function in individuals with RD (Duffy & McAnulty, 1985; Flowers et al., 1991; Kraus, McGee, Carrell, Zecker, Nicol, & Koch, 1996; Kubova, Kuba, Peregrin, & Novakova, 1995; Lehmkuhle, Garzia, Turner, Hash, & Baro, 1993; Livingstone, Rosen, Drislane, & Galaburda, 1991; Salmelin, Service, Kiesila, Uutela, & Salonen, 1996). Several investigations have reported slowed visual evoked potenials in dyslexics (Kubova et al., 1995; Lehmkuhle et al., 1993). In another study, Salmelin and co-workers conducted a *magnetic source imagining* (MSI) experiment with adult dyslexics. MSI combines the (sub)millisecond temporal resolution of intracranial electrical recordings provided by magnetoencephalogy with the millimeter-precision anatomic images of MRI (Poeppel & Rowley, 1996). Salmelin and colleagues found that in a reading task, dyslexic adults, as compared to controls, failed to show appropriate cortical activity in the left occipital and temporal lobes. They proposed that these differences were a reflection of deficits in phonological and visual processes involved in reading.

In summary, numerous differences have been found in the brain structure and function of individuals with RD as compared to normal readers. Although group differences have been uncovered, considerable individual variation exists. Furthermore, the abnormalities that have been observed are unlike the focal lesions found in acquired reading disorders. Rather, abnormalities appear to be more diffuse, involving a variety of structures in the brain. These findings are consistent with the view that individual differences in neurological development, not neurological deficits, contribute to many cases of developmental reading disabilities. These individual brain differences, which appear to be present in many RD children, make it difficult (but not impossible) for them to learn to read.

It is still unclear how the observed brain anomalies are related to reading disabilities and to the cognitive-perceptual abilities associated with them (e.g., language or visual processes). Explanations of this relationship are quite speculative in nature (Heilman, Voeller, & Alexander, 1996; Paulesu et al., 1996; Rumsey, Zametkin, Andreason, Hanahan, Hamburger, Aquino, King, Pikus, & Cohen, 1994). Most assume that the observed brain differences are causally linked to reading disabilities. Researchers who find differences in posterior regions of the brain often propose that visual impairments cause reading problems. On the other hand, researchers who identify anterior and temporal differences have argued that language impairments underlie reading problems. Alternatively, it may well be that some of the observed differences are more the result of reading problems rather than the cause. Learning to read in a different way likely results in differences in brain function and structure. The brain differences that have been observed in some poor readers, especially older poor readers, thus may reflect years of poor reading rather than the cause of the poor reading. Clearly more research is necessary to understand the neurological basis of reading disabilities. As new technologies are combined with appropriate research designs (e.g., longitudinal, reading-age match), we will gain a better understanding of the influence of brain differences in reading disabilities.

Visual-Based Deficits

Neurological factors that influence reading disabilities must have their immediate effect on cognitive-perceptual abilities that are not specific to reading because reading is an acquired skill. There is no aspect of cognition or a specific region of the brain that could fail to develop and just cause a reading disability (Ellis, 1985). If a reading disability is instrinsically motivated, it must be caused by differences in perceptual, cognitive, or linguistic abilities that have evolved to serve more primary human functions. We believe that the primary deficit underlying many reading disabilities is linguistic in nature. Later in this chapter, we will review the extensive body of research supporting the language basis of reading disabilities. First, however, we will consider the evidence that deficits in visual or attentional processes play a causal role in reading disabilities.

Because the visual system is the primary sensory system involved in reading, it should not be surprising that visual-based explanations of reading disabilities have a long history in the field (Bronner, 1917; Fildes, 1922; Frostig, 1968; Hermann, 1959). Many early reported cases of reading disabilities were seen by ophthalmologists, who explained these problems in terms of visual difficulties. As noted in Chapter 3, the term "word blindness" was frequently used to refer to reading disabilities. Several early clinics for reading difficulties also bore the name "Word Blind" in their title. Since these early accounts, there have been numerous attempts to uncover the visual deficits that might cause reading disabilities. These attempts have considered reversal errors, problems in visual memory, erratic eye movements, light sensitivity, and visual timing deficits.

Reversal Errors

Over the years, much attention has been focused on the reversal errors made by children with RD. These errors, which involve, for example, the reading/writing of *b* for *d* or *was* for *saw,* have traditionally been linked closely with dyslexia. Even today, most people still think of dyslexia as a problem reading letters or words backwards. Despite this view, there is surprisingly little research that has systematically investigated reversal errors. The few studies that have examined reversal errors have found that these errors do not actually occur that often in children with RD (Fischer, Liberman, & Shankweiler, 1978; Liberman, Shankweiler, Orlando, Harris, & Berti, 1971). Furthermore, when considered in terms of percentage of overall errors, reversal errors may be no more prevalent in young poor readers than they are in young good readers (Holmes & Peper, 1977). In other words, all beginning readers occasionally make reversal errors, just as all children learning to talk make errors involving grammatical morphemes (e.g., past tense *-ed,* third person *-s*). Just as children with language delays continue to have difficulty with grammatical morphemes beyond the developmental period, children with RD often continue to make reversal errors in later grades.

When reversal errors do occur, they generally are not the result of perceptual problems. Children who write *saw* as *was* or *girl* as *gril* typically do not have trouble perceiving letter sequences. Vellutino and his colleagues (Vellutino, Pruzek, Steger, & Meshoulam, 1973; Vellutino, Steger, DeSetto, & Phillips, 1975) found that children with RD could accurately copy what they sometimes failed to read correctly. Rather than having problems perceiving letter sequences, poor readers more likely have difficulties remembering the order of letters in words. Because of the spatial orientation of words, a primary way a word can be misspelled/misread is to fail to remember the correct order of its letters.

Visual Memory

Apparent problems in the memory for the letters in words led some early investigators to propose that poor readers had generalized deficits in visual memory (Fildes, 1922). Vellutino (1979), however, maintained that most of the early work showing deficits in visual memory was confounded by the use of stimuli that could be verbally labeled. Consequently, children with RD might have performed poorly because of verbal memory deficits rather than visual deficits. In support of this possibility, Vellutino and his colleagues (Vellutino, et al., 1975) showed that poor readers scored comparably to good readers on a visual memory task involving stimuli that could not be easily labeled (but see Willows, Kruk, & Corcos, 1993).

Rather than focusing on a generalized problem in visual memory, some researchers have investigated the possibility that poor readers have specific problems in orthographic processing. As discussed in Chapter 2, orthographic knowledge involves the knowledge of letter sequences or spelling patterns. This knowledge allows the reader to directly access semantic memory without going through the intermediate step of phonetic decoding. Orthographic processing has often been tested by tasks that ask subjects to choose which of two letter sequences (*goat, gote*) is a real word. Because the foil in each word pair (*gote*) can be pronounced like a real word, the subject must rely on orthographic knowledge to answer correctly. Research using this task has shown that orthographic processing ability is related to reading achievement in that children with good orthographic knowledge read better than those with limited orthographic knowledge (Conners & Olson, 1990; Stanovich & West, 1989). Researchers have been quick to point out, however, that orthographic processing skills may be heavily influenced by phonological processing abilities (Share & Stanovich, 1995). Children who have mastered the use of sound-letter correspondence rules should develop richer orthographic knowledge by virtue of many successful trials reading words. Nevertheless, some studies show that orthographic processing may make an independent contribution to reading ability (Barker, Torgesen, & Wagner, 1992; Conners & Olson, 1990; Stanovich & West, 1989). Such findings suggest the possibility that some children with RD may have specific deficits in remembering the letters in words.

Erratic Eye Movements

When reading, we get the impression that our eyes are moving smoothly and continuously across the printed page. Actually, eye movements for reading (and many other visual activities) involve a series of rapid jerks, called *saccades*, that move from left to right, and occasionally from right to left (i.e., regressions). Each of these saccades is followed by a short fixation period averaging 200 to 250 milliseconds. It is during these fixations that information is obtained for the purpose of recognizing words.

Could problems in eye movements be a cause of reading disabilities? Poor readers have been noted to have more fixations per line, longer fixations, shorter saccades, and more regressions than good readers (Rayner, 1978). Rayner (1985) and others point out, however, that these differences in eye movements may actually be a reflection of cognitive processing difficulties during reading rather than problems in oculomotor control. For example, because poor readers take longer to recognize words and often need to go back to refresh their memory, they may show longer fixations and more regressions. In opposition to such a conclusion, Pavlidis (1981, 1985) has reported that dyslexics demonstrated abnormal eye movements in non-reading tasks (also see Eden, Stein, Wood, & Wood, 1994, 1995). Olson, Conners, and Rack (1991), however, have argued that even such findings could be a consequence of a reading problem and not a cause. They demonstrated that when poor readers were matched for reading skill with younger normal readers, no differences were observed in eye movements during non-reading tasks. (but see Eden et al., 1994).

The belief that erratic eye movements are a cause of reading disabilities has often led to the popularity of visually oriented treatment approaches that involve "eye movement training" devices (Metzer & Werner, 1984). The assumption is that if poor readers could learn to move their eyes in a smoother, less erratic fashion, reading would improve. But as we pointed out above, the basic premise that skilled reading involves smooth eye movements is false. Not surprisingly, these training programs have not proven to be effective. Today, most professionals agree that oculomotor exercises, and behavioral optometry in general, have little to offer in the treatment of reading disabilities (Clark & Uhry, 1995; Keogh & Pelland, 1985; Silver, 1995).

Scotopic Sensitivity Syndrome

In 1983 Irlen introduced a visual-perceptual condition called *scotopic sensitivity syndrome* (SSS) (Irlen, 1983). This condition was argued to result from an oversensitivity to particular frequencies of light. Individuals with SSS were noted to experience a variety of problems during reading, including perceptual distortions, reduced visual field, poor focus, eye strain, and/or headaches. Irlen reported that colored eyeglass lenses or tinted plastic overlays could eliminate troublesome wavelengths of light and reduce the symptoms of SSS. The use of colored lenses/overlays soon became part of a commercial enterprise. Colored lenses/ overlays can now be purchased at clinics, and even through advertisements in *Reading Today*, a publication of the International Reading Association. Because it is often claimed in promotional materials that many dyslexics suffer from SSS, colored filters have become an alternative, but controversial, treatment for reading disabilities (Silver, 1995).

Despite heavy press coverage, supportive testimonials, and some research, little is still known about SSS and its role in reading disabilities (Stanley, 1994). As Stanley (1994) points out, the condition is probably misnamed since most reading involves the photopic, rather than the scotopic visual system. Futhermore, it is unclear what mechanisms may be responsible for the symptoms associated with SSS and how colored lenses may affect these mechanisms. Deficits in visual timing (discussed in the next section) have been linked with SSS (Breitmeyer, 1989; Weiss, 1990), but the relationship between these deficits, SSS, and improvements with the use of colored filters is far from clear (Stanley, 1994). Of more significance is the fact that there is still little empirical evidence to show a causal link between SSS and reading disabilities. Despite what is claimed in promotional materials and publications (Irlen & Lass, 1989), it is unclear if children with RD have a higher incidence of SSS than non-disabled readers. It is also unresolved whether SSS, if present, is a cause of reading disabilities or an associated problem.

Notwithstanding the above concerns, recent studies have begun to examine the effectiveness of colored filters. Some investigations have found significant improvements in vision and/or reading with the use of colored lenses or overlays (Adler & Atwood, 1987; Fletcher & Martinez, 1994; O'Connor, Sofo, Kendall, & Olsen, 190; Robinson & Conway, 1990; but see Blaskey, Scheiman, Parisi, Ciner, Gallaway, & Selznick, 1990 & Cotton & Evans, 1989). However, much of this improvement could be due to a placebo effect or an arousal effect. Wearing colored glasses or using tinted overlays could motivate some poor readers to improve or could affect their mood, and thus, their performance (Cotton & Evans, 1989; Stanley, 1991, 1994). These and other problems make it difficult to recommend the use of colored lens or overlays as a viable treatment alternative for reading disabilities (Parker, 1990; Solan, 1990; Stanley, 1991).

Transient Processing Deficits

Scotopic sensitivity syndrome and problems in eye movements have both been suggested to be the result of more primary deficits in visual processing. Researchers have identified two basic visual processing systems, the transient and sustained systems (Campbell, 1974; Graham, 1980). Each system appears to specialize in the processing of particular visual information. The transient system seems to be especially sensitive to global visual features and is thought to play an important role in guiding eye movement. The sustained system, on the other hand, responds to fine detail and is used in visual feature identification (e.g., letter/word recogntion). Both of these systems must operate efficiently to meet the visual perceptual demands of reading.

Lovegrove and his colleagues (Lovegrove, 1992; Lovegrove, Martin, & Slaghuis, 1986) have observed that individuals with RD have significant difficulties on a number of nonverbal visual tasks believed to involve the transient system. They proposed that individuals with RD may have a sluggish transient processing system. The slowed processing of the transient visual system could disrupt parallel operation with the sustained system, which in turn might lead to visual distortions and other visual problems during reading.

Others have also found individuals with RD to have deficits on visual tasks related to transient processing (Eden et al., 1995; Lehmkuhle et al., 1993; Livingstone et al., 1991; Solman & May, 1990; Williams, Molinet, & LeCluyse, 1989; but see Hayduk, Bruck, & Cavanagh, 1992). In addition, these behavioral findings are consistent with reports of recent anatomical and physiological findings in dyslexia (Eden et al., 1996; Livingstone et al., 1991). Livingstone and colleagues (1991), for example, found in postmortem examinations that dyslexics may have less organized and smaller neurons in the brain regions associated with transient visual processing than do normal individuals. Also, as noted above, Eden and colleagues (1996) reported that dyslexics show less task-related activation in these brain regions.

Although evidence has begun to converge in support of transient visual processing deficits in poor readers, it is still not clear what role these deficits may play in reading disabilities. Are these problems sufficient causes of a reading disability, or do they co-occur with other more primary causal factors? At least some evidence suggests that transient processing deficits often occur in concert with phonological processing deficits (e.g., Eden et al., 1995). A visually based explanation of reading disabilities would be better supported if a group of children with RD could be identified who have a documented history of visual deficits but no impairments in phonological processing or other known causal factors (Share & Stanovich, 1995). If such children do exist, they will represent an important subgroup of children with RD.

Attention-Based Deficits

Attention problems have often been associated with reading disabilities. Interest in this relationship has increased recently. *Attention deficit hyperactivity disorder* (ADHD), the clinical classification for problems in inattention, implusivity, and overactivity, has become a prominant clinical diagnosis for children with behavioral and academic problems. Because reading requires considerable attentional resources, many practitioners think that most children with ADHD have reading/learning problems and vice versa. Initial accounts seemed to support the co-occurrence of these disorders (Safer & Allen, 1976; Silver, 1981). However, these reports were largely based on clinic-referred samples of children with RD or ADHD. Such samples often overestimate the co-occurrence of disorders. When more representative samples of children were examined, the association between reading disabilities and ADHD has been shown to be much weaker. Specifically, Shaywitz and colleagues found that in a research-identified sample of children with ADHD, only 36 percent of the children had reading problems (Shaywitz, Fletcher, & Shaywitz, 1994). More significantly, in a similarly identified sample of children with RD, they found that only 15 percent of the subjects had ADHD.

In further support of the distinction between ADHD and reading disabilities, researchers have identified distinct cognitive profiles associated with these disorders. For example, in one study, children with RD were found to perform poorly on phonological processing tests, whereas children with ADHD generally performed well on these tasks, but poorly on visual memory tasks (Shaywitz, Fletcher, Holahan, Shneider, Marchione, Stuebing, Francis, Shankweiler, Katz, Liberman, & Shaywitz, 1995). In another study, conducted in Finland, children with ADHD had problems on tasks involving inhibition and control, whereas children with RD had deficits on various language-based measures (e.g., phonological awareness, verbal memory, story retelling) (Korkman and Pesonen, 1994). Twin studies also suggest that ADHD is genetically distinct from reading disabilities (Gilger, Pennington, & DeFries, 1992).

Researchers have also examined the relative contribution of attentional factors to reading achievement (Shaywitz et al., 1995). In an investigation of children from the Connecticut Longitudinal Study, Shaywitz and colleagues found that measures of attention failed to explain significant variance in word recognition once language measures had been considered (also see Felton & Wood, 1989). Attention variables did, however, account for a small but significant percentage of the variance in silent reading comprehension over and above that explained by language variables.

In summary, research clearly indicates that attentional deficits are not a primary cause of reading disabilities. Although reading disabilities and ADHD often occur together in children, they appear to be distinct developmental disorders, each with its own set of causal factors. In cases where reading disabilities and ADHD co-occur, attentional deficits may contribute to reading problems, but this contribution is likely to be relatively small and confined primarily to higher-level aspects of reading comprehension.

Language-Based Deficits

In Chapter 3, we argued that reading disabilities are best defined as developmental language disorders. From a theoretical perspective, such a claim is well founded. Reading is first and foremost a language activity. Reading relies heavily on one's knowledge of the phonologic, semantic, syntactic, and pragmatic aspects of language. As such, deficiencies in one or more of these aspects of language could significantly disrupt one's ability to read. Not only is a language-based account of reading disabilities theoretically sound, considerable evidence has accumulated over the last twenty-five years to support this view.

Longitudinal Study of Language-Impaired Children

The relationship between language deficits and reading disabilities has been examined from several different perspectives. One approach has been the longitudinal study of children with early spoken language impairments (Aram, Ekelman, & Nation, 1984; Bishop & Adams, 1990; Catts, 1993; Menyuk, Chesnick, Liebergott, Korngold D'Agostino, & Belanger, 1993; Silva, McGree, & Williams, 1987; Stark, Bernstein Condino, Bender, Tallal, & Catts, 1984; Stothard et al., 1996; Tallal, Curtiss, & Kaplan, 1989; Wilson & Risucci, 1988). In this work, children displaying significant impairments in language (generally in semantic-syntactic aspects) have been identified in preschool or kindergarten and tested for reading and academic achievement in the later grades. Evidence that children with language impairments (LI) are more likely than typically developing children to have subsequent reading disabilities indicates that language deficits precede and play a causal role in reading disabilities.

The results of longitudinal studies have consistently shown that children with LI often have reading disabilities. In general, research indicates that 50 percent or more of children with LI in preschool or kindergarten go on to have reading disabilities in primary or secondary grades. In the most comprehensive study to date, the first author and a colleague (Catts, Fey, Zhang, & Tomblin, in preparation) are investigating the reading outcomes of 225 children with LI. These children are a subsample of children who participated in an epidemiological study of developmental language impairments in children (Tomblin, Records, Buckwalter, Zhang, Smith, & O'Brien, 1997). In kindergarten, the participants were administered tests of language and nonverbal abilities. Language abilities were assessed by the *Test of Language Development-Primary 2* (Newcomer & Hammill, 1988) and a measure of narrative production and comprehension (Culatta, Page, & Ellis, 1983). The Block Design and Picture

Completion subtests of the *Weschler Preschool and Primary Intelligence Scale-Revised* (Wechsler, 1967) was used to measure nonverbal abilities. Children with LI demonstrated a mean language composite score that was at least one SD below the mean of a normative sample of children (average score was 1.7 SD below normal). Fifty-five percent of the children had normal or above normal nonverbal abilities, while the remaining had moderately low nonverbal IQs. None of the latter children had been diagnosed as mentally retarded. In second grade, reading was assessed by two tests of word recognition and three tests of reading comprehension. The Word Identification and Word Attack subtests of the *Woodcock Reading Mastery Tests - Revised* (WRMT-R, Woodcock, 1987) were employed as measures of word recognition. Reading comprehension was measured by the Passage Comprehension subtest of the *WRMT-R*, the *Gray Oral Reading Test-Revised* (Wierdholt & Bryant, 1986), and the Reading Comprehension subtest of the *Diagnostic Achievement Battery-2* (Newcomer, 1990).

Our preliminary results indicate that, as a group, the children with LI read well below expected levels in second grade. Approximately 52 percent of the children with LI performed one or more standard deviations below the mean on a composite measure of reading comprehension, whereas about 44 percent scored one or more standard deviations below the mean on a composite measure of word recognition. Children with low nonverbal abilities in addition to an LI performed significantly less well in reading than did those with normal nonverbal IQs. Severity of language impairment and degree of nonverbal deficit each accounted for a small, but independent amount of variance in reading outcome. Further analysis showed that letter identification was a good predictor of reading achievement. Specifically, LI children who had limited knowledge of letters in kindergarten were among the poorest readers in second grade.

Language Problems in Poor Readers
The fact that many children with LI exhibit reading disabilities does not necessarily mean that most children with RD have a history of language impairments. To better draw such a conclusion, studies have directly examined the language abilities of children with RD. In one body of research, investigators have selected school-age children identified as reading disabled (or in some cases, learning disabled) and studied their performance on traditional measures of language development. This work has shown that children with RD often have problems in receptive and/or expressive vocabulary (Fry, Johnson, & Muehl, 1970; Wiig & Semel, 1975) or in the use and/or comprehension of morphology and syntax (Doehring, Trites, Patel, & Fiedorowitcz, 1981; Fletcher, 1981; Morice & Slaghuis, 1985; Semel & Wiig, 1975; Stanovich & Siegel, 1994; Vogel, 1974). Deficits have also been reported in the production and/or comprehension of text-level language (Donahue, 1984; Feagans & Short, 1984; McConnaughy, 1985; Roth & Spekman, 1986; Smiley, Oakley, Worthen, Campione, & Brown, 1977; Stothard & Hulme, 1992; Yuill & Oakhill, 1991).

Although this research clearly shows that children with RD have language deficits, it does not necessarily indicate that these deficits are causally related to reading disabilities. A major problem for the interpretation of this work is that in most cases language abilities were examined in children who had reading problems for several years. This makes it difficult to determine if the observed language deficits were the cause or the consequence of a reading problem. Recall that earlier in the chapter we argued that Matthew effects can lead to language deficits in children with RD. Thus, at least some of the language problems observed in children with RD will be the consequence and not the initial cause of their reading difficulties.

Not all studies of language problems in children with RD have examined reading and language abilities concurrently. Some studies have investigated language deficits in children with RD prior to their learning to read. Scarborough (1990, 1991), for example, investigated the early language development of children who later developed reading disabilities. In this study, the language abilities of children with a family history of dyslexia (N = 34) and children without a family history (N = 44) were assessed at age 2 1/2 years, and at six- or twelve-month intervals through age 5. Language assessments included measurements of receptive and expressive vocabulary, sentence comprehension, and grammatical production (not all measurements were administered at each age). In second grade, children's reading abilities were assessed. Of the 34 children with a family history of dyslexia, 22 were themselves diagnosed as dyslexic in second grade. The early language abilities of these dyslexic children through 4 years of age were found to be significantly poorer than those of the children without a family history of dyslexia. By age 5, however, only expressive vocabulary differentiated the two groups.

In an ongoing study, the first author and colleagues (Catts, Fey, Zhang, & Tomblin, in preparation) are investigating the language abilities of a large group of poor readers. In this work, we identified 180 second-grade children who performed at least one SD below normal on a composite measure of reading comprehension. We did not exclude subjects on the basis of low IQ (except for those with mental retardation) as others have done in the past. The latter practice may bias results concerning language deficits in poor readers because IQ tests often measure verbal abilities. We compared the poor readers' performance on a battery of kindergarten language tests to that of a normal control group. We also used weighted scores based on epidemiological data (Tomblin et al., 1997) to ensure that our results were representative of poor readers from the population at large. Our findings indicated that the poor readers performed significantly less well than the good readers on tests of vocabulary, grammar, and narration. In addition, we observed that more than half of the poor readers (54%) had a language composite score in kindergarten that was at least one SD below normal. These results thus indicate that problems in vocabulary, grammar, and narration are quite prevalent in poor readers.

Our results further indicated that the poor reader's early language deficits extended beyond vocabulary, grammar, and narration. Poor readers were also found to have difficulties in phonological awareness and phonological retrieval in the kindergarten assessment. Specifically, 55 percent of the poor readers performed at least one SD below that of the normative sample on a measure of phonological awareness (syllable/phoneme deletion) and 43 percent performed below that level on a test of phonological retrieval (rapid naming). These deficits, however, rarely occurred in isolation from problems in vocabulary, grammar, and narration. Our findings concerning deficits in phonological awareness and retrieval are consistent with a large body of research that has documented the prevalence of phonological processing deficits in children with RD. Phonological processing deficits refer to difficulties in linguistic operations that make use of information involving the sounds of speech (e.g., verbal short-term memory, phonological awareness) (see Catts, 1989b; Rack, Hulme, Snowling, & Wightman, 1994; Wagner & Torgesen, 1987). As discussed in Chapter 3, phonological processing deficits are the primary language problems associated with dyslexia and a prominent characteristic of language-learning disabilities. In the sections that follow, the research findings concerning the relationship between phonological processing deficits and reading disabilities will be reviewed.

Phonological Awareness.   Phonological awareness is the explicit awareness of, or sensitivity to, the sound structure of speech (Stanovich, 1988; Torgesen, 1996). It is one's ability to attend to, reflect on, or manipulate the speech sounds in words. Over the last twenty-five years, no variable has proven to be as consistently related to reading (at least word recognition) as phonological awareness. Children who are aware of the sounds of speech appear to more quickly and accurately acquire sound-letter correspondence knowledge and learn to use this knowledge to decode printed words. Evidence of a relationship between phonological awareness and reading has been demonstrated across a wide range of ages (Calfee & Lindamood, 1973; Torgesen, Wagner, Rashotte, Burgess, & Hecht, 1997), experimental tasks (Catts, Wilcox, Wood-Jackson, Larrivee, & Scott, 1997), and languages (Cossu, Shankweiler, Liberman, Katz, & Tolar, 1988; Hu & Catts, 1997; Lundberg, Olofsson, & Wall, 1980).

Numerous studies have shown that children with RD have deficits in phonological awareness (Bradley & Bryant, 1983; Fletcher, Shaywitz, Shankweiler, Katz, Liberman, Stuebing, Francis, Fowler, & Shaywitz, 1994; Fox & Routh, 1980; Katz, 1986; Olson, Wise, Conners, Rack, & Fulker, 1989). In fact, Torgesen (1996) argues that "dyslexic children are consistently more impaired in phonological awareness than any other single ability" (p. 6). In one of the earliest studies in the area, Bradley and Bryant (1978) documented just how impaired the phonological awareness abilities are in some children with RD. In their study, they compared a group of 10-year-old children with RD to a group of 6 1/2-year-old normal children matched for reading ability. Children were administered a task in which they were asked to choose the odd member from a list of spoken words, such as *lot, cot, hat, pot.* Even though the children with RD were three and one-half years older than the normal children, they performed significantly less well on this task than did the normal readers.

It is possible that the deficits in phonological awareness observed in children with RD are due, at least in part, to their reading problems (Morais, 1991). Because of the abstract nature of phonology, children are often unaware of some phonological aspects of language until their attention is directly drawn to these features of language. For example, the fact that words are composed of individual phonemes does not become apparent to most language users until these units are explicitly highlighted through instruction and practice in an alphabetic orthography. Support for this view comes from studies that show that preschoolers, as well as illiterate adults, are generally unable to perform tasks that require the explicit segmentation of words into individual phonemes (Lundberg & Hoien, 1991; Morais, Bertelson, Cary, & Alegria, 1986; Morais, Cary, Alegria, & Bertelson, 1979; Read & Ruyter, 1985).

Findings such as these suggest that children with RD might be expected to have some deficits in phonological awareness as a result of their poor reading abilities. Because children with RD have less experience and skill in using the alphabet, they may not acquire the same level of speech sound awareness as their normal reading peers. Not all deficits in phonological awareness, however, are a consequence of reading problems. Research clearly demonstrates that some phonological awareness deficits are apparent in at-risk children prior to beginning reading instruction, and that these deficits are related to subsequent problems in learning to read. As reported above, we found that over half of a group of second grade poor readers had deficits in phonological awareness in kindergarten (Catts & Fey, 1995). In further analyses, we found that phonological awareness was the best predictor among our kindergarten language and cognitive measures of word recognition abilities in second grade children in general. Our results also showed that phonological awareness was significantly related to reading even after kindergarten letter naming ability, a measure of alphabetic experience, was taken into consideration. Thus, it is not simply limited exposure to the alphabet during the preschool years that causes phonological awareness and subsequent readng problems. Other studies have also shown a strong relationship between phonological awareness in preschool or kindergarten and reading in the primary grades (Badian, 1994; Catts, 1993; Felton, 1992; Lundberg et al., 1980; Mann, 1993; Scarborough, 1989; Torgesen, Wagner, & Rashotte, 1994; Wagner, Torgesen, & Rashotte, 1994).

The best evidence of the causal role of phonological awareness in reading comes from training studies (Alexander, Andersen, Heilman, Voeller, & Torgesen, 1991; Ball & Blachman, 1988; Byrne & Fielding-Barnsley, 1990; Fox & Routh, 1983; Hatcher, Hulme, & Ellis, 1994; Hurford, Johnston, Nepote, Hampton, Moore, Neal, Mueller, McGeorge, Huff, Awad, Tatro, Juliano, & Huffman, 1994; Lie, 1991; Lundberg, Frost, & Peterson, 1988; Torgesen, Morgan, & Davis, 1992; Warrick, Rubin, & Rowe-Walsh, 1993; Wise & Olson, 1995). In these studies, children are provided with instruction in phonological awareness and are subsequently evaluated for phonological awareness ability and reading achievement. In general, this work has found that phonological awareness training can increase speech sound awareness and, in turn, improve reading achievement. Because the greatest gains are made when phonological awareness training is combined with explicit phonics instruction, Share and Stanovich (1995) argue that phonological awareness is better described as a corequisite to learning to read. Torgesen (this volume) provides further discussion concerning the relationship between phonological awareness training and reading achievement.

Phonological Retrieval. Clinical observations have shown that children with RD frequently have word-finding difficulties and are sometimes described as dysnomic (Rudel, 1985). Word-finding problems include substitutions (e.g., "knife" for "fork"), circumlocutions (e.g., "you know, what you eat with"), and overuse of words lacking specificity (e.g., stuff, thing). It is often assumed that because individuals with RD seem to know the words they are looking for, that these naming problems are due to difficulties in remembering phonological information.

The word-finding difficulties observed clinically in individuals with RD have also been borne out in research. Studies have consistently found that poor readers perform less well than good readers on tasks involving confrontation picture naming (Catts, 1986; Denckla, 1976; German, 1979; Katz, 1986; Scarborough, 1989; Wolf, 1984). For example, Denckla and Rudel (1976) administered the Oldfield-Wingfield Picture-Naming Test to dyslexic, nondyslexic learning disabled (LD), and normal achieving children. Dyslexic children were slower and made more errors on this naming task than nondyslexic LD and normal children. Because the dyslexic and normal children performed similarly on a test of receptive vocabulary, the naming deficits observed in dyslexic children were most likely due to retrieval problems (also see Swan & Goswami, 1997b; Wolf & Goodglass, 1986). How-ever, equating reading groups on receptive vocabulary may control for semantic knowl-edge and name recognition, but it does not assure that reading groups are comparable in expressive lexical knowledge. In fact, differences in the quality of phonological memory codes (see next section) probably explain a portion of the reading group differences in naming abilities (Kamhi, Catts, & Mauer, 1990; Katz, 1986).

Perhaps the best evidence of phonological retrieval deficits in children with RD comes from studies using continuous naming tasks. These tasks, often referred to as *rapid naming* or *rapid automatic naming* tasks, require the individual to quickly and automatically say the name of a series of letters, numbers, familiar objects, or colors. Because the names of the items are quite common, it is assumed that storage factors play little role in these tasks. As a result, rapid naming tasks may be thought of as a "purer" measure of naming retrieval than other confrontation naming tasks.

Children with RD have been found to be slower on rapid naming tasks than are normal children (Denckla & Rudel, 1976; Vellutino, Scanlon, & Spearing, 1995; Wolf, 1991).[1] Studies also indicate that variability in rapid naming during the preschool years is predictive of reading achievement during the school years (Badian, 1994; Catts, 1993; Ellis & Large, 1987; Felton, 1992; Wolf, Bally, & Morris, 1986). Research further indicates that the rela-tionship between rapid naming and reading remains after controlling for variability in phonological awareness (Badian, 1994; Bowers & Swanson, 1991; Catts, 1993).

Bowers and Wolf (1993) suggest that children at risk for RD may have deficits in either or both phonological awareness and rapid naming. If a child has problems in both areas, what is called a *double deficit*, he or she will have more pronounced difficulty learning to read than if problems are limited to one area. Children with naming problems in addition to deficits in phonological awareness will have difficulties not only in phonetic decoding, but also in orthographic processing. While there is some support for the "double deficit" hypoth-esis (Doi & Manis, 1996; Sundeth & Bowers, 1997), not all evidence supports it (Torgesen et al., 1997).

Phonological Memory. Children with RD also demonstrate problems in phonological memory (Hulme, 1988; Jorm & Share, 1983; Torgesen, 1985). Phonological memory or what some call phonological coding, refers to the encoding and storage of phonological information in memory. Phonological memory has typically been assessed by memory span tasks involving meaningful or nonmeaningful strings of verbal items (e.g., digits, letters, words). Poor readers have been found to perform more poorly than good readers on these tasks (Cohen & Netley, 1981; Mann & Ditunno, 1990; Mann, Liberman, & Shankweiler, 1980; Rapala & Brady, 1990; Shankweiler, Liberman, Mark, Fowler, & Fischer, 1979; Stone & Brady, 1995; Vellutino & Scanlon, 1982). Reading group differences have been observed for verbal stimuli even when they are presented visually. As noted earlier in this chapter,

---

[1]Reading group differences in speed of retrieval in discrete trial tasks have been less consistent. For a discussion of this work and its implications for conclusions concerning retrieval problems, see Bowers, Golden, Kennedy, and Young (1994), Catts (1989a), or Share (1995).

studies typically have failed to find differences between good and poor readers when stimuli are nonverbal and cannot be phonologically labeled (Brady, 1986; Holmes & McKeever, 1979; Katz, Shankweiler, & Liberman, 1981; Liberman, Mann, Shankweiler, & Werfelman, 1982; Rapala & Brady, 1990; Vellutino, Steger, Harding, & Phillips, 1975).

These findings suggest that poor readers have particular problems using phonological memory codes to store verbal information. Speech-sound based memory codes are the most efficient way to hold verbal information in memory (Baddeley, 1986). These codes are automatically activated in listening and in skilled reading. Further evidence of poor readers' difficulties using phonological memory codes comes from comparisons of good and poor readers' memory for lists of rhyming and nonrhyming words. Good readers generally have been found to perform more poorly in recalling rhyming than nonrhyming words. This difficulty is presumed to be the result of interference or confusion caused by similar phonological memory codes being activated in the rhyming condition. Poor readers typically have not shown a performance difference on rhyming and nonrhyming word lists, suggesting that they utilize phonological memory codes to a lesser extent than good readers (Brady, Shankweiler, & Mann, 1983; Shankweiler et al., 1979; but see Holligan & Johnston, 1988).

Good and poor readers have also been compared on tasks involving memory of single items rather than strings of items (Catts, 1986; Kamhi, Catts, Mauer, Apel, & Gentry, 1988; Snowling, 1981; Stone & Brady, 1995). These tasks have usually required participants to repeat multisyllablic nonwords spoken by the examiner. Because nonword repetition is less influenced by attentional factors and rehearsal strategies, it may be a more direct measure of the ability to use phonogical codes in memory. In an early investigation, Snowling (1981) reported that dyslexic children made more errors than reading-age matched children in the repetition of nonwords such as *bagmivishent*. In a follow-up study, Snowling and colleagues (Snowling, Goulandris, Bowlby, & Howell, 1986) had dyslexic, age-matched, and reading-age matched children repeat high- and low-frequency real words and nonwords. They found that high-frequency words were repeated equally well by the three groups. However, dyslexic children performed worse in the repetition of low-frequency real words and nonwords than both the other groups. Subsequent studies have further confirmed these results (Catts, 1986; Kamhi et al., 1988; Kamhi et al., 1990; Stone & Brady, 1995).

Deficits in phonological memory do not seem to be a consequence of reading problems since performance on memory tasks in kindergarten is predictive of reading achievement in the primary grades (Ellis & Large, 1987; Mann & Liberman, 1984; Torgesen et al., 1994). Measures of phonological memory, however, do not account for variability in reading achievement independent of measures of phonological awareness (Torgesen et al., 1994; Wagner, Balthazor, Hurley, Morgan, Rashotte, Shaner, Simmons, & Stage, 1987; Wagner et al., 1994). These findings have led Wagner and Torgesen to speculate that the problems children with RD have on tasks of phonological memory and phonological awareness stem from a common cause, namely, deficiencies in the quality of phonological representations.

Other researchers have also hypothesized that difficulty in developing phonological representations underlies poor readers' phonological processing problems (Brady et al., 1983; Catts, et al., 1997; Elbro, Nielsen, & Petersen, 1994; Swan & Goswami, 1997a). Some have further speculated that auditory perceptual deficits, specifically temporal processing problems, may lead to poorly specified phonological representations in RD children (Farmer & Klein, 1995; Tallal, 1980). Most empirical evidence, however, indicates that poor readers do not have general auditory processing problems, but may have perceptual problems related to processing speech (Brady et al., 1983; Mody, Studdert-Kennedy, & Brady, 1997; Studdert-Kennedy & Mody, 1995). Brady and colleagues (1983), for example, investigated good and poor readers' perception of speech (monosyllabic real words) and nonspeech stimuli (environmental sounds) in quiet and noise conditions. Poor readers made significantly more errors than good readers in identifying the speech stimuli in noise. No group differences were observed in the perception of nonspeech stimuli. More recently, Mody and colleagues (1997) reported that children with RD had more difficulty than normal children in the discrimination of stop consonants, but showed no impairment in distinguishing nonspeech stimuli that were acoustically similar to stop consonants. Other studies have also shown that poor readers have problems in speech discrimination/categorization (Brandt & Rosen, 1980; Godfrey, Lasky, Millag, & Knox, 1981; Hurford, Gilliland, & Ginavan, 1992; Manis, McBride-Chang, Seidenberg, Keating, Doi, Manson, & Petersen, 1997; Werker & Tees, 1987).

While studies indicate that children with RD have problems in speech perception, these problems seem to be quite subtle in nature, generally involving inconsistency in phonetic classification of speech stimuli. It is unclear how these subtle differences might be related to the large differences found between good and poor readers in phonological memory. Clearly, further research is necessary to understand the difficulties children with RD may have in the perception of speech. This research needs to consider poor readers' speech perception in highly structured and controlled stimulus conditions (e.g., Mody et al., 1997) as well as in situations more akin to everyday speech perception (e.g. Kamhi et al., 1990).

Phonological Production.   A final area of phonological processing that has been empirically linked to reading achievement is speech production abilities. Clinical accounts of poor readers' difficulty producing complex speech sound sequences (Blalock, 1982; Johnson & Myklebust, 1967; Miles, 1983) have been confirmed by a number of empirical studies (Apthorp, 1995; Catts, 1986; Catts, 1989c; Kamhi et al., 1988; Rapala & Brady, 1990; Snowling, 1981; Taylor, Lean, & Schwartz, 1989). Catts (1986), for example, found that adolescents with RD made significantly more speech production errors than age-matched peers in naming pictured objects with complex names (e.g., ambulance, thermometer) and repeating phonologically complex words (e.g., specific, aluminum) and phrases (e.g., brown and blue plaid pants). In a follow-up study, Catts (1989c) examined the ability of college students with and without a history of RD to rapidly repeat simple (e.g., small wristband) and complex phrases (e.g., Swiss wristwatch). Students with a history of RD repeated the complex phrases at a significantly slower rate and made more errors than students without a history of RD.

The difficulty individuals with RD have in producing complex phonological sequences may be due, in part, to problems in phonological memory. In fact, some of this work converges well with research involving nonword repetition. That is, in the former studies individuals with RD are asked to produce real, but novel words. Like nonword production tasks, the repetition of these stimuli rests heavily on the formation and storage of accurate phonological memory codes. However, individuals with RD have also been shown to have problems producing words/phrases with which they were clearly familiar. For example, Catts (1989c) showed that college students with a history of RD had little difficulty correctly producing complex phrases in isolation (thus demonstrating accurate memory for the words), but had significant problems in the rapid repetition of these sequences. These findings suggest that deficits in speech planning may contribute to the speech production problems in individuals with RD, a suggestion that has been supported by work showing that the relationship between production of complex stimuli and reading remains after statistically controlling for memory factors (Apthorp, 1995).

The link between complex speech production and reading has led some researchers to consider a possible association between expressive phonological disorders and reading disabilities. Children with expressive phonological disorders display difficulties in the development of the speech sound system. Unlike the problems noted above, these children have difficulties with sound segments in both complex and simple contexts. Initial investigations seemed to indicate that children with expressive phonological disorders had reading problems only if they also had an LI (Bishop & Adams, 1990; Catts, 1993; Lewis & Freebairn, 1992). Recent investigations have more directly tested this conclusion by examining reading outcome in phonologically disordered children with and without accompanying LIs (Bird, Bishop, & Freeman, 1995). Results of this work indicate that reading achievement in children with expressive phonological disorders is more closely associated with the severity of the phonological disorder, level of phonological awareness, and nonverbal intelligence than it is with language abilities. Children with severe phonological disorders and accompanying problems in phonological awareness and nonverbal IQ appear to be at particular risk for reading disabilities.

Language Deficits: Causes or Consequences

The research reviewed in these studies clearly demonstrates that language deficits are closely associated with reading disabilities. In many cases, these language deficits precede and are causally linked to reading problems. Reading is a linguistic behavior and, as such, it depends on adequate language development. Many children with RD have developmental language disorders that become manifested as reading problems upon entering school. While language problems often play a causal role in reading disabilities, they may also be a consequence of reading difficulties. As noted in the section on Matthew effects, poor readers do not read as much as good readers and, as a result, gain less language experience. Over time this limited experience can lead to less well developed language abilities. For example, poor readers would be expected to fall behind their peers in knowledge and use of vocabulary, advanced grammar, and text-level structures (e.g., story grammar). These and other aspects of language are dependent on rich literacy experiences that poor readers seldom encounter during the school years.

The fact that language deficits are both a cause and consequence of reading disabilities ensures that language problems will be a major component of almost all cases of reading disabilities. In some instances, it may be possible to differentiate between those language problems that are causal and those that are consequences of reading disabilities. However, in other cases, intrinsic and extrinsic factors will interact to such an extent that causes and consequences become quite obscured, especially in older poor readers. Regardless of whether language problems are causes or consequences, they will need to be addressed in intervention. Early problems in phonological awareness and language development will need to be considered in order to ensure that at-risk children get off to a good start in reading. Practitioners will also have to address problems in vocabulary, grammar, and discourse that arise as a lack of reading experience. Although these problems may emerge as a consequence of reading difficulties, once present, they will interfere with further reading development. In the following chapters, specific suggestions will be provided concerning language intervention for poor readers.

References

Adams, M.J. (1990). *Beginning to read: Thinking and learning about print.* Cambridge, MA: MIT Press.

Adler, L., & Atwood, M. (1987). *Poor readers: What do they really see on the page?* CA: East San Gabriel Valley Regional Occupational Program.

Alexander, A., Andersen, H.G., Heilman, P.C., Voeller, K.K.S., & Torgesen, J.K. (1991). Phonological awareness training and remediation of analytic decoding deficits in a group of severe dyslexics. *Annals of Dyslexia, 41,* 193–27.

Apthorp, H.S. (1995). Phonetic coding and reading in college students with and without learning disabilities. *Journal of Learning Disabilities, 28,* 342–352.

Aram, D.M., Ekelman, B.L., & Nation, J.E. (1984). Preschoolers with language disorders: 10 years later. *Journal of Speech and Hearing Research, 27,* 232–244.

Baddeley, A. (1986). Working memory, reading and dyslexia. In E. Hjelmquist & L. Nilsson (Eds.), *Communication and handicap: Aspects of psychological compensation and technical aids* (pp. 141–152). North Holland: Elsevier.

Badian, N.A. (1994). Preschool prediction: Orthographic and phonological skills, and reading. *Annals of Dyslexia, 44,* 3–25.

Ball, E.W., & Blachman, B.A. (1988). Phoneme segmentation training: Effect on reading readiness. *Annals of Dyslexia, 38,* 208–224.

Barker, K., Torgesen, J.K., & Wagner, R.K. (1992). The role of orthographic processing skills on five different reading tasks. *Reading Research Quarterly, 27,* 334–345.

Bird, J., Bishop, D.V.M., & Freeman, N.H. (1995). Phonological awareness and literacy development in children with expressive phonological impairments. *Journal of Speech and Hearing Research, 38,* 446–462.

Bisgaard, M.L., Eiberg, H., Moller, N., Neihbar, E., & Mohr, J. (1987). Dyslexia and chromosome 15 heteromorphism: Negative load scores in a Danish sample. *Clinical Genetics, 32,* 118–119.

Bishop, D.V.M. (1990). *Handedness and developmental disorder.* Oxford: Blackwell Scientific.

Bishop, D.V.M., & Adams, C. (1990). A prospective study of the relationship between specific language impairment, phonological disorders and reading retardation. *Journal of Child Psychology and Psychiatry, 31,* 1027–1050.

Blalock, J.W. (1982). Persistent auditory language deficits in adults with learning disabilities. *Journal of Learning Disabilities, 15,* 604–609.

Blaskey, P., Scheiman, M., Parisi, M., Ciner, E.B., Gallaway, M., & Selznick, R. (1990). The effectiveness of Irlen filters for improving reading performance: A pilot study. *Journal of Learning Disabilities, 23,* 604–610.

Bowers, P.G., Golden, J., Kennedy, A., & Young, A. (1994). Limits upon orthographic knowledge due to processes indexed by naming speed. In V. Berninger (Ed.), *The varieties of orthographic knowledge. I: Theoretical and developmental issues* (pp. 173–218). Dordecht: Klüwer.

Bowers, P.G., & Swanson, L.B. (1991). Naming speed deficits in reading disability: Multiple measures of a singular process. *Journal of Experimental Child Psychology, 51,* 195–219.

Bowers, P.G., & Wolf, M. (1993). Theoretical links among naming speed, precise timing mechanisms and orthographic skill in dyslexia. *Reading and Writing: An Interdisciplinary Journal, 5,* 69–85.

Bradley, L., & Bryant, P. (1983). Categorizing sounds and learning to read: A causal connection. *Nature, 301,* 419–421.

Brady, S. (1986). Short-term memory, phonological processing, and reading ability. *Annals of Dyslexia, 36,* 138–153.

Brady, S., Shankweiler, D., & Mann, V. (1983). Speech perception and memory coding in relation to reading ability. *Journal of Experimental Child Psychology, 35,* 345–367.

Brandt, J., & Rosen, J.J. (1980). Auditory phonemic perception in dyslexia: Categorical identification and discrimination of stop consonants. *Brain and Language, 9,* 324–337.

Breitmeyer, B. (1989). A visually based deficit in specific reading disability. *The Irish Journal of Psychology, 10,* 534–541.

Bronner, A. (1917). *The psychology of special abilities and disabilities.* Boston: Little, Brown.

Bus, A., van Ijzendoorn, M. & Pellegrini, A. (1995) Joint book reading makes success in learning to read: A meta-analysis on intergenerational transmission of literacy. *Review of Educational Research, 65,* 1–21.

Bryden, M.P. (1982). *Laterality: Functional asymmetry in the intact brain.* New York: Academic Press.

Byrne, B., & Fielding-Barnsley, R. (1990). Acquiring the alphabetic principle: A case for teaching recognition of phoneme identity. *Journal of Educational Psychology, 82,* 805–812.

Calfee, R.C., & Lindamood, P. (1973). Acoustic-phonetic skills and reading—kindergarten through twelfth grade. *Journal of Educational Psychology, 64,* 293–298.

Campbell, F.W. (1974). The transmission of spatial information through the visual system. In F.O. Schmidt & F.S. Worden (Eds.), *The neurosciences third study program* (pp. 95–103). Cambridge, MA: MIT Press.

Cardon, L.R., & Fulker, D.W. (1994). A sibling pair approach to internal mapping of quantitative trait loci. *American Journal of Human Genetics, 55,* 825–831.

Catts, H.W. (1986). Speech production/phonological deficits in reading-disordered children. *Journal of Learning Disabilities, 19,* 504–508.

Catts, H.W. (1989a). Phonological processing deficits and reading disabilities. In A. Kamhi & H. Catts (Eds.), *Reading disabilities: A developmental language perspective.* Boston: Allyn & Bacon.

Catts, H.W. (1989b). Defining dyslexia as a developmental language disorder. *Annals of Dyslexia, 39,* 50–64.

Catts, H.W. (1989c). Speech production deficits in developmental dyslexia. *Journal of Speech and Hearing Disorders, 54,* 422–428.

Catts, H.W. (1993). The relationship between speech-language impairments and reading disabilities. *Journal of Speech and Hearing Research, 36,* 948–958.

Catts, H.W., Fey, M.E., Zhang, X., & Tomblin, J.B. (in preparation). Language basis of reading and reading disabilities: Evidence from a longitudinal investigation.

Catts, H.W., Wilcox, K.A., Wood-Jackson, C., Larrivee, L., & Scott, V.G. (1997). Toward an understanding of phonological awareness. In C.K. Leong & R.M. Joshi (Eds.), *Cross-language studies of learning to read and spell: Phonologic and orthographic processing.* Dordrecht: Klüwer.

Clark, D.B., & Uhry, J.K. (1995). *Dyslexia: Theory and practice of remedial instruction.* Baltimore, MD: York Press.

Cohen, R.L., & Netley, C. (1981). Short-term memory deficits in reading disabled children in the absence of opportunity for rehearsal strategies. *Intelligence, 5,* 69–76.

Cole, G. (1987). *The learning mystique.* New York: Pantheon.

Conners, F., & Olson, R.K. (1990). Reading comprehension in dyslexic and normal readers: A component skills analysis. In D.A. Balota, G.B. Flores d'Arcais, & K. Rayner (Eds.), *Comprehension processes in reading* (pp. 557–579). Hillsdale, NJ: Erlbaum.

Cossu, G., Shankweiler, D., Liberman, I.Y., Katz, L., & Tolar, G. (1988). Awareness of phonological segments and reading ability in Italian children. *Applied Psycholinguistics, 9,* 1–16.

Cotton, M.M., & Evans, K.M. (1989). *An evaluation of the Irlen lenses as a treatment for specific learning disorders.* Prepublication manuscript, University of Newcastle.

Critchley, M. (1970). *The dyslexic child.* Springfield, IL: Thomas.

Culatta, B., Page, J., & Ellis, J. (1983). Story retelling as a communicative performance screening tool. *Language, Speech, and Hearing Services in Schools, 14,* 66–74.

DeFries, J.C. Fulker, D.W., & LaBuda, M.C. (1987). Reading disability in twins: Evidence for a genetic etiology. *Nature, 329,* 537–539.

Denckla, M.B. (1976). Naming of object-drawings by dyslexic and other learning disabled children. *Brain and Language, 3,* 1–15.

Denckla, M.B., & Rudel, R.G. (1976). Rapid automatized naming (RAN): Dyslexia differentiated from other learning disabilities. *Neuropsychologia, 14,* 471–479.

Doehring, D., Trites, R., Patel, P., & Fiedorowitcz, C. (1981). *Reading difficulties: The interaction of reading, language, and neuropsychological deficits.* New York: Academic Press.

Doi, L.M., & Manis, F.R. (1996). *The impact of speeded naming ability on reading performance.* Paper presented at the Society for the Scientific Study of Reading, New York.

Donahue, M. (1984). Learning disabled children's comprehension and production of syntactic devices for marking given versus new information. *Applied Psycholinguistics, 5,* 101–116.

Duara, R., Kushch, A., Gross-Glenn, K., et al. (1991). Neuroanatomic differences between dyslexic and normal readers on magnetic resonance imaging scans. *Archives of Neurology, 48,* 410–416.

Duffy, F.H., & McAnulty, G.B. (1985). Brain electrical activity mapping (BEAM): The search for the physiology signature of dyslexia. In F.H. Duffy & N. Geschwind (Eds.), *Dyslexia: A neuroscientific approach to clinical evaluation* (pp. 105–122). Boston: Little, Brown.

Eden, G.F., Stein, J.F., Wood, M.H., & Wood, F.B. (1994). Differences in eye movements and reading problems in reading disabled and normal children. *Vision Research, 34,* 1345–1358.

Eden, G.F., Stein, J.F., Wood, M.H., & Wood, F.B. (1995). Verbal and visual problems in reading disability. *Journal of Learning Disabilities, 28,* 272–290.

Eden, G.F., VanMeter, J., Rumsey, J., Maisog, J., Woods, R., & Zeffiro, T. (1996). Abnormal processing of visual motion in dyslexia revealed by functional brain imaging. *Nature, 382,* 66–69.

Elbro, C., Nielsen, I., & Petersen, D.K. (1994). Dyslexia in adults: Evidence for deficits in non-word reading and in the phonological representation of lexical items. *Annals of Dyslexia, 44,* 205–226.

Ellis, A.W. (1985). The cognitive neuropsychology of developmental (and acquired) dyslexia: A critical survey. *Cognitive Neuropsychology, 2,* 196–205.

Ellis, N., & Large, B. (1987). The development of reading: As you seek so shall you find. *British Journal of Psychology, 78,* 1–28.

Farmer, M.E., & Klein, R.M. (1995). The evidence for a temporal processing deficit linked to dyslexia: A review. *Psychonomic Bulletin & Review, 2,* 460–493.

Feagans, L., & Short, E. (1984). Developmental differences in the comprehension and production of narratives by reading disabled and normally achieving children. *Child Development, 55,* 1727–1736.

Felton, R.H. (1992). Early identification of children at risk for reading disabilities. *TECSE, 12,* 212–229.

Felton, R.H., & Wood, F.B. (1989). Cognitive deficits in reading disability and attention deficit disorder. *Journal of Learning Disabilities, 22,* 3–13.

Fildes, L. (1922). A psychological inquiry into the nature of the condition known as congenital word blindness. *Brain, 44,* 286–307.

Filipek, P.A., MD (1995). Neurobiologic correlates of developmental dyslexia: How do dyslexics' brains differ from those of normal readers? *Journal of Child Neurology, 10,* S62–S69.

Finucci, J.M., Gutherie, J.T., Childs, A.L., Abbey, H., & Childs, B. (1976). The genetics of specific reading disability. *Annual Review of Human Genetics, 40,* 1–23.

Fischer, F.W., Liberman, I.Y., & Shankweiler, D. (1978). Reading reversals and developmental dyslexia: A further study. *Cortex, 14,* 496–510.

Fletcher, J., & Martinez, G. (1994). An eye-movement analysis of the effects of scotopic sensitivity correction on parsing and comprehension. *Journal of Learning Disabilities, 27*(94/01), 67–70.

Fletcher, J.M. (1981). Linguistic factors in reading acquisition: Evidence for developmental changes. In *Neuropsychological and Cognitive Processes in Reading* (pp. 261–294) New York: Academic Press.

Fletcher, J.M., Shaywitz, S.E., Shankweiler, D.P., Katz, L., Liberman, I.Y., Stuebing, K.K., Francis, D.J., Fowler, A.E., & Shaywitz, B.A. (1994). Cognitive profiles of reading disability: Comparisons of discrepancy and low achievement definitions. *Journal of Educational Psychology, 86,* 6–23.

Flowers, D.L., Wood, F.B., & Naylor, C.E. (1991). Regional cerebral blood flow correlates of language processes in reading disability. *Archives of Neurology, 48,* 637–643.

Foundas, A.L., Leonard, C.M., Gilmore, R., et al. (1994). Planum temporal asymmetry and language dominance. *Neuropsychologia, 32,* 1225–1231.

Fox, B., & Routh, D.K. (1980). Phonemic analysis and severe reading disability in children. *Journal of Psycholinguistic Research, 9,* 115–119.

Fox, B., & Routh, D.K. (1983). Reading disability, phonemic analysis, and dysphonic spelling: A follow-up study. *Journal of Clinical Child Psychology, 12,* 28–32.

Frostig, M. (1968). Education for children with learning disabilities. In H. Myklebust (Ed.), *Progress in learning disabilities* (pp. 234–266). New York: Grune & Stratton.

Fry, M.A., Johnson, C.S., & Muehl, S. (1970). Oral language production in relation to reading achievement among select second graders. In D. Baker & P. Satz (Eds.), *Specific reading disability: Advances in theory and method* (pp. 123–159). Rotterdam: Rotterdam University Press.

Galaburda, A.M. (1988). The pathogenesis of childhood dyslexia. In F. Plum (Ed.), *Language, Communication, and the Brain.* New York: Raven Press.

Galaburda, A.M. (1991). Anatomy of dyslexia: Argument against phrenology. In D.D. Duane & D.B. Gray (Eds.), *The reading brain: The biological basis of dyslexia.* Parkton, MD: York Press.

Galaburda, A.M., Corsiglia, J., Rosen, G.D., & Sherman, G.F. (1987). Planum temporale asymmetry: Reappraisal since Geschwind and Levitsky. *Neuropsychologia, 28,* 314–318.

Galaburda, A.M., Sherman, G.F., Rosen, G.D., Aboitiz, F., & Geschwind, N. (1985). Developmental dyslexia: Four consecutive patients with cortical anomalies. *Annals of Neurology, 18*(85), 222–233.

Gerber, A. (1993). *Language-related learning disabilities: Their nature and treatment.* Baltimore: Paul H. Brooks.

German, D.J. (1979). Word-finding skills in children with learning disabilities. *Journal of Learning Disabilities, 12,* 43–48.

Gilger, J.W., Pennington, B.F., & DeFries, J.C. (1991). Risk for reading disability as a function of parental history in three family studies. *Reading and Writing: An Interdisciplinary Journal, 3,* 205–217.

Gilger, J.W., Pennington, B.F., & DeFries, J.C. (1992). A twin study of the etiology of comorbidity: Attention-deficit hyperactivity disorder and dyslexia. *Journal of the American Academy of Child and Adolescent Psychiatry, 31,* 343–348.

Godfrey, J.J., Lasky, A.K., Millag, K.K., & Knox, C.M. (1981). Performance of dyslexic children on speech perception tests. *Journal of Experimental Child Psychology, 32,* 401–424.

Graham, N. (1980). Spatial frequency channels in human vision. Detecting edges without edge detectors. In C.S. Harris (Ed.), *Visual coding and adaptability* (pp. 215–262). Hillsdale, NJ: Erlbaum.

Grigorenko, E., Wood, F., Meyer, M., Hart., L.A., Speed, W.C., Shuster, A., & Pauls, D. (1997). Susceptibility loci for distinct components of developmental dyslexia on chromosomes 6 and 15. *American Journal of Human Genetics, 60,* 27–39.

Hallgren, B. (1950). Specific dyslexia (congenital word blindness): A clinical and genetic study. *Acta Psychiatrica et Neurologica Supplement, 65,* 1–287.

Hatcher, P., Hulme, C., & Ellis, A.W. (1994). Ameliorating early reading failure by integrating the teaching of reading and phonological skills: The phonological linkage hypothesis. *Child Development, 65,* 41–57.

Hayduk, S., Bruck, M., & Cavanagh, P. (1992). *Do adult dyslexics show low level visual processing deficits?* Paper presented at the Rodin Remediation Society, New York Academy of Sciences, New York.

Heilman, K.M., Voeller, K., & Alexander, A.W. (1996). Developmental dyslexia: A motor-articulatory feedback hypothesis. *Annals of Neurology, 39,* 407–412.

Hermann, K. (1959). *Reading disability: A medical study of word-blindness and related handicaps.* Copenhagen: Munksgarrd.

Hinshelwood, J. (1917). *Congenital word blindness.* London: H.K. Lewis.

Holligan, C., & Johnston, R.S. (1988). The use of phonological information by good and poor readers in memory and reading tasks. *Memory & Cognition, 16,* 522–532.

Holmes, D., & McKeever, W. (1979). Material-specific serial memory deficit in adolescent dyslexics. *Cortex, 15,* 51–62.

Holmes, D., & Peper, R. (1977). An evaluation of the use of spelling error analysis in the diagnosis of reading disabilities. *Child Development, 48,* 1708–1711.

Hu, C., & Catts, H.W. (1997). The role of phonological processing in early reading ability: What we can learn from Chinese. *Scientific Studies in Reading, 2,* 55–79.

Hulme, C. (1988). Short-term memory development and learning to read. In M. Gruneberg, P. Morris, & R. Sykes (Eds.), *Practical aspects of memory: Current research and issues. Vol. 2: Clinical and educational implications* (pp. 234–271). Chichester, England: Wiley.

Hurford, D.P., Gilliland, C., & Ginavan, S. (1992). Examination of the intrasyllable phonemic discrimination deficit in children with reading disabilities. *Contemporary Educational Psychology, 17,* 83–88.

Hurford, D.P., Johnston, M., Neopote, P., Hampton, S., Moore, S., Neal, J., Mueller, A., McGeorge, K., Huff, L., Awad, A., Tatro, C., Juliano, C., & Huffman, D. (1994). Early identification and remediation of phonological-processing deficits in first-grade children at risk for reading disabilities. *Journal of Learning Disabilities, 27,* 647–659.

Hynd, G.W., Hall, J., Novey, E.S., Eliopulos, D., Black, K., Gonzalez, J.J., Edmonds, J.E., Riccio, C., & Cohen, M. (1995). Dyslexia and corpus callosum morphology. *Archives of Neurology, 52,* 32–38.

Hynd, G.W., Semrud-Clikeman, M., Lorys, A.R., Novey, E.S., & Eliopulos, D. (1990). Brain morphology in developmental dyslexia and attention deficit disorder/hyperactivity. *Archives of Neurology, 47,* 919–926.

Irlen, H. (1983). *Successful treatment of learning disabilities.* Paper presented at the 91st Annual Convention of the American Psychological Association, Anaheim, CA.

Irlen, H., & Lass, M.J. (1989). Improving reading problems due to symptoms of scotopic sensitivity using Irlen lenses and overlays. *Education, 109,* 413–417.

Jernigan, T.L., Hesselink, J.R., Sowell, E., & Tallal, P.A. (1991). Cerebral structure on magnetic resonance imaging in language- and learning-impaired children. *Archives of Neurology, 48,* 539–545.

Johnson, D., & Myklebust, H. (1967). *Learning disabilities: Educational principles and practice.* New York: Grune & Stratton.

Jorm, A.F., & Share, D.L. (1983). Phonological recoding and reading acquisition. *Applied Psycholinguistics, 4,* 103–147.

Jorm, A.F., Share, D.L., Maclean, R., & Matthews, R. (1986). Cognitive factors at school entry predictive of specific reading retardation and general reading backwardness: A research note. *Journal of Child Psychology and Psychiatry, 27,* 45–54.

Kamhi, A.G., Catts, H.W., & Mauer, D. (1990). Explaining speech production deficits in poor readers. *Journal of Learning Disabilities, 23,* 632-636.

Kamhi, A.G., Catts, H.W., Mauer, D., Apel, K., & Gentry, B. (1988). Phonological and spatial processing abilities in language and reading impaired children. *Journal of Hearing and Speech Disorders, 3,* 316–327.

Katz, R.B. (1986). Phonological deficiencies in children with reading disability: Evidence from an object-naming task. *Cognition, 22,* 225–257.

Katz, R.B., Shankweiler, D., & Liberman, I. (1981). Memory for item order and phonetic recoding in the beginning reader. *Journal of Experimental Child Psychology, 32,* 474–484.

Keefe, B., & Swinney, D. (1979). On the relationship of hemispheric specialization and developmental dyslexia. *Cortex, 15,* 471–481.

Keogh, B.K., & Pelland, M. (1985). Vision training revisited. *Journal of Learning Disabilities, 18.*

Korkman, M., & Pesonen, A.-E. (1994). A comparison of neuropsychological test profiles of children with attention deficit-hyperactivity disorder and/or learning disorder. *Journal of Learning Disabilities, 27,* 383–392.

Kraus, N., McGee, T.J., Carrell, T.D., Zecker, S.G., Nicol, T.G., & Koch, D.B. (1996). Auditory neurophysiologic responses and discrimination deficits in children with learning problems. *Science, 273,* 971–973.

Kubova, Z., Kuba, M., Peregrin, J., & Novakova, V. (1995). Visual evoked potential evidence for magnocellular system deficit in dyslexia. *Physiological Research, 44,* 87–89.

Larsen, J.P., Hoien, T., & Odegaard, H. (1992). Magnetic resonance imaging of the corpus callosum in developmental dyslexia. *Cognitive Neuropsychology, 9,* 123–134.

Lehmkuhle, S., Garzia, R.P., Turner, L., Hask, T., & Baro, J.A. (1993). A defective visual pathway in children with reading disability. *New England Journal of Medicine, 328,* 989–996.

Lewis, B., & Freebairn, L. (1992). Residual effects of preschool phonology disorders in grade school, adolescence, and adulthood. *Journal of Speech and Hearing Research, 35,* 819-831.

Liberman, I.Y., Mann, V.A., Shankweiler, D., & Werfelman, M. (1982). Children's memory for recurring linguistic and nonlinguistic material in relation to reading ability. *Cortex, 18,* 367–375.

Liberman, I.Y., Shankweiler, D., Orlando, C., Harris, K., & Berti, F. (1971). Letter confusion and reversal of sequence in the beginning reader: Implications for Orton's theory of developmental dyslexia. *Cortex, 7,* 127–142.

Lie, A. (1991). Effects of a training program for stimulating skills in word analysis in first-grade children. *Reader Research Quarterly, 26,* 234–250.

Light, J.G., & DeFries, J.C. (1995). Comorbidity of reading and mathematics disabilities: Genetic and environmental etiologies. *Journal of Learning Disabilities, 28,* 96–106.

Livingstone, M., Rosen, G., Drislane, F., & Galaburda, A. (1991). Physiological and anatomical evidence for a magnocellular defect in developmental dyslexia. *Proceedings of the National Academy of Science, 88,* 7943–7947.

Lovegrove, W. (1992). The visual deficit hypothesis. In N. Singh & I. Beale (Eds.), *Learning disabilities: Nature, theory, and treatment.* New York: Springer-Verlag.

Lovegrove, W., Martin, F., & Slaghuis, W. (1986). The theoretical and experimental case for a visual deficit in specific reading disability. *Cognitive Neuropsychology, 3,* 225–267.

Lubs, H., Duara, R., Levin, B., Jallad, B., Lubs, M., Rabin, M., Kushch, A., & Gross-Glenn, K. (1991). Dyslexia subtypes: Genetics, behavior, and brain imaging. In D.D. Drake & D.B. Gray (Eds.), *The reading brain: The biological basis of dyslexia.* Parkton, MD: York Press.

Lundberg, I., Frost, J., & Peterson, O. (1988). Effects of an extensive program for stimulating phonological awareness in young children. *Reading Research Quarterly, 23,* 263–284.

Lundberg, I., & Hoien, T. (1991). Initial enabling knowledge and skills in reading acquisition: Print awareness and phonological segmentation. In D.J. Sawyer & B.J. Fox (Eds.), *Phonological awareness in reading: The evolution of current perspectives* (pp. 74–95). New York: Springer-Verlag.

Lundberg, I., Olofsson, A., & Wall, S. (1980). Reading and spelling skills in the first school years predicted from phonemic awareness skills in kindergarten. *Scandinavian Journal of Psychology, 21,* 159–173.

Manis, F., McBride-Chang, C., Seidenberg, M., Keating, P., Doi, L., Munson, B, & Petersen, A. (1997). Are speech perception deficits associated with developmental dyslexia? *Journal of Experimental Child Psychology, 66,* 211–235.

Mann, V.A. (1993). Phoneme awareness and future reading ability. *Journal of Learning Disabilities, 26,* 259–269.

Mann, V.A., & Ditunno P. (1990). Phonological deficiencies: Effective predictors of future reading. In G.T. Pavlidis (Ed.), *Perspectives on dyslexia: Cognition, language and treatment* (Vol. 2, pp. 105–131). New York: Wiley.

Mann, V.A., & Liberman, I.Y. (1984). Phonological awareness and verbal short-term memory. *Journal of Learning Disabilities, 17,* 592–599.

Mann, V.A., Liberman, I.Y., & Shankweiler, D. (1980). Children's memory for sentences and word strings in relation to reading ability. *Memory & Cognition, 8,* 329–335.

Marcel, T., Katz, K., & Smith, M. (1974). Laterality and reading proficiency. *Neuropsychologia, 12,* 131–139.

McConnaughy, S. (1985). Good and poor readers' comprehension of story structure across different input and output modalities. *Reading Research Quarterly, 20,* 219–232.

Menyuk, P., Chesnick, M., Liebergott, J., Korngold, B., D'Agostino, R., & Belanger, A. (1993). Predicting reading problems in at-risk children. *Journal of Speech and Hearing Research, 34,* 893–903.

Metzer, R.I., & Werner, D.B. (1984). Use of visual training for reading disabilities: A review. *Pediatrics, 73,* 824–829.

Miles, T. (1983). *Dyslexia: The pattern of difficulties.* Springfield, IL: Charles C. Thomas.

Mody, M., Studdert-Kennedy, M., & Brady, S. (1997). Speech perception deficits in poor readers: Auditory processing or phonological coding. *Journal of Experimental Child Psychology, 64,* 199–231.

Morais, J. (1991). Phonological awareness: A bridge between language and literacy. In D. Sawyer & B. Fox (Eds.), *Phonological awareness and reading acquisition* (pp. 31–71). New York: Springer-Verlag.

Morais, J., Bertelson, P., Cary, L., & Alegria, J. (1986). Literacy training and speech segmentation. *Cognition, 24,* 45–64.

Morais, J., Cary, L., Alegria, J., & Bertelson, P. (1979). Does awareness of speech as a sequence of phones arise spontaneously? *Cognition, 7,* 323–331.

Morice, R., & Slaghuis, W. (1985). Language performance and reading ability at 8 years of age. *Applied Psycholinguistics, 6,* 141–160.

Newcomer, P. (1990). *Diagnostic Achievement Battery.* Austin, TX: Pro-Ed.

Newcomer, P., & Hammill, D. (1988). *Test of Language Development-2 Primary.* Austin, TX: Pro-Ed.

Obrzat, J.E. (1979). Dichotic listening and bisensory memory in qualitatively dyslexic readers. *Journal of Learning Disabilities, 12,* 304–313.

Obrzat, J.E., Hynd, G.W., & Boliek, C.A. (1986). Lateral asymmetries in learning disabled children: A review. In S.J. Ceci (Ed.), *Handbook of cognitive, social, and neuropsychological aspects of learning disabilities* (Vol. 1). Hillsdale, NJ: Erlbaum.

O'Connor, P.D., Sofo, F., Kendall, L., & Olsen, G. (1990). Reading disabilities and the effects of colored filters. *Journal of Learning Disabilities, 23,* 597–603.

Olson, M.E. (1973). Laterality differences in Tachistoscopic word recognition in normal and delayed readers in elementary school. *Neuropsychologia, 11,* 343–350.

Olson, R.K., Conners, F.A., & Rack, J.P. (1991). Eye movements in normal and dyslexic readers. In J.F. Stein (Ed.), *Vision and visual dyslexia.* London: Macmillan.

Olson, R.K., Wise, B., Conners, F., Rack, J., & Fulker, D. (1989). Specific deficits in component reading and language skills: Genetic and environmental influences. *Journal of Learning Disabilities, 22,* 339–348.

Orton, S. (1937). *Reading, writing and speech problems in children.* London: Chapman Hall.

Parker, R.M. (1990). Power, control, and validity in research. *Journal of Learning Disabilities, 23,* 613–620.

Paulesu, E., Connelly, A., Frith, C.D., Friston, K.J., Heather, J., & Myers, R. (1995). Functional MRI correlations with positron emission tomography: Initial experience using a cognitive activation paradigm on verbal working memory. *Neuroimaging and Clinical N A., 5,* 207–212.

Paulesu, E., Frith, C.D., & Frackowiak, R.S. (1993). The neural correlates of the verbal component of working memory. *Nature, 362,* 342–345.

Paulesu, E., Frith, U., Snowling, M., Gallagher, A., Morton, J., Frackowiak, R., & Frith, C.D. (1996). Is developmental dyslexia a disconnection syndrome? *Brain, 119,* 143–157.

Pavlidis, G.T. (1981). Do eye movements hold the key to dyslexia? *Neuropsychologia, 19,* 57–64.

Pavlidis, G.T. (1985). Eye movement differences between dyslexics, normal and slow readers while sequentially fixating digits. *American Journal of Optometry and Physiological Optics, 62,* 820–822.

Pennington, B.F., & Gilger, J.W. (1996). How is dyslexia transmitted? In C.H. Chase, G.D. Rosen, & G.F. Sherman (Eds.), *Developmental dyslexia: Neural, cognitive, and genetic mechanisms* (pp. 41–62). Baltimore: York Press.

Pennington, B.F., Gilger, J.W., Pauls, D., Smith, S.A., Smith, S.D., & DeFries, J.C. (1991). Evidence for major gene transmission of developmental dyslexia. *Journal of American Medical Association, 266,* 1527–1534.

Poeppel, D., & Rowley, H.A. (1996). Magnetic source imaging and the neural basis of dyslexia. *Annals of Neurology, 40,* 137–138.

Rack, J., Hulme, C., Snowling, M., & Wightman, J. (1994). The role of phonology in young children learning to read words: The direct-mapping hypothesis. *Journal of Experimental Child Psychology, 57*(1994), 42–71.

Rapala, M.M., & Brady, S. (1990). Reading ability and short-term memory: The role of phonological processing. *Reading and Writing: An Interdisciplinary Journal, 2,* 1–25.

Rayner, K. (1978). Eye movements in reading and information processing. *Psychological Bulletin, 85,* 618–660.

Rayner, K. (1985). Do faulty eye movements cause dyslexia? *Developmental Neuropsychology, 1,* 3–15.

Read, C., & Ruyter, L. (1985). Reading and spelling skills in adults of low literacy. *Remedial and Special Education, 6,* 43–52.

Robinson, G.L.W., & Conway, R.N.F. (1990). The effects of Irlen colored lenses on students' specific reading skills and their perception of ability: A 12-month validity study. *Journal of Learning Disabilities, 23,* 589–596.

Roth, P., & Spekman, N.J. (1986). Narrative discourse: Spontaneously generated stories of learning-disabled and normally achieving students. *Journal of Speech and Hearing Disorders, 51,* 8–23.

Rudel, R. (1985). The definition of dyslexia: Language and motor deficits. In F.H. Duffy & N. Geschwind (Eds.), *Dyslexia: A neuroscientific approach to clinical evaluation* (pp. 33–53). Boston: Little, Brown.

Rumsey, J.M., Andreason, P., Zametkin, A.J., Aquino, T., King, A.C., Hamburger, S.D., Pikus, A., Rapoport, J.L., & Cohen, R. (1992). Failure to activate the left temporoparietal cortex in dyslexia. *Archives of Neurology, 49,* 527–534.

Rumsey, J.M., Nace, K., Donohue, B., Wise, D., Maisog, J., & Andreason, P. (1997). A positron emission tomographic study of impaired word recognition and phonological processing in dyslexic men. *Archives of Neurology, 54,* 562–573.

Rumsey, J.M., Zametkin, A.J., Andreason, P., Hanahan, A.P., Hamburger, S.D., Aquino, T., King, C., Pikus, A., & Cohen, R.M. (1994). Normal activation of frontotemporal language cortex in dyslexia, as measured with Oxygen 15 Positron Emission Tomography. *Archives of Neurology, 51,* 27–38.

Safer, D.J., & Allen, R.D. (1976). *Hyperactive children: Diagnosis and management.* Baltimore: University Park Press.

Salmelin, R., Service, E., Kiesila, P., Uutela, K., & Salonen, O. (1996). Impaired visual word processing in dyslexia revealed with magnetoencephalography. *Annals of Neurology, 40,* 157–162.

Satz, P. (1977). Laterality tests: An inferential problem. *Cortex, 13,* 208–212.

Satz, P., & Sparrow, S.S. (1970). Specific developmental dyslexia: A theoretical formulation. In D.J. Bakker & P. Satz (Eds.), *Specific reading disability: Advances in theory and method.* Rotterdam: Rotterdam University Press.

Scanlon, D.M., & Vellutino, F.R. (1996). Prerequisite skills, early instruction and success in first grade reading: Selected results from a longitudinal study. *Mental Retardation and Developmental Disabilities, 2,* 54–63.

Scanlon, D.M., & Vellutino, F.R. (1997). A comparison of the instructional backgrounds and cognitive profiles of poor, average, and good readers who were initially identified as at risk for reading failure. *Scientific Studies of Reading, 1,* 191–216.

Scarborough, H.S. (1989). Prediction of reading disability from familial and individual differences. *Journal of Educational Psychology, 81,* 101–108.

Scarborough, H.S. (1990). Very early language deficits in dyslexic children. *Child Development, 61,* 1728–1743.

Scarborough, H.S. (1991). Early syntactic development of dyslexic children. *Annals of Dyslexia, 41,* 207–220.

Scarborough, H.S., & Dobrich, W. (1994). On the efficacy of reading to preschoolers. *Developmental Review, 14,* 245–302.

Semel, E., & Wiig, E. (1975). Comprehension of syntactic structures and critical verbal elements by children with learning disabilities. *Journal of Learning Disabilities, 8,* 53–58.

Shankweiler, D., Liberman, I.Y., Mark, L.S., Fowler, C.A., & Fischer, F.W. (1979). The speech code and learning to read. *Journal of Experimental Psychology: Human Learning and Memory, 5,* 531–545.

Share, D.L. (1995). Phonological recoding and self-teaching: Sine qua non of reading acquisition. *Cognition, 55,* 151–218.

Share, D.L., & Stanovich, K.E. (1995). Cognitive processes in early reading development: Accommodating individual differences into a model of acquisition. *Issues in Education, 1,* 1–57.

Shaywitz, B.A., Fletcher, J.M., Holahan, J.M., Shneider, A.E., Marchione, K.E., Stuebing, K.K., Francis, D.J., Shankweiler, D.P., Katz, L., Liberman, I.Y., & Shaywitz, S.E. (1995). Interrelationships between reading disability and attention-deficit/hyperactivity disorder. *Cognitive Neuropsychology, 1,* 170–186.

Shaywitz, S.E., Fletcher, J.M., & Shaywitz, B.A. (1994). Issues in the definition and classification of attention deficit disorder. *Topics in Language Disorders, 14,* 1–25.

Silva, P.A., McGree, R., Williams, S.M. (1987). Developmental language delay from three to seven and its significance for low intelligence and reading difficulties at age seven. *Developmental Medicine and Clinical Neurology, 25,* 783–793.

Silver, L.B. (1981). The relationship between learning disabilities, hyperactivity, distractibility, and behavioral problems. *Journal of the American Academy of Child Psychiatry, 20,* 385–397.

Silver, L.B. (1995). Controversial therapies. *Journal of Child Neurology, 10,* S96–S100.

Smiley, S.S., Oakley, D.D., Worthen, D., Campione, J.C., & Brown, A.L. (1977). Recall of thematically relevant material by adolescent good and poor readers as a function of written versus oral presentation. *Journal of Educational Psychology, 69*, 381–387.

Smith, S.D., Kimberling, W.J., & Pennington, B.F. (1991). Screening for multiple genes influencing dyslexia. *Reading and Writing: An Interdisciplinary Journal, 3*, 285–298.

Smith, S.D., Kimberling, W.J., Pennington, B.F., & Lubs, H.A. (1983). Specific reading disability: Identification of an inherited form through linkage analysis. *Science, 219*(83), 1345–1347.

Snowling, M. (1981). Phonemic deficits in developmental dyslexia. *Psychological Research, 43*, 219–234.

Snowling, M.J., Goulandris, N., Bowlby, M., & Howell, P. (1986). Segmentation and speech perception in relation to reading skill: A developmental analysis. *Journal of Experimental Child Psychology, 41*, 489–507.

Solan, H.A. (1990). An appraisal of the Irlene technique of correcting reading disorders using tinted overlays and tinted lenses. *Journal of Learning Disabilities, 23*, 621–623.

Solman, R.T., & May, J.G. (1990). Spatial localization discrepancies: A visual deficiency in poor readers. *American Journal of Psychology, 103*, 243–263.

Spear-Swerling, L., & Sternberg, R.J. (1994). The road not taken: An integrative theoretical model of reading disability. *Journal of Learning Disabilities, 27*, 91–103, 122.

Spear-Swerling, L., & Sternberg, R.J. (1996). *Off track: When poor readers become "learning disabled."* Boulder, CO: Westview Press.

Stanley, G. (1991). Glare, scotopic sensitivity and colour therapy. In J.F. Stein (Ed.), *Vision and visual dyslexia.* London: Macmillan.

Stanley, G. (1994). Visual deficit models of dyslexia. In G. Hales (Ed.), *Dyslexia matters.* San Diego, CA: Singular.

Stanovich, K.E. (1986). Matthew effects in reading: Some consequences of individual differences in the acquisition of literacy. *Reading Research Quarterly, 86*, 360–406

Stanovich, K.E. (1988). *Children's reading and the development of phonological awareness.* Detroit: Wayne State University Press.

Stanovich, K.E., & Siegel, L.S. (1994). The phenotypic performance profile of reading-disabled children:

A regression-based test of the phonological-core variable-difference model. *Journal of Educational Psychology, 86*, 24–53.

Stanovich, K.E., & West, R.F. (1989). Exposure to print and orthographic processing. *Reading Research Quarterly, 24*, 402–433.

Stark, R.E., Bernstein, L.E., Condino, R., Bender, M., Tallal, P., & Catts, H. (1984). Four-year follow-up study of language impaired children. *Annals of Dyslexia, 34*, 49–67.

Stellern, J., Collins, J., Bayne, M. (1987). A dual-task investigation of language-spatial lateralization. *Journal of Learning Disabilities, 20*, 551–556.

Stephenson, S. (1907). Six cases of congenital word-blindness affecting three generations of one family. *Ophthalmoscope, 5*, 482–484.

Stone, B., & Brady, S. (1995). Evidence for phonological processing deficits in less-skilled readers. *Annals of Dyslexia, 95*, 51–78.

Stothard, S., & Hulme, C. (1992). Reading comprehension difficulties in children: The role of language comprehension and working memory skills. *Reading and Writing: An Interdisciplinary Journal, 4*, 245–256.

Stothard, S., Snowling, M., & Bishop, D.V.M. (1996). *Language-impaired preschoolers: A follow-up into adolescence.* Paper presented at the Annual Conference of the American Speech-Language Hearing Association, Seattle, WA.

Studdert-Kennedy, M., & Mody, M. (1995). Auditory termporal perception deficits in reading-impaired: A critical review of the evidence. *Psychonomic Bulletin & Review, 2*, 508–514.

Sundeth, K., & Bowers, P.G. (1997). *The relationship between digit naming speed and orthography in children with and without phonological deficits.* Paper presented at the Society for the Scientific Study of Reading, Chicago, IL.

Swan, D.M., & Goswami, U. (1997a). Phonological awareness deficits in developmental dyslexia and the phonological representations hypothesis. *Journal of Experimental Child Psychology, 66*, 18–41.

Swan, D.M., & Goswami, U. (1997b). Picture naming deficits in developmental dyslexia: The phonological representations hypothesis. *Brain and Language, 56*, 334–353.

Tallal, P. (1980). Auditory temporal perception, phonics, and reading disabilities in children. *Brain and Language, 9*, 182–198.

Tallal, P., Curtiss, S., & Kaplan, R. (1989). *The San Diego longitudinal study: Evaluating the outcomes of preschool impairments in language development.* Bethesda, MD: NINCDS.

Taylor, H.G., Lean, D., & Schwartz, S. (1989). Pseudoword repetition ability in learning-disabled children. *Applied Psycholinguistics, 10,* 203–219.

Thomson, M.E. (1976). Laterality effects in dyslexics and controls using verbal dichotic listening tasks. *Neuropsychologia, 14,* 243–246.

Tomblin, J.B., Records, N.L., Buckwalter, P., Zhang, X, Smith, E., & O'Brien, M. (1997). The prevalence of specific language impairment in kindergarten children. *Journal of Speech, Language, and Hearing Research, 40,* 1245–1260.

Torgesen, J.K. (1985). Memory processes in reading disabled children. *Journal of Learning Disabilities, 18,* 350–357.

Torgesen, J.K. (1996). *Phonological awareness: A critical factor in dyslexia.* Baltimore: Orton Dyslexia Society.

Torgesen, J.K., Morgan, S.T., & Davis, C. (1992). Effects of two types of phonological awareness training on word learning in kindergarten children. *Journal of Educational Psychology, 84,* 364–370.

Torgesen, J.K., Wagner, R.K., & Rashotte, C.A. (1994). Longitudinal studies of phonological processing and reading. *Journal of Learning Disabilities, 27,* 276–286.

Torgesen, J.K., Wagner, R.K., Rashotte, C.A., Burgess, S., & Hecht, S. (1997). Contributions of phonological awareness and rapid naming to the growth of word-reading skills in second- and fifth-grade children. *Scientific Studies in Reading, 1,* 161–185.

Vellutino, F.R. (1979). *Dyslexia: Theory and research.* Cambridge, MA: MIT Press.

Vellutino, F.R., Pruzek, R., Steger, J.A., & Meshoulam, U. (1973). Immediate visual recall in poor and normal readers as a function of orthographic-linguistic familiarity. *Cortex, 9,* 368–384.

Vellutino, F.R., & Scanlon, D.M. (Eds.). (1982). *Verbal processing in poor and normal readers.* New York: Springer-Verlag.

Vellutino, F.R., Scanlon, D.M., Sipay, E.R., Small, S.G., Chen, R., Pratt, A., & Denckla, M.B. (1996). Cognitive profiles of difficult-to-remediate and readily remediated poor readers: Early intervention as a vehicle for distinguishing between cognitive and experiential deficits as basic causes of specific reading disabilities. *Journal of Educational Psychology, 88,* 601–638.

Vellutino, F.R., Scanlon, D.M., & Spearing, D. (1995). Semantic and phonological coding in poor and normal readers. *Journal of Experimental Child Psychology, 59,* 76–123.

Vellutino, F.R., Steger, J.A., DeSetto, L., & Phillips, F. (1975). Immediate and delayed recognition of visual stimuli in poor and normal readers. *Journal of Experimental Child Psychology, 19,* 223–232.

Vellutino, F.R., Steger, J.A., Harding, C.J., & Phillips, F. (1975). Verbal vs. non-verbal paired-associate learning in poor and normal readers. *Neuropsychologia, 13,* 75–82.

Vogel, S.A. (1974). Syntactic abilities in normal and dyslexic children. *Journal of Learning Disabilities, 7,* 47–53.

Vogler, G.P., DeFries, J.C., & Decker, S.N. (1985). Family history as an indicator of risk for reading disability. *Journal of Learning Disabilities, 18,* 419–421.

Wagner, R., Balthazor, M., Hurley, S., Morgan, S., Rachotte, C., Shaner, R., Simmons, K., & Stage, S. (1987). The nature of prereaders' phonological processing abilities. *Cognitive Development, 2,* 355–373.

Wagner, R.K., & Torgesen, J.K. (1987). The nature of phonological processing and its causal role in the acquisition of reading skills. *Psychological Bulletin, 101,* 1–21.

Wagner, R.K., Torgesen, J.K., & Rashotte, C.A. (1994). Development of reading-related phonological processing abilities: New evidence of bidirectional causality from a latent variable longitudinal study. *Developmental Psychology, 30,* 73–87.

Warrick, N., Rubin, H., & Rowe-Walsh, S. (1993). Phoneme awareness in language-delayed children: Comparative studies and intervention. *Annals of Dyslexia, 43,* 153–173.

Wechsler, D. (1967). *Wechsler Preschool and Primary Scale of Intelligence.* Cleveland: Psychological Cooperation.

Weiss, R. (1990). Dyslexics read better with blues. *Science News, 138,* 196.

Werker, J.F., & Tees, R.C. (1987). Speech perception in severely disabled and average reading children. *Canadian Journal of Psychology, 41,* 48–61.

Wierdholt, J.L., & Bryant, B.R. (1986). *Gray Oral Reading Test-Revised.* Austin, TX: Pro-Ed.

Wiig, E.H., & Semel, E.M. (1975). Productive language abilities in learning disabled adolescents. *Journal of Learning Disabilities, 8*(9), 578–586.

Williams, M., Molinet, K., & LeCluyse, K. (1989). Visual masking as a measure of temporal processing in normal and disabled readers. *Clinical Vision Sciences, 4*, 137–144.

Willows, D.M., Kruk, R., & Corcos, E. (Eds.). (1993). *Visual processes in reading and reading disabilities.* San Diego: Academic Press.

Wilson, B., & Risucci, D. (1988). The early identification of developmental disorders and the prediction of the acquisition of reading skills. In R. Masland & M. Masland (Eds.), *Preschool prediction of reading failure.* Parkton, MD: York Press.

Wise, B.W., & Olson, R.K. (1995). Computer-based phonological awareness and reading instruction. *Annals of Dyslexia, 45*, 99–122.

Wolf, M. (1984). Naming, reading, and the dyslexias: A longitudinal overview. *Annals of Dyslexia, 34*, 87–136.

Wolf, M. (1991). Naming speed and reading: The contribution of the cognitive neurosciences. *Reading Research Quarterly, 26*, 123–141.

Wolf, M., Bally, H., & Morris, R. (1986). Automaticity, retrieval processes, and reading: A longitudinal study in average and impaired readers. *Child Development, 57*, 988–1000.

Wolf, M., & Goodglass, H. (1986). Dyslexia, dysnomia, and lexical retrieval: A longitudinal investigation. *Brain and Language, 28*, 154–168.

Woodcock, R. (1987). *Woodcock Reading Mastery Tests—Revised.* Circle Pines, MN: American Guidance Service.

Yuill, N., & Oakhill, J. (1991). *Children's problems in test comprehension.* Cambridge, England: Cambridge University Press.

Chapter *6*

Assessment and Instruction for Phonemic Awareness and Word Recognition Skills

JOSEPH K. TORGESEN

This chapter provides an overview of procedures for assessment and instruction of phonemic awareness and word recognition skills. It assumes that the reader has already learned from other chapters about the nature of reading disabilities and reading acquisition processes. The reader should also understand that the ultimate goal of reading instruction is to help children acquire all the skills required to comprehend the meaning of text, and that the acquisition of effective word-level reading skills is critical to the attainment of that goal. The reader should also have a good understanding of the kind of language abilities that directly influence the acquisition of word recognition skills.

One of the most critical of these language skills is phonemic awareness. Since the development of phonemic awareness is critical to the subsequent acquisition of good word recognition skills, it seems logical to discuss assessment and instruction in this area first, and then to continue the discussion to the more complex issues involved in the assessment and instruction of word recognition skills.

Acknowledgments

The research reported in this chapter was supported by grants numbered HD23340 and HD30988 from the National Institute of Child Health and Human Development and by grants from the National Center for Learning Disabilities and the Donald D. Hammill Foundation.

Assessment and Instruction in Phonemic Awareness

There are several general issues related to assessment of phonological awareness that must be considered before information about specific tests is presented. Perhaps the most central of these issues is the matter of definition. Before any construct can be assessed, it should be defined, and phonemic awareness is a construct that is not easy to pin down to a simple definition. One issue is whether we should consider phonemic awareness to be a kind of conceptual understanding about language, or whether it should be considered a skill. What do we mean, precisely, when we say that a child's phonemic awareness has increased from the last time we measured it?

Certainly, part of what we mean by phonemic awareness is that it involves an understanding, or awareness, that a single-syllable word such as *cat*, which is experienced by the listener as a single beat of sound, actually can be subdivided into beginning, middle, and ending sounds. It also involves the idea, or understanding, that individual segments of sound at the phonemic level can be combined together to form words. Otherwise, the child would not be able to make sense out of the request to blend the sounds represented by the letters *c - a - t* together to make a word.

However, a complete understanding of phonemic awareness must also account for the fact that it behaves like a skill. That is, children seem to acquire an increasing ability to notice, think about, and manipulate the phonemes in words as they attend school from kindergarten through elementary school. At the beginning of first grade, for example, a child might be able to isolate and pronounce the first sound in a word like *cat*, but by the beginning of second grade, children can commonly segment all the sounds in three and four phoneme words. Children also show regular improvements during this same period of time in their ability to blend individually presented sounds together to form words (Torgesen & Morgan, 1990).

In order to account for both the conceptual and skill components of the construct we need a definition of phonemic awareness such as the following: It involves a more or less explicit understanding that words are composed of segments of sound smaller than a syllable, as well as knowledge, or awareness, of the distinctive features of individual phonemes themselves. It is this latter knowledge of the identity of individual phonemes themselves that continues to increase after an initial understanding of the phonemic structure of words is acquired. For example, children must acquire a knowledge of the distinctive features of a phoneme such as /l/ so they can recognize it when it occurs with slightly varied pronunciation at the beginning of a word such as *last*, as the second sound in a consonant blend as in *flat*, in the middle of a word, such as *shelving*, or when it occurs in a final blend such as in *fault*.

Sometimes the term *phonological awareness* is used to refer to the construct we are discussing here, but it actually implies a more general level of awareness than *phonemic awareness*. For example, awareness of the syllabic structure of words would qualify as a form of phonological awareness, because it involves awareness of part of the sound structure in words. Additionally, rhyme awareness is a beginning form of phonological awareness, because it involves an ability to analyze words at the level of the onset and rime (*c-at*, *m-at*). The distinction between these more general forms of phonological awareness and the more specific form of phonemic awareness is supported in factor analyses of groups of these tasks, and it is important because measures of phonemic awareness appear to be more predictive of individual differences in reading growth (Hoien, Lundberg, Stanovich, & Bjaalid, 1995).

The Importance of Phonemic Awareness in Learning to Read

In addition to understanding the concept of phonemic awareness, assessment must also be informed by an understanding of why phonemic awareness is important to the growth of word reading ability. There are at least three ways that phonemic awareness contributes to the growth of early reading skills.

1. *It helps children understand the alphabetic principle.* In order to take advantage of the fact that English is an alphabetic language, a child must be aware that words have sound segments that are represented by the letters in print. Without at least emergent levels of phonemic awareness, the rationale for learning individual letter sounds, and "sounding out" words is not understandable.

2. *It helps children notice the regular ways that letters represent sounds in words.* If children can "hear" four sounds in the word *clap*, it helps them to notice the way the letters correspond to the sounds. The ability to notice the correspondence between the sounds in a word and the way it is spelled has two potential benefits. First, it reinforces knowledge of individual sound-letter correspondences, and second, it helps in forming mental representations of words that involve a close amalgamation of their written and spoken forms. Linnea Ehri (1992, in press) has shown how this specific association of the sounds in words to their letters creates the kind of whole word representations that facilitate fluent reading.

3. *It makes it possible to generate possibilities for words in context that are only partially "sounded out."* For example, consider the child who comes to a sentence such as "The boy r_ _ _ his bike to the store," and cannot recognize the third word, but knows the sound represented by the first letter. An early level of phonemic awareness supports the ability to search the lexicon for words that begin with similar sounds. That is, in addition to being categorized by their meanings, words can be categorized by their beginning, middle, or ending sounds. So, some degree of phonemic awareness is usually required to utilize partial phonetic decodings in combination with context to arrive at the fully correct pronunciation of unfamiliar words in text.

This analysis suggests that phonemic awareness has its primary impact on reading growth through its contribution to children's ability to use sound-letter correspondences to decode words in text. Although the ability to phonetically decode words is not an end in itself (phonetic decoding is too slow and effortful to support fluent reading and good comprehension), recent accounts of reading growth indicate that phonetic reading skills play a critical role in supporting overall reading growth, particularly the growth of a rich vocabulary of words that can be recognized orthographically, or "by sight" (Ehri, in press; Share & Stanovich, 1995).

As an empirical illustration of the impact of deficient phonemic awareness on the growth of early phonetic decoding ability, Figure 6-1 presents data on growth of phonetic

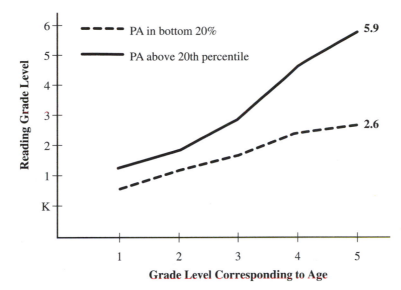

FIGURE 6-1   Growth in phonetic reading ability from first to end of fifth grade in children selected to be low in phonological awareness at the beginning of first grade.

reading ability in a sample of children selected at the beginning of first grade to be in the bottom 20 percent of a random sample of 200 children in performance on measures of phonemic awareness. Phonemic awareness was assessed by three tasks that asked children either to blend sounds together or to identify individual sounds in words presented orally.

In this study (Torgesen, Wagner, & Rashotte, 1994), our measure of phonetic decoding skills was the Word Attack subtest from the *Woodcock Reading Mastery Test-Revised* (Woodcock, 1987). This test requires children to read phonetically regular nonwords of increasing difficulty. The numbers at the right of the graphs represent average grade level score at the end of fifth grade of children above and below the 20th percentile in phonemic awareness at the beginning of first grade. Children with weak phonemic awareness skills ended up about three and one-half grade levels below their peers in phonetic decoding ability at the end of fifth grade!

Purposes for Assessment of Phonemic Awareness

The relationship illustrated in Figure 6-1 and the high correlation that has been reported in many studies (see Share & Stanovich, 1995, for a recent review) between emerging phonemic awareness and later growth of reading skills suggests one of the two reasons why we should be concerned about assessment of this construct. At present, phonemic awareness is being assessed both to identify children at risk for reading failure before reading instruction actually begins and to help describe level of phonological impairment in children being diagnosed with RD.

Although these are both promising areas for the development of useful assessment procedures, we are still some distance away from being able to precisely identify future reading-disabled children on the basis of their performance on measures of phonemic awareness in kindergarten. There have been a number of recent attempts to use measures of early phonemic awareness administered either in kindergarten or at the beginning of first grade to identify children at risk for reading failure (Catts, 1996). With the exception of two studies that measured phonological and early reading skills at the beginning of first grade, however, these studies have universally had high numbers of false positives (children who are predicted to be poor, but turn out to be good readers), with rates ranging from 23 to 69 percent.

In our own work (Torgesen, Burgess, & Rashotte, 1996) we have used measures of phonological awareness in combination with measures of letter name knowledge and rapid naming ability (Wolf, 1991) to predict which children are likely to fall in the bottom 10 percent in word recognition ability at the beginning of second grade. Although we can do this with an overall accuracy rate (with measures taken at the beginning of kindergarten) of 91 percent, with a false positive rate of only 5 percent, our false negative rate (children who were not identified as at-risk, but who ended in the bottom 10%) was 48 percent. This false negative rate means that approximately half the children who eventually ended up in the bottom 10 percent of readers were not included in the 10 percent of children we had identified as "at risk" in kindergarten. However, when we allowed our prediction equation to identify 20 percent of the kindergarten children as "at risk," the false negative rate was reduced to only 8 percent, while the false positive rate climbed to 14 percent. These rates suggest that if schools had the resources to provide preventive interventions for 20 percent of kindergarten children, only about one in ten children destined to fall in the bottom 10 percent of readers by second grade would be missed in that early screening.

As an aid in the diagnosis of reading disabilities, measures of phonemic awareness are consistently more reliable than any other measure of nonreading skills (Fletcher, Shaywitz, Shankweiter, Katz, Liberman, Stuebing, Francis, Fowler, & Shaywitz, 1994). However, the issue here is whether they actually add any precision to the diagnosis of reading disability beyond the information that is provided by direct measures of phonetic decoding ability. In one study that addressed this question (Torgesen, Wagner, Rashotte, Burgess, & Hecht, 1997), we did find that measures of phonemic awareness in second- and third-grade children provided a small amount of useful information beyond that provided by reading measures. However, the amount of additional information may not have been large enough to warrant the additional time it took to administer the phonemic tests. The principle reason why assessment of phonemic awareness may not add to the diagnosis of reading disability once children have begun to learn to read is that phonetic decoding skills and phonemic awareness are very highly correlated with one another. However, it is far too early to rule out the use of phonemic awareness measures as part of a diagnostic battery for older children with reading disability. In individual cases, these measures may have clinical or educational implications that go substantially beyond those derived from measures of nonword reading.

Procedures Used to Assess Phonemic Awareness

In a review of methods used to assess phonemic awareness, Catts and his colleagues (Catts, Wilcox, Wood-Jackson, Larrivee, & Scott, 1997) found over twenty different tasks that have been used by researchers to measure awareness of phonemes in words. In their analysis, they grouped these measures into three broad categories: phoneme segmentation, phoneme synthesis, and sound comparison. *Phoneme segmentation* tasks require a relatively explicit level of awareness of phonemes because they involve counting, pronouncing, deleting, adding, or reversing the individual phonemes in words. Common examples of this type of task require pronouncing the individual phonemes in words ("Say the sounds in *cat* one at a time."), deleting sounds from words ("Say *card* without saying the /d/ sound."), or counting sounds ("Put one marker on the line for each sound you hear in the word *fast*.")

There is really only one kind of task that can be used to measure *phoneme synthesis*. This is the sound blending task in which the tester attempts to pronounce a series of phonemes in isolation and asks the child to blend them together to form a word (i.e., "What word do these sounds make, /f/ - /a/ - /t/?). Easier variants of the sound blending task can be produced by allowing the child to choose from two or three pictures the word that is represented by a series of phonemes (Torgesen & Bryant, 1993).

Sound comparison tasks use a number of different formats that have a common requirement to make comparisons between the sounds in different words. For example, a child might be asked to indicate which word (of several) begins or ends with the same sound as a target word. Additionally, tasks that require children to generate words that have the same first, last, or middle sound as a target word would fall in this category.

An important point about these different kinds of tasks is that they all appear to be measuring essentially the same construct. Although some research (Yopp, 1988) has indicated that the tasks may vary in the complexity of their overall cognitive requirements, and there may be some differences between analysis and synthesis tasks at certain ages (Wagner, Torgesen, & Rashotte, 1994), for the most part, they all seem to be measuring different levels of growth in the same general ability (Hoien et al., 1995; Stanovich, Cunningham, & Cramer, 1984). Differences among these tasks in their level of difficulty seem primarily related to the extent to which they require explicit manipulation of individual phonemes. For example, most kindergarten children have difficulty with phoneme segmentation tasks, but many can perform sound comparison tasks successfully.

Currently Available Measures of Phonemic Awareness

There are a number of readily available measures to assess phonemic awareness, and more are currently under development. It is beyond the scope of this chapter to critically evaluate each of the available tests, so we will simply provide a brief description along with information about where each instrument can be obtained. Only three of these tests have normative data, but they all have well-established predictive relationships with the growth of word recognition skills. For screening purposes, local norms may prove to be more useful than norms based on performance of a nationally representative sample of children.

Rosner Test of Auditory Analysis

This is the oldest published test of phonemic awareness, and it has been widely used in research. It is a relatively brief test (13 items) involving the deletion of phonemes from words and is available in a book titled *Helping Children Overcome Learning Difficulties* (Rosner, 1975). It is suitable for children kindergarten age through the end of elementary school. The author provides suggested levels of performance for kindergarten through second grade based on his clinical experience with the test.

Lindamood Auditory Conceptualization Test (Lindamood & Lindamood, 1979)

This test has been used widely in clinical work with reading-disabled children. The test provides "recommended minimum scores" for grades kindergarten through sixth grade, with a separate estimate for the range of seventh grade to adult. These estimates are based on the author's extensive clinical experience with the test, and they suggest that children who score below these levels will likely have difficulties acquiring phonetic decoding skills. The test requires children to indicate the number, identity, and order of phonemes in words using colored blocks.

Test of Invented Spelling

This test is suitable for administration for groups, although it measures more than simple phoneme analysis. Since it requires children to "represent as many of the sounds in words as they can" by spelling them, it also assesses knowledge of sound-letter correspondences. It is included here because it is very sensitive to individual differences in phonemic awareness and may actually be more predictive of later reading growth than many purely oral measures of phonemic awareness (Mann, 1993). It is available, along with information about scoring, in an article by Mann, Tobin, and Wilson (1987) published in an issue of the *Merrill-Palmer Quarterly*. This kind of test may not be appropriate once children begin formal instruction in spelling, as many of the words would simply be spelled correctly because they had been memorized.

Test of Phonological Awareness (Torgesen & Bryant, 1993)

This simple test contains two subtests that both involve sound comparison activities. It was developed with support of a grant from the National Institute of Child Health and Human Development and is nationally normed and has excellent psychometric characteristics. There is a version for kindergarten children involving comparisons of the first sounds in words, while the first-grade version involves comparison of the last sounds in words. Both the kindergarten and first-grade versions of the TOPA can be given to groups of children, and the items were developed to be most sensitive to individual differences in phonemic awareness at lower levels of ability.

Yopp-Singer Test of Phoneme Segmentation

This twenty-two-item test is suitable for kindergarten and first-grade children. It requires children to pronounce the individual phonemes in two- and three-phoneme words. It is available in an article (Yopp, 1995) in *The Reading Teacher*, along with information about its predictive relationships to reading growth.

The Phonological Awareness Test (Robertson & Salter, 1995)

This is a norm-referenced test that provides a broad assessment of phonological and phonemic awareness through six different subtests. It is designed for children from kindergarten through fifth grade, and it is individually administered. The subtests, which all have good psychometric characteristics, include measures of children's ability to: (1) discriminate and produce rhymes; (2) segment sentences, compound words, syllables, and phonemes; (3) pronounce separately the beginning, ending, or medial sound in short words; (4) delete a syllable or a phoneme from a word and pronounce the word that remains; (5) use colored blocks to show the number and order of phonemes in words; and (6) blend together separately presented syllables or phonemes to make words.

The Comprehensive Test of Phonological Processes in Reading (Wagner & Torgesen, 1997)

This test provides several different measures of phonological awareness that are normed for children from kindergarten through high school. Its development was supported by a grant from the National Institute of Child Health and Human Development. For children in kindergarten and first grade, phonological awareness is measured by sound comparison tests as well as measures involving segmentation and phoneme blending. For children second grade and older, measures of phoneme segmentation and blending are employed. This test is intended for use as an individually administered diagnostic/predictive battery, and it also includes four measures of rapid naming ability (objects, colors, digits, and letters) and two measures of short-term memory for phonological information.

Instruction in Phonemic Awareness

There is now a very strong consensus among professionals who study reading and reading disability that instruction in phonological awareness is important as part of any good reading curriculum (Adams, 1990; Blachman; 1989, NCLD, 1996). This consensus derives not only from longitudinal-correlational research showing causal relationships between individual differences in phonemic awareness and subsequent reading growth (Wagner et al., 1994), but also, and more importantly, from demonstrations that training in phonemic awareness actually produces a positive effect on subsequent reading growth (Ball & Blachman, 1991; Bradley & Bryant, 1985; Lundberg, Frost, & Peterson, 1988). Before actual methods and materials used to stimulate the growth of phonemic awareness are considered, there are two very important questions to address. First, what do we know about maximizing the influence of training in phonemic awareness on subsequent growth in reading, and second, do we know how to train phonemic awareness so that it will help improve reading in children with the *most severe* phonological processing disabilities?

The answer to the first question has one main answer: Methods that integrate instruction in sound-letter correspondences in a way that directly links newly acquired phonemic awareness to reading and spelling produce stronger effects on reading than those that do not. While most instructional programs in phonemic awareness begin with oral language activities, most also conclude by leading children to apply their newly developed ability to think about the phonemic segments in words in relation to reading and spelling activities.

The importance of this progression from oral to written language activities was illustrated in the first major demonstration of the effectiveness of training in phonemic awareness reported by Bradley and Bryant (1985). In this study, phonemic awareness was stimulated by using activities that required children to categorize words on the basis of similarities in their beginning, middle, and ending sounds (sound comparison tasks). However, in one of the conditions, this training was supplemented by work with individual plastic letters to illustrate the way new words could be made by changing only one letter (or sound) in a word. It was children in this latter condition who showed the largest benefit from the phonemic awareness training program. While training in phonemic awareness, by itself, can produce significant improvement in subsequent reading growth (Lundberg et al., 1988), programs that directly illustrate the relevance of the training to reading and spelling activities consistently produce the largest gains in reading (Blachman, Ball, Black, & Tangel, 1994; Byrne & Fielding-Barnsley, 1993; Cunningham, 1990).

It is recommended, therefore, that practitioners combine training in phonological awareness with instruction in how the alphabet works. This integration of orally based instruction in phonological awareness with activities involving print does not mean that training in phonological awareness is useful only if it precedes systematic and complete "phonics"-oriented reading instruction. These activities should be included simply to help children learn to apply their newly acquired phonological awareness to reading and spelling tasks. The print-based activities that should accompany instruction in phonological awareness are necessarily very simple. For example, children who have been taught a few letter sounds, and who have achieved a beginning level of phonemic awareness, should be able to identify the first letter of a word when they hear it pronounced. They might also be led to substitute different letters at the beginning or end of a word like *cat* to make different words. They could also be asked to pronounce the "sounds" of the letters *c - a - t* and then blend them together to form a word. If children have learned to blend orally presented sounds together, they can be led to perform the same process when the phonemes are represented by letters.

The answer to the second question about our ability to improve phonemic awareness in children with the most severe disabilities has two parts. The first part of the answer comes from research that has examined individual differences in response to training in phonemic awareness itself (Blachman, 1997; Lundberg, 1988) This research has consistently shown that there is always a small proportion of children whose improvement in phonemic awareness as a result of training is very small. In the most extensive investigation of this question to date, Torgesen and Davis (1996) provided small group (4-5 students) training in phonemic segmentation and blending skills to a large number (60) of high-risk kindergarten children in a twelve-week program that provided a total of about sixteen hours of training. About a third of the children failed to show any measurable improvement in phonemic segmentation skills, while about 10 percent showed negligible growth in blending skills. When average improvement of the whole group was considered, the training appeared to be very effective, producing growth in phonemic awareness that was slightly above average for this type of study. Since the training procedures used in this study, as well as the overall group effects, were very similar to most other instructional studies in the research literature, we may need to experiment with either more intensive or more explicit training procedures to build the phonemic awareness skills of our most phonologically impaired children.

The second part of the answer to this question comes from studies that have examined individual differences in reading growth in response to reading instruction that contains activities to stimulate phonemic awareness. The answer is that, once again, there is always a small proportion of children in the at-risk samples (ranging from 15 to 25% of the sample) that shows unsatisfactory growth in word recognition ability as a result of instruction (Brown

& Felton, 1990; Torgesen, 1997a; Vellutino, Scanlon, Sipay, Small, Pratt, Chen, & Denckla, 1996). Of course, the growth of word recognition ability requires knowledge and skill other than phonemic awareness. Nevertheless, the overall answer to our question must be that we still do not know the conditions that need to be in place for *all* children to acquire phonemic awareness of sufficient strength to facilitate acquisition of normal phonetic reading abilities.

Programs and Materials to Stimulate Growth of Phonemic Awareness

As in the earlier discussion of assessment procedures, programs and materials that are currently available for instruction in phonemic awareness will be described without critically evaluating them. As Table 6-1 indicates, the materials fall roughly into two categories: those that are meant primarily for regular class instruction in kindergarten and first grade as a supplement to beginning reading instruction, and those that are designed for more in-depth instruction of at-risk or reading-disabled children. Where prices are provided, these should be taken as estimates, as they are likely to change over time.

TABLE 6-1   Sources of Curriculum Materials to Stimulate Growth of Phonological Awareness

Materials for Whole Class Instruction

Sounds Abound by Hugh Catts and Tina Vartiainen	LinguiSystems, Inc. 3100 4th Avenue East Moline, IL 61244 800-776-4332	$31.95 (manual)

Description: This is a collection of materials and activities that can be used to teach phonemic awareness to young children. It contains wordlists that can be used in rhyming, sound comparison, and phonemic analysis and synthesis activities. Most of these wordlists are supplemented with pictures for visual support during the instructional activities. It is not a systematic curriculum, but rather a collection of materials and activities that can be adapted by the teacher to support a curriculum in phonemic awareness.

DaisyQuest & Daisy's Castle by Gina Erickson, Kelly Foster, David Foster, & Joseph Torgesen	PRO-ED Publishing 8700 Shoal Creek Blvd. Austin, Texas 78757-6897 (512) 451-3246	$89.00 (both) $49.00 (each)

Description: These computer programs require a McIntosh computer as a platform. They contain activities to build rhyme awareness, sound comparison skills, and phoneme analysis and synthesis skills. They were developed with support from a grant from the National Institute of Child Health and Human Development, and several research studies have shown their effectiveness in stimulating phonemic awareness in young children. They do not contain integrated sound-letter activities, so those would have to be added by the teacher after children finish the program.

Phonemic Awareness in Young *Children: A Classroom Curriculum* Marilyn Adams, Barbara Foorman, Ingvar Lundberg, & Terri Beeler.	Brooks Publishing Co. P.O. Box 10624 Baltimore, MD 21285-0624 800-638-3775	$22.95 (manual)

(continued)

TABLE 6-1   Continued

Description: This is a carefully sequenced series of activities that will stimulate phonemic awareness through 15-20 minutes of teacher-led activities each day. It is a complete curriculum that provides detailed guidance about how to sequence and deliver the activities to groups of children. It starts with basic listening activities and takes children through basic word and syllable awareness, rhyme awareness, and into sound comparison and segmenting and blending activities, then to the transition to print. It is most appropriate for kindergarten children, but could also be used with at-risk children in first grade.

The Phonological Awareness Kit by Carolyn Robertson & Wanda Salter	Linguisystems 3100 4th Avenue East Moline, IL 61244 800-776-4332	$69.95 (kit)

Description: This set of materials is designed as a companion to the Phonological Awareness Test described earlier. It contains activities and supporting visual materials to stimulate phonological awareness through several different levels as well as assist in the transition to early decoding skills.

The Waterford Early Reading Program: Level 1	Waterford Institute 2500 N. University Ave. Suite 200 Provo, Utah 84604 800-669-4533	Relatively expensive

Description: A complete kindergarten computer-based program that stimulates phonological awareness, teaches letter names and sounds, and builds print awareness. Very high quality and very comprehensive. Provides enough content for 165 fifteen-minute lessons for every child.

Materials Specifically Designed for At-Risk Children

Phonological Awareness Training for Reading by Joseph Torgesen & Brian Bryant	PRO-ED Publishing 8700 Shoal Creek Blvd Austin, Texas 78757-6897 (512) 451-3246	$129 (kit)

Description: This program is suitable for small group instruction and requires minimal teacher training to use. It was developed with support from a grant from the National Institute of Child Health and Human Development, and there is research evidence to show its effectiveness in stimulating phonemic awareness in at-risk children. It is an organized curriculum that takes children from rhyme awareness, through sound comparison and analysis and synthesis activities, to beginning work with letters in reading and spelling.

Auditory Discrimination in Depth by Patricia Lindamood & Charles Lindamood	PRO-ED 8700 Shoal Creek Blvd Austin, Texas 78757-6897 (512) 451-3246	$329 (kit)

Description: This instructional program builds phonological awareness by helping children to discover and feel the articulatory gestures associated with each phoneme in the English language. Children are taught to "feel" the sounds in words as well as hear them. There is extensive overlap between phonemic awareness activities and reading and spelling exercises. Because of the intensity and explicitness of this program, as well as its multisensory base, it may be particularly appropriate for children with more severe phonological disabilities. It has been used primarily for one-on-one instruction, although newly developed computer software that supports the program may allow it to be used effectively in small groups as well. The program requires special teacher training for maximal effectiveness.

As with any instructional materials, most of the instructional programs and materials described in Table 6-1 can be adapted for uses other than those for which they seem most clearly appropriate. That is, skillful teachers should be able to adapt "whole class" materials to support instruction for small groups of at-risk children, and the more intensive material can also be adapted for whole class instruction (Howard, 1986). In addition, it should be noted that many activities that teachers already engage in can be used to build phonemic awareness. Spelling and writing activities can be used to stimulate phonemic awareness (Ehri, 1992), and any teacher-led reading activities that involved direct instruction in sound-letter correspondences, blending skills, or that draw attention to similarities between the way words are spelled and the way they sound can be used to improve children's awareness of the phonemic structure of words. In general, instruction to stimulate phonological awareness should begin by providing exposure to rhyming songs, books, and activities for children in preschool and the early part of kindergarten. Once children begin to understand the concept of rhyme (as shown by their ability to decided whether words rhyme or to generate rhyming words), they can begin to do a variety of sound comparison activities involving the first, last, and middle sounds of words. Tasks that require children to manipulate, segment, or blend individual phonemes would come next and are most appropriate for use immediately prior to or in conjunction with instruction in sound-letter correspondences and phonemic reading and writing.

Assessment and Instruction of Word Recognition

Assessment of word recognition skills is considerably more complex than assessment of phonemic awareness because readers can identify words in a number of different ways as they process text. Words in text can be identified in at least five different ways (Ehri, 1992, in press):

1. By identifying and blending together the individual phonemes in words
2. By noticing and blending together familiar spelling patterns (i.e., *pre, in*), which is a more advanced form of decoding
3. By recognizing words as whole units or reading them "by sight"
4. By making analogies to other words that are already known
5. By using clues from the context to guess a word's identity

Different processes and knowledge are required to use each of these word identification methods, and these methods play roles of varying importance during different stages of learning to read.

A method that is of primary importance during early stages of learning to read is *phonetic decoding*. To use this method, readers must know the sounds that are usually represented by letters in words, then they must blend together the individual sounds that are identified in each word. This method is important to early reading success because it provides a relatively reliable way to identify words that have not been seen before. As children become more experienced readers, they begin to process letters in larger chunks called *spelling patterns*. This improves decoding speed, because it allows children to process groups of letters as units, rather than having to decode each grapho-phonic unit individually.

Some common spelling patterns found at the end of single syllable words in English are *-ack, -ight, -unk, -eat, -ay, -ash, -ip, -ore,* and *-ell.* Common affixes for longer words include *-able, -ing, -ous, -ize, pro-, con-, pre-,* and *un-.* A number of studies have shown that words that contain common spelling patters like those above are easier to decode if children are familiar with the patterns (Bowey & Hansen, 1994; Trieman, Goswami, & Bruck, 1990).

As children repeatedly read the same word several times, it eventually becomes stored in memory as a *sight word.* No analysis is required to read sight words. A single glance at these words is sufficient to activate information about their pronunciation and meaning. Sight words are read rapidly (within one second) with no pauses between different parts of the word. Sight words are not recognized on the basis of shape or just some of the letters, but rather information about all the letters in a word is used to accurately identify it as a sight word (Adams, 1990).

Those who conduct research on word recognition use the term *orthographic processing* (Ehri, in press) to refer to the way that words are recognized "by sight." The orthography of a language refers to the way it is represented visually. Hence, when researchers indicate that words are processed as *orthographic units,* they are implying that they are recognized on the basis of an integrated visual representation.

When sight words are well practiced (and hence orthographic representations are well established), they can be identified automatically, with almost no expenditure of attention or effort (LaBerge & Samuels, 1974). Having a large vocabulary of sight words that can be recognized automatically is the key to fluent text reading. Because so little effort is required to identify sight words, the reader is able to concentrate effectively on the complex processes involved in constructing the meaning of text (Perfetti, 1985).

Words can also be read by *analogy to known words* (Glushko, 1981; Laxon, Coltheart, & Keating, 1988). For example, the word *cart* might be read by noticing the word *car* and then adding to it the /t/ sound at the end. Longer words like *fountain* might be initially read by noticing its similarity to a known word like *mountain* and making the slight adjustment to pronunciation required for the different initial phoneme. Recent research has shown that children need to have at least a beginning level of phonetic decoding skill before they can effectively use an analogy strategy to identify unknown words (Ehri & Robbins, 1992).

A very different way to identify words in text is to *guess their identity from the context* in which they occur. This context may include pictures on the page or the meaning of the passage. When children make errors in their oral reading, the errors are often consistent with the context, which indicates that this is one source of information they are using to help them identify the words (Biemiller, 1970).

There are three important facts to understand about the use of context to aid word identification. First, skilled readers do not rely on context as a major source of information about words in text (Share & Stanovich, 1995). Second, poor readers actually rely on context clues for identifying words more than good readers do (Briggs, Austin, & Underwood, 1984; Simpson, Lorsback, & Whitehouse, 1983). And third, context, by itself, is not a very accurate way to identify words in text. For example, Gough and Walsh (1991) have shown that only about 10 percent of the words that are most important to the meaning of passages can be guessed correctly from context alone.

These facts do not, however, mean that skill in using context as an aid in word identification is not important to reading and reading growth (Tunmer & Chapman, 1995). When children phonetically decode words, often they do not arrive at the fully correct pronunciation unless they can use contextual constraints to suggest a real word that sounds like their decoding and makes sense in the context (Share & Stanovich, 1995). Furthermore, good readers do appear to use contextual clues as a check on reading accuracy, and they will usually correct their reading if they mispronounce a word that does not fit the context (Adams, 1990).

Issues in the Assessment of Word Recognition

As has been documented in other parts of this book, the word recognition processes most impaired in children with reading disabilities are those that involve identifying words from the visual information in the text (the first four of the five processes in the list just discussed). These children are most frequently impaired in both the ability to apply alphabetic strategies in reading new words (phonetic decoding) and in the ability to retrieve sight words from memory (orthographic processing). They not only have difficulty becoming accurate in the application of these processes, but they frequently have additional special difficulties with becoming fluent in their application. Before discussing specific methods for the diagnostic assessment of these word recognition skills, two general issues require discussion.

First, the assessment that will be outlined here is very different than the "authentic literacy assessment" that is currently advocated by many reading professionals (Paris, Clafee, Filby, Hiebert, Pearson, Valencia, & Wolf, 1992). Authentic assessment is different in at least two ways from the reading assessment measures we will be discussing. First, authentic assessment seeks to measure children's application of broad literacy skills to authentic tasks like gathering information for a report, use of literacy as a medium for social interactions, or ability to read a selection and then write a response to it. It also seeks to measure children's enjoyment, ownership, and involvement in literacy activities both at school and at home. Second, authentic assessment attempts to align assessment directly with instructional goals in the classroom. It is an approach to direct assessment of the kinds of literacy activities that are frequently emphasized particularly in whole language instructional settings.

This kind of assessment is an important complement to the type of diagnostic assessments that will be described for word-level reading skills in this chapter. All of the literacy outcomes that are part of authentic assessment are essential parts of a total literacy assessment program. After all, if a child *can* read, but does not enjoy reading and does not apply important literacy skills to everyday tasks, then some important goals of literacy instruction have not been attained. Furthermore, it is important for teachers to know how children are responding to elements of their instruction that go beyond basic reading skills, and "authentic assessment" procedures are useful for that purpose.

However, since these procedures are focused on high-level reading outcomes, they cannot provide precise information about level of performance on important subskills in reading. If a child's overall performance on authentic literacy tasks is limited, it is frequently difficult to obtain from the work samples used a precise estimate of the specific component processes that are weak. The goal of the kind of assessments that will be discussed in this chapter is to quantify the degree of skill a child possesses in word identification processes that have been shown in many research studies to be critical contributors to overall reading success.

The second issue is that the type of diagnostic assessments described are different from the more informal and comprehensive assessments of word recognition skills that can help to guide instruction. Assessment for diagnoses is different than assessment for teaching. Assessment for instruction would involve use of informal inventories to measure very specific aspects of word-level reading skills such as: what sound-letter correspondences are already known to the child, ability to blend sounds together, knowledge of common prefixes and suffixes, knowledge of syllabification strategies, extent of sight vocabulary for high-frequency words, and so on. All these specific pieces of information are important for instruction, but they are not provided by the general indices of word recognition ability that are part of diagnostic tests.

Commonly Used Diagnostic Measures of Word Recognition Ability

It is beyond the scope of this chapter to identify all the available tests of word recognition skills. Rather, examples of measurement strategies from the most commonly used measures will be provided.

Sight-Word Reading Ability

Two measures are widely used in this area and both involve the same assessment strategy. The Word Identification subtest from the *Woodcock Reading Mastery Test-Revised* (Woodcock, 1987), and the reading subtest of the *Wide Range Achievement Test-3* (Wilkinson, 1995) both require children to read lists of words that gradually increase in length and complexity while decreasing in frequency of occurrence in printed English. For example, the easiest three words on the Word Identification subtest are *go, the,* and *me.* Words of mid-level difficulty are *pioneer, inquire*, and *wealth,* and the hardest three are *epigraphist, facetious,* and *shillelagh.* Of the first 50 words on the test, 31 follow normal phonetic spelling patterns and 39 occur in a list of the 1000 most frequent words in English (Fry, Kress, & Fountoukidis, 1993). After about third-grade level, none of the words on the list are among the 1000 most frequent.

Neither of these widely used tests places stringent time pressure on students, so both phonetic decoding processes and sight-word processes can be used to identify words on these lists. Both tests have been normed nationally, so that they provide age-equivalent, grade-equivalent, percentile, and standard score estimates of children's ability to read words out of context. The strength of these measures is that they allow a direct assessment of children's ability to identify words solely on the basis of the word's spelling. When reading text, children also have context clues available to assist word identification. Thus, text-based measures, although more "authentic" in one sense, are less direct in their assessment of the kinds of word processing skills that are particularly deficient in children with RD.

Phonetic Decoding Ability

The single best measure of children's ability to apply grapho-phonetic knowledge in decoding words is provided by measures of nonword reading (Share & Stanovich, 1995). The Word Attack subtest of the *Woodcock Reading Mastery Test-Revised* (Woodcock, 1987) is a good example of this kind of diagnostic test. It consists of a series of increasingly complex nonwords that children are asked to "sound out as best they can." The three easiest items on the test are *ree, ip,* and *din,* items of moderate difficulty are *rejune, depine,* and *viv,* and the three hardest items are *pnir, ceisminadolt,* and *byrcal.* Because the words are presented out of context, they stress the child's ability to fully analyze each word to produce the correct pronunciation. On the other hand, measures such as this do not allow an assessment of children's ability to combine phonetic decoding with use of context to arrive at a word's correct pronunciation. However, since both good and poor readers appear able to use context equally well (as long as the context is understood, [Share & Stanovich, 1995]), this is not an important omission on a diagnostic measure of word recognition ability.

Word Recognition Fluency

Measures of word recognition fluency have typically assessed the rate of reading connected text. One of the more widely used measures in this area is the *Gray Oral Reading Test-3rd Edition* (Wiederholt & Bryant, 1992). This test consists of thirteen increasingly difficult passages, each followed by five comprehension questions. A measure of oral reading rate is obtained by recording the time it takes for the child to read each passage. The test provides procedures to combine the rate score with a score for word reading accuracy to form a Passage score. The Passage score reflects the combination of reading speed and accuracy, and typical normed reference comparisons are available for this score.

One potential problem with the *Gray Oral Reading Test* is that it does not provide a very sensitive measure of individual differences in word recognition ability at very low levels of performance, such as those found in beginning first graders, or disabled readers through second grade. The passages simply begin at too high a level for children with very poor or undeveloped reading skills to display the word recognition skills they actually possess. In an effort to provide measures of fluency and accuracy in word recognition skill that are simple to administer and sensitive to individual differences across a broad range of reading skills, we (Torgesen & Wagner, 1997) have developed simple measures of *Word Reading Efficiency* and *Nonword Reading Efficiency.* In both of these measures, children are shown lists of increasingly difficult words and nonwords and asked to read as many words as possible in 45 seconds. There are two forms to each test, and the child's score is simply the average number of words read in 45 seconds. Initial evaluations indicate that these measures are very reliable (parallel form reliabilities vary between .97 and .98 for kindergarten through fifth grade). They are also highly correlated with corresponding measures from the *Woodcock Reading Mastery Test-Revised* at early grades (when children often run out of words they can read before they run out of time, correlations range from .89 to .94) and slightly less correlated (.86 to .88) at fourth grade, when fluency of word recognition processes becomes more important to performance on the tests.

To summarize, an adequate diagnostic assessment of children's word recognition abilities should include out-of-context measures of word recognition ability, phonetic decoding ability (as measured by ability to read nonwords), and word recognition fluency. The fluency measures become more important after about second to third grade, after children have acquired a fund of word recognition skills they can apply with reasonable accuracy. Measures that involve out-of-context word reading more directly assess the kinds of word recognition skills that are particularly problematic for children with RD because they eliminate the contextual support on which these children rely heavily. To obtain a *complete* picture of overall reading development, however, it is also important to observe the way that children integrate all sources of information about words in text, and this can only be estimated by carefully observing children as they read connected passages.

Instruction in Word Recognition

It is possible to combine what is known about reading growth with knowledge of the factors that specifically limit reading growth in some children to construct a hierarchy of instructional issues for children with RD (Torgesen, 1997a). First, can these children be taught to utilize grapho-phonic information accurately and fluently in reading novel words? In other words, can children with serious phonological processing disabilities be taught effective phonetic decoding skills? Second, if they can be taught good phonetic decoding ability, does this skill lead to the development of a rich vocabulary of words that can be recognized fluently by sight? That is, will orthographic (sight-word) reading skills develop normally in RD children if they can be taught reliable phonetic decoding skills? And, finally, can these children utilize newly taught phonetic and orthographic word reading skills to produce acceptable levels of reading comprehension?

Answers to the first two of these questions are related to one another, because we really do not know how well developed one's phonetic decoding abilities must be in order to facilitate the growth of a sight-word vocabulary. It is likely that the influence of one's phonetic reading skill on the growth of fluent word recognition processes will be affected by a number of other factors such as size of oral vocabulary, amount of reading practice and breadth of print exposure, and effective use of context. Weaknesses in phonetic decoding ability may be compensated for by strengths in one of these latter factors, while extra strength in phonetic reading ability may enable growth in orthographic skills even in the presence of weakness in one of these other variables. It is also possible that many children with phonologically based reading disabilities may have additional weaknesses that interfere specifically with the formation of orthographic representations for words (e.g., phonological retrieval [Bowers & Wolf, 1993]).

As a starting point, however, it seems clear that instructional methods must have a significant impact on the phonetic reading skills of these children if they are going to have a lasting long-term effect on reading growth. This inference creates a dilemma of sorts for those who are interested in preventing or remediating reading disabilities. Instruction to build phonetic decoding skills, which are seen as essential in normal reading growth, is instruction directed toward the primary cognitive/linguistic *weakness* of most children with severe reading disabilities. There is a strong component of instructional theory in the area of learning disabilities (Hammill & Bartel, 1995) that emphasizes teaching to children's strengths rather than their weaknesses. Thus, we sometimes see recommendations to teach reading disabled children using sight-word or visually based approaches that do not overly stress limited phonological abilities.

Experienced reading clinicians have favored multisensory, phonetically based approaches to instruction for children with RD from very early in the history of the field (Clark & Uhry, 1995). Until fairly recently, however, research and case study information tended to emphasize how extremely difficult it is to teach these children generalized phonetic reading skills (Lovett, Warren-Chaplin, Ransby, & Borden, 1990; Lyon, 1985; Snowling &

Hulme, 1989). In contrast to these earlier results, more recent work by Lovett and her associates (Lovett, Borden, Deluca, Lacerenza, Benson, & Brackstone, 1994) and by others (Alexander, Andersen, Heilman, Voeller, & Torgesen, 1991; Brown & Felton, 1990; Foorman, Francis, Fletcher, Schatschneider, & Menta, in press, Vellutino et al., 1996; Wise & Olsen, 1995) has reported significant success in building generalized phonetic reading skills in children with phonologically based reading disabilities. In two ongoing studies in which we are involved (Torgesen, Wagner, Rashotte, Alexander, & Conway, in press), we are also obtaining very encouraging results about the ability of children with phonologically based reading disabilities to acquire functional phonetic decoding abilities when exposed to the right instructional conditions.

In one of our studies, for example, we are working with 8 to 10-year-old children who have already been identified by the public school system as learning disabled. Children were initially identified by their teachers as those having the greatest difficulties acquiring word recognition skills, and then we verified their difficulties in phonetic decoding and phonological awareness through a series of tests of our own.

One of the more unusual things about this study is the intensity of the instruction provided to the children. Students are seen individually in two-hour sessions, five days a week, for about eight weeks, or a total of eighty hours of instruction. Following the intensive instruction, students are seen in their learning disabilities classroom by the project teacher for one hour a week for eight weeks. The purpose of this follow-up instruction is to help the children generalize their newly developed reading skills to the kinds of assignments they receive in the classroom.

The children are being randomly assigned to two different instructional conditions. Although each of the instructional programs contain relatively explicit instruction in "phonics," this instruction is provided in two different ways. The *Auditory Discrimination In-Depth Program* (ADD) (Lindamood & Lindamood, 1984) stimulates phonological awareness by helping children discover the articulatory positions and movements associated with the different phonemes in the English language. For example, they learn to label the sounds represented by the letters *p* and *b* as *lip poppers* because of the way the lips pop open and air pops out when they are pronounced. The sounds represented by *t* and *d* are labeled *tip tappers* because of the way the tip of the tongue taps against the roof of the mouth when they are pronounced. After discovering the articulatory gestures associated with each phoneme, students are able to "feel" the identity, order, and number of sounds in words as well as hear them. They can also identify the phonemes in words by observing their mouths in a mirror as they pronounce the word. This curriculum also provides explicit instruction in letter-sound correspondences along with extensive instruction and practice in the application of these correspondences to decoding words, both out of context and within meaningful text. This approach is designed to provide a level of instruction and experience in phonological processing of words that is much deeper than most reading instructional methods.

The other approach, which we call *Embedded Phonics* (EP), provides less intensive, but still explicit and systematic, phonics training in the context of meaningful experiences in reading and writing text. Both approaches acknowledge that the children being instructed have special difficulties processing phonological information. However, the ADD program attempts to directly attack these difficulties through an intensive program of oral and phonological awareness training, while the EP program seeks to reduce the demands on these skills by using an approach to phonics instruction that does not place as much emphasis on full phonological decoding, but rather emphasizes the early integration of partial phonological decodings with context clues to identify unknown words. The EP method also focuses on direct instruction in a core sight-word vocabulary to support fluent reading in the texts that children read during their instructional sessions.

Thus far, we have immediate posttest data on 50 children, 24 in the ADD group and 26 in the EP condition, and one-year follow-up data on 27 children (Torgesen, 1997a, b). The most striking feature of the immediate posttest results so far is the large gains that children in both instructional conditions are making in the accuracy of their phonetic decoding skills. Children in both groups have moved from below the 2nd percentile in performance on measures of phonetic reading up into the average range. This change represents from about one and a half (EP group) to two years (ADD group) of growth in this skill over the eighty hours of instruction. The children have also experienced substantial growth in their ability to recognize real words and to comprehend what they read, although these changes have not been as dramatic as those for phonetic reading skills. Table 6-2 shows the changes in standard score experienced by the children in each group on five reading measures. Another important observation from these results is that changes in fluency of word recognition processes were not nearly as great as those for accuracy. The comprehension scores at the end of the intervention are roughly consistent with the children's general verbal ability.

Figure 6-2 provides a graphic illustration of the dramatic change in growth rate caused by this intensive intervention, and it also shows that the students are continuing to improve their reading skills in the following year. This figure simply plots growth in raw score on

TABLE 6-2   Changes in Standard Score on Reading Measures Resulting from 80 Hours of Intensive Instruction

	Group					
	ADD (n=24)			EP (n=26)		
	pre	post	gain	pre	post	gain
Word Attack[1]	68	95	27	69	90	21
Nonword Efficiency[2]	72	83	11	79	86	7
Word Identification[1]	69	82	13	65	81	16
Word Efficiency[3]	67	74	7	67	76	9
Passage Comprehension[1]	82	92	10	84	91	7

*Note. This table contains scores for each test in standard score units (Mean = 100, SD = 15.)

[1]Word Attack, Word Identification and Passage Comprehension subtests from the *Woodcock Reading Mastery Test-Revised* (Woodcock, 1987)

[2]*Nonword Reading Efficiency* —a measure of fluency in alphabetic reading that requires children to read as many nonwords as possible in 45 seconds from a list that increases from two phoneme nonwords to 10 phoneme words (locally normed).

[3]*Word Reading Efficiency* —a measure of fluency in word reading that requires children to read as many words as possible in 45 seconds from a word list that gradually increases in difficulty (locally normed).

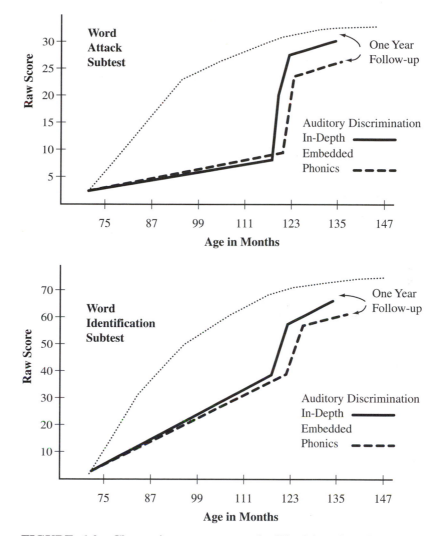

FIGURE 6-2 **Change in raw scores on the Word Attack and Word Identification subtests as a function of age for children receiving eighty hours of intensive intervention in reading.**

the Word Attack and Word Identification measures as a function of age in months. The dotted line at the top of each graph represents normal growth on these measures.

The most appropriate conclusion from recent instructional research with children who have phonologically based reading disabilities is that it is clearly possible to have a substantial impact on the growth of their phonetic decoding skills if the proper instructional conditions are in place. These conditions appear to involve instruction that is more *explicit*, more *intensive*, and more *supportive* than that which is usually offered in most public and private school settings.

It is more *explicit* in that it makes fewer assumptions about pre-existing skills or children's abilities to make inferences about sound-letter regularities on their own. For example, most successful programs have involved some form of direct instruction designed to stimulate children's awareness of the phonological segments in words. Although some form of instruction in phonological awareness characterizes all successful programs, there has been substantial variability in the way this instruction is provided.

A second way in which successful instruction for children with RD must be explicit involves direct instruction in sound-letter correspondences and in strategies for using these correspondences to decode words while reading text. Explicit instruction and practice in these skills is characteristic of *all* programs that have produced substantial growth in phonetic reading skills in children with RD. In a direct test of the utility of this type of instruction, Iversen and Tunmer (1993) added explicit training in phonological decoding to the popular *Reading Recovery* (Clay, 1979) program, which has traditionally placed less emphasis on instruction and practice in these skills. This carefully controlled study showed that a small amount of explicit instruction in phonics increased the efficiency of the *Reading Recovery* program by approximately 37 percent.

In addition to being more explicit, effective reading instruction for children with RD must be more *intensive* than regular classroom instruction. Increased intensity involves more teacher-student instructional interactions, or reinforced learning trials, per unit of time. Intensity of instruction can be increased either by lengthening total instructional time, or by reducing teacher-pupil ratios. Children with the most severe phonological processing disabilities will almost certainly require a substantial amount of individual or small group instruction in order to attain adequate reading skills.

A third way in which instruction for children with reading disabilities must be modified in order to be successful involves the level of *support* provided within the instructional interactions. At least two kinds of special support are required. First, because acquiring word recognition skills is more difficult for these children than others, they will require more *emotional* support in the form of encouragement, positive feedback, and enthusiasm from the teacher in order to maintain their motivation to learn. Second, instructional interactions must be more supportive in the sense that they involve carefully *scaffolded* interactions with the child. In a recent investigation of the characteristics of effective reading tutors, Juel (1996) identified the number of scaffolded interactions during each teaching session as one of the critical variables predicting differences in effectiveness across tutors. A scaffolded interaction is one in which the teacher enables the student to complete a task (i.e., read a word) by directing the student's attention to a key piece of information or breaking the task up into smaller, easier to manage ones. The goal of these interactions is to provide just enough support so the child can go through the processing steps necessary to find the right answer. In essence, the teacher leads the child to do all the thinking required to accomplish a task (decoding or spelling a word) that he or she could not do without teacher support. With enough practice, the child becomes able to go through the processing steps independently. Juel's finding about the importance of carefully scaffolded instructional interactions is consistent with the emphasis on these types of interactions in the teacher's manuals that accompany two instructional programs shown to be effective with children who have severe reading disabilities (Lindamood & Lindamood, 1984; Wilson, 1988).

Issues for Future Research and Development

Although research over the past twenty years has made enormous progress in helping to develop appropriate diagnostic and instructional procedures for children who experience difficulties acquiring good word recognition skills, there are many important issues remaining for further research and development. For example, we still do not understand fully the amount and type of instruction and practice that will be required for *all* RD children to attain normal word-level reading. Even in studies that produce very large gains in phonetic reading ability, some children remain significantly impaired in this area at the conclusion of the study. Furthermore, even in a remedial effort such as ours that produced very large improvements in the accuracy of children's word recognition skills, the children still obtained an average standard score of approximately 75 on the Word Reading Efficiency measure. Whether word reading efficiency will improve simply with more practice, or whether RD children need to be explicitly taught to process words in chunks larger than individual phonemes (cf. Gaskins, Ehri, Cress, O'Hara, & Donnelly, 1997; Henry & Redding, 1996), is still an open question.

We also need to understand more about the range of individual differences in the level of word recognition ability required for good reading comprehension. We know that, in general, better phonetic reading ability and more fluent word recognition skills are associated with better reading comprehension (Share & Stanovich, 1995). We also know that better phonetic reading skills are reliably associated with more accurate and fluent word recognition ability (Adams, 1990; Beck & Juel, 1995; Chall, 1983). However, cases have been reported in which students seem able to develop good word recognition ability in the absence of strongly developed phonetic skills. In one particular case (Campbell & Butterworth, 1985), the student was highly motivated to learn to read, had substantially above average general intellectual ability, and was particularly strong on measures of visual memory. If there prove to be certain limits on fluency of phonological processes in reading for many children, it will be very helpful to understand more fully what other routes to effective reading may be available.

In addition to the content of instruction (the skills and knowledge that are taught), we also need to learn more about the critical "arts" of good instruction for children with RD. For example, there is fairly wide agreement that scaffolded interactions between teachers and children is a very effective way to build complex information processing skills (Brown & Palincsar, 1987; Stone, 1989). Connie Juel's (1996) beginning demonstration of the utility of scaffolded interactions during instruction in word recognition skills is an example of the kind of research on the process of instruction that is needed. As teachers are trained to help children with RD, they need to learn not only what they should teach, but also how they should teach it.

References

Adams, M., Foorman, B., Lundberg, I. & Beeler, C. (1997). *Phonemic awareness in young children: A classroom curriculum.* Baltimore, MD: Brooks Publishing Co.

Adams, M.J. (1990). *Beginning to read: Thinking and learning about print.* Cambridge, MA: MIT Press.

Alexander, A., Anderson, H., Heilman, P.C., Voeller, K.S., & Torgesen, J.K. (1991). Phonological awareness training and remediation of analytic decoding deficits in a group of severe dyslexics. *Annals of Dyslexia, 41,* 193–206.

Ball, E.W., & Blachman, B. A. (1991). Does phoneme awareness training in kindergarten make a difference in early word recognition and developmental spelling? *Reading Research Quarterly, 26,* 49–66.

Beck, I.L. & Juel, C. (1995) The role of decoding in learning to read. *American Educator, 19,* 8–42.

Biemiller, A. (1970). The development of the use of graphic and contextual information as children learn to read. *Reading Research Quarterly, 6,* 75–96.

Blachman, B. (1989). Phonological awareness and word recognition: Assessment and intervention. In A. G. Kamhi & H.W. Catts (Eds.), *Reading disabilities: A developmental language perspective* (133–158). Boston: Allyn & Bacon.

Blachman, B. (1997). Early intervention and phonological awareness: A cautionary tale. In B. Blachman (Ed.) *Foundations of reading acquisition and dyslexia, implications for early intervention.* Mahwah, NJ: Erlbaum.

Blachman, B., Ball, E., Black, S. & Tangel, D. (1994). Kindergarten teachers develop phoneme awareness in low-income, inner-city classrooms: Does it make a difference? *Reading and Writing: An Interdisciplinary Journal, 6,* 1–17.

Bowers, P.G., & Wolf, M. (1993). Theoretical links between naming speed, precise timing mechanisms and orthographic skill in dyslexia. *Reading and Writing: An Interdisciplinary Journal, 5,* 69–85.

Bowey, J., & Hansen, J. (1994). The development of orthographic rimes as units of word recognition. *Journal of Experimental Child Psychology. 58,* 465–488.

Bradley, L., & Bryant, P. (1985). *Rhyme and reason in reading and spelling.* Ann Arbor: University of Michigan Press.

Briggs, A., Austin, R., & Underwood, G. (1984). Phonological coding in good and poor readers. *Reading Research Quarterly, 20,* 54–66.

Brown, I. S., & Felton, R.H. (1990) Effects of instruction on beginning reading skills in children at risk for reading disability. *Reading and Writing: An Interdisciplinary Journal, 2,* 223–241.

Brown, A.L., & Palincsar, A.S. (1987). Reciprocal teaching of comprehension strategies: A natural history

of one program for enhancing learning. In L. Borkowski & L.D. Day (Eds.), *Intelligence and exceptionality: New directions for theory, assessment, and instructional practices.* (pp. 81–132) New York: Ablex.

Byrne, B., & Fielding-Barnsley, R. (1993). Evaluation of a program to teach phonemic awareness to young children: A 1-year follow-up. *Journal of Educational Psychology, 85,* 104–111.

Campbell, R., & Butterworth, B. (1985). Phonological dyslexia and dysgraphia in a highly literate subject: A developmental case with associated deficits of phonemic processing and awareness. *The Quarterly Journal of Experimental Psychology, 37,* 435–475.

Catts, H.W. (1996). *Phonological awareness: A key to detection.* Paper presented at conference titled The Spectrum of Developmental Disabilities XVIII: Dyslexia. Johns Hopkins Medical Institutions, Baltimore, March.

Catts, H.W., & Vartianen, T. (1993). *Sounds abound: Listening rhyming, and reading.* East Moline, IL: LinguiSystems, Inc.

Catts, H.W., Wilcox, K.A., Wood-Jackson, C., Larrivee, L.S., & Scott, V.G. (1997) Toward an understanding of phonological awareness. In C.K. Leong & R.M. Joshi (Eds.). *Cross-language studies of learning to read and spell: Phonologic and orthographic processing.* Dordecht: Klüwer Academic Press.

Chall, J.S. (1983). *Stages of reading development.* New York: McGraw Hill.

Clark, D.B., & Uhry, J.K. (1995). *Dyslexia: Theory and practice of remedial instruction, (2nd ed.).* Baltimore, MD: York Press.

Clay, M.M. (1979). *Reading: The patterning of complex behavior.* Auckland, New Zealand: Heinemann.

Cunningham, A.E. (1990). Explicit versis implicit instruction in phonemic awareness. *Journal of Experimental Child Psychology, 50,* 429–444.

Ehri, L.C. (1992). Reconceptualizing the development of sight word reading and its relationship to recoding. In P.B. Gough, L.C. Ehri, & R. Trieman (Eds.), *Reading acquisition* (pp. 107–143). Hillsdale, NJ: Erlbaum.

Ehri, L.C. (in press). Grapheme-phoneme knowledge is essential for learning to read words in English. In J. Metsala & L. Ehri (Eds.), *Word recognition in beginning reading.* Hillsdale, NJ: Erlbaum.

Ehri, L.C., & Robbins, C. (1992). Beginners need some decoding skill to read words by analogy. *Reading Research Quarterly, 27,* 12–26.

Erickson, G.C., Foster, K.C., Foster, D.F., & Torgesen, J.K. (1992). *DaisyQuest.* Austin, TX: PRO-ED, Inc.

Erickson, G.C., Foster, K.C., Foster, D.F., & Torgesen, J.K. (1993). *Daisy's castle.* Austin, TX: PRO-ED, Inc.

Fletcher, J.M., Shaywitz, S.E., Shankweiler, D.P., Katz, L., Liberman, I.Y., Stuebing, K.K., Francis, D.J., Fowler, A.E., & Shaywitz, B.A. (1994). Cognitive profiles of reading disability: Comparisons of discrepancy and low achievement definitions. *Journal of Educational Psychology, 86,* 6–23.

Foorman, B.R., Francis, D.J., Fletcher, J.M., Schatschneider, C., & Mehta, P. (in press). The role of instruction in learning to read: Preventing reading failure in at-risk children. *Journal of Educational Psychology.*

Foorman, B.R., & Schatschneider, C. (1997). Beyond alphabetic reading: Comments on Torgesen's prevention and intervention studies. *Journal of Academic Language Therapy, 1,* 59–65.

Fry, E.B., Kress, J.E., & Fountoukidis, D.L. (1993). *The reading teacher's book of lists.* Englewood Cliffs, NJ: Prentice Hall.

Gaskins, I.W., Ehri, L.C., Cress, C. O'Hara, C., & Donnelly, K. (1997). Procedures for word learning: Making discoveries about words. *The Reading Teacher, 50,* 312–327.

Glushko, R.J. (1981). Principles for pronouncing print: The psychology of phonography. In A.M. Lesgold & C.A. Perfetti (Eds.), *Interactive processing in reading* (pp. 61–84). Hillsdale, NJ: Erlbaum.

Gough, P., & Walsh , S. (1991). Chinese, Phoenicians, and the orthographic cipher of English. In S. Brady & D. Shankweiler (1991), *Phonological processes in literacy: A tribute to Isabelle Y. Liberman.* Hillsdale, NJ: Erlbaum.

Hammill, D.D., & Bartel, M.R. (1995). *Teaching children with learning and behavior problems.* Boston: Allyn & Bacon.

Henry, M.K., & Redding, N.C. (1996). *Patterns for success in reading and spelling: A multisensory approach to teaching phonics and word analysis.* Austin, TX: PRO-ED, Inc.

Hoien, T., Lundberg, I., Stanovich, K.E., & Bjaalid, I. (1995). Components of phonological awareness. *Reading and Writing: An Interdisciplinary Journal, 7,* 171–188.

Howard, M. (1986). *Effects of pre-reading training in auditory conceptualization on subsequent reading achievement.* Ph.D. dissertation, Brigham Young University.

Iversen, S., & Tunmer, W.E. (1993) Phonological processing skills and the reading recovery program. *Journal of Educational Psychology, 85,* 112–126.

Juel, C. (1996). What makes literacy tutoring effective? *Reading Research Quarterly, 31,* 268–289.

LaBerge, D., & Samuels, S.J. (1974). Toward a theory of automatic information processing in reading. *Cognitive Psychology, 6,* 293–323.

Laxon, V., Coltheart, V., & Keating, C. (1988). Children find friendly words friendly too: Words with many orthographic neighbours are easier to read and spell. *British Journal of Educational Pyschology, 58,* 103–119.

Lindamood, C.H., & Lindamood, P.C. (1979). *Lindamood Auditory Conceptualization Test.* Austin, TX: PRO-ED.

Lindamood, C.H., & Lindamood, P.C. (1984). *Auditory Discrimination in Depth.* Austin, TX: PRO-ED.

Lovett, M.W., Borden, S.L., Deluca T., Lacerenza, T.D, Benson, N.J., & Brackstone, D. (1994). Treating the core deficits of developmental dyslexia: Evidence of transfer of learning after phonologically and strategy-based reading training programs. *Developmental Psychology, 30,* 805–822.

Lovett, M.W., Warren-Chaplin, P.M., Ransby, M.J., & Borden, S.L. (1990). Training the word recognition skills of reading disabled children: Treatment and transfer effects. *Journal of Educational Psychology, 82,* 769–780.

Lundberg, I. (1988). Preschool prevention of reading failure: Does training in phonological awareness work? In R.L. Masland and M.W. Masland (Eds.), *Prevention of reading failure* (pp. 163–176). Parkton, MD: York Press.

Lundberg, I., Frost, J., & Peterson, O. (1988). Effects of an extensive program for stimulating phonological awareness in pre-school children. *Reading Research Quarterly, 23,* 263–284.

Lyon, G.R. (1985). Identification and remediation of learning disability subtypes: Preliminary findings. *Learning Disabilities Focus, 1,* 21–35.

Mann, V.A. (1993). Phoneme awareness and future reading ability. *Journal of Learning Disabilities, 26,* 259–269.

Mann, V.A. Tobin, P., & Wilson, R. (1987). Measuring phonological awareness through the invented spellings of kindergarten children. *Merrill-Palmer Quarterly, 33,* 365–389.

National Center for Learning Disabilities (NCLD) (1996, Summer). Learning to read, reading to learn: NCLD joins in a national campaign to prevent reading failure among young children. *NCLD News*, p. 6.

Paris, S.G., Clafee, R.C., Filby, N., Hiebert, E.H., Pearson, P.D., Valencia S.W., & Wolf, K.P. (1992). A framework for authentic literacy assessment. *The Reading Teacher, 46,* 88–98.

Perfetti, C.A. (1985). *Reading ability.* New York: Oxford University Press,

Robertson, C., & Salter, W. (1995). *The Phonological Awareness Kit.* East Moline, IL: Linguisystems.

Robertson, C., & Salter, W. (1997). *Phonological Awareness Test.* East Moline, I.: LinguiSystems.

Rosner, J. (1975). *Helping children overcome learning difficulties.* New York: Walker and Company.

Share, D.L., & Stanovich, K.E. (1995). Cognitive processes in early reading development: A model of acquisition and individual differences. *Issues in Education: Contributions from Educational Psychology, 1,* 1–57.

Simpson, G.B., Lorsbach, T., & Whitehouse, D. (1983). Encoding and contextual components of word recognition in good and poor readers. *Journal of Experimental Child Psychology, 35,* 161–171.

Snowling, M., & Hulme, C. (1989). A longitudinal case study of developmental phonological dyslexia. *Cognitive Neuropsychology, 6,* 379–401.

Stanovich, K.E., Cunningham, A.E., & Cramer, B.B. (1984). Assessing phonological awareness in kindergarten children: Issues of task comparability. *Journal of Experimental Child Psychology, 38,* 175–190.

Stone, A. (1989). Improving the effectiveness of strategy training for learning disabled students: The role of communicational dynamics. *Remedial and Special Education, 10,* 35–41.

Torgesen, J.K. (1997a). The prevention and remediation of reading disabilities: Evaluating what we know from research. *Journal of Academic Language Therapy, 1,* 11–47.

Torgesen, J.K. (1997b). *Conclusions from intervention research with children who have phonologically based reading disabilities: What we have learned from 10 years of research.* Invited paper presented at Conference titled, "Progress and Promise in Research and Education for Individuals with Learning Disabilities." Sponsored by the National Institutes of Health and the Learning Disabilities Association of America, Washington, D.C., May.

Torgesen, J.K., & Bryant, B. (1993). *Phonological awareness training for reading.* Austin, TX: PRO-ED.

Torgesen, J.K., & Bryant, B. (1994). *Test of Phonological Awareness.* Austin, TX: PRO-ED.

Torgesen, J.K., Burgess, S., & Rashotte, C.A. (1996). *Predicting phonologically based reading disabilities: What is gained by waiting a year?* Paper presented at the annual meetings of the Society for the Scientific Study of Reading, New York, April, 1996.

Torgesen, J.K., & Davis, C. (1996). Individual difference variables that predict response to training in phonological awareness. *Journal of Experimental Child Psychology, 63,* 1–21.

Torgesen, J.K., & Morgan, S. (1990). Phonological synthesis tasks: A developmental, functional, and componential analysis. In H.L. Swanson & B. Keogh (Eds.) *Learning disabilities: Theoretical and research issues.* Hillsdale, NJ: Erlbaum.

Torgesen, J.K., & Wagner, R.K. (1997). *Test of Word and Nonword Reading Efficiency.* Austin, TX: PRO-ED.

Torgesen, J.K., Wagner, R.K., & Rashotte, C.A. (1994). Longitudinal studies of phonological processing and reading. *Journal of Learning Disabilities, 27.* 276–286.

Torgesen, J.K., Wagner, R.K., & Rashotte, C.A., Alexander, A. W., & Conway, T. (in press). Preventive and remedial interventions for children with severe reading disabilities. *Learning Disabilities: An Interdisciplinary Journal.*

Torgesen, J.K., Wagner, R.K., Rashotte, C.A., Burgess, S.R., & Hecht, S.A. (1997). The contributions of phonological awareness and rapid automatic naming ability to the growth of word reading skills in second to fifth grade children. *Scientific Studies of Reading*, 1, 161–185.

Trieman, R., Goswami, U., & Bruck, M. (1990). Not all nonwords are alike: Implications for reading development and theory. *Memory and Cognition, 18,* 559–567.

Tunmer, W.E., & Chapman, J.W. (1995). Context use in early reading development: Premature exclusion of a source of individual differences? *Issues in Education, 1,* 97–100.

Vellutino, F. R., Scanlon, D.M., Sipay, E.R., Small S. G., Pratt, A., Chen R., & Denckla, M.B. (1996). Cognitive profiles of difficult-to-remediate and readily remediated poor readers: Early intervention as a vehicle for distinguishing between cognitive and experiential deficits as basic causes of specific reading disability. *Journal of Educational Psychology, 88,* 601–638.

Wagner, R.K. & Torgesen, J.K. (1997). *The Comprehensive Test of Phonological Processes in Reading.* Austin, TX: PRO-ED.

Wagner, R.K., Torgesen, J.K., & Rashotte, C.A. (1994). The development of reading-related phonological processing abilities: New evidence of bi-directional causality from a latent variable longitudinal study. *Developmental Psychology, 30,* 73–87.

Wiederholt, J.L. Y Bryant, B.R. (1992). *Gray Oral Reading Tests—III.* Austin, TX: PRO-ED.

Wilkinson, G.S. (1995). *The Wide Range Achievement Test-3.* Wilmington, DE: Jastak Associates.

Wilson, B.A. (1988). *Instructor manual.* Millbury, MA: Wilson Language Training.

Wise, B.W., & Olsen, R.K. (1995). Computer-based phonological awareness and reading instruction. *Annals of Dyslexia, 45,* 99–122.

Wolf, M. (1991). Naming speed and reading: The contribution of the cognitive neurosciences. *Reading Research Quarterly, 26,* 123–141.

Woodcock, R.W. (1987). *Woodcock Reading Mastery Tests-Revised.* Circle Pines, MN: American Guidance Service.

Yopp, H.K. (1988) The validity and reliability of phonemic awareness tests. *Reading Research Quarterly, 23,* 159–177.

Yopp, H.K. (1995). A test for assessing phonemic awareness in young children. The *Reading Teacher, 49,* 20–29.

Chapter 7

Assessing and Facilitating Text Comprehension Problems

CAROL E. WESTBY

In a culture where written language is prominent and readily available, basic literacy is a natural extension of an individual's linguistic development.
—*(FILLION & BRAUSE, 1987, p. 216)*

All language processes are dependent on the same superordinate cognitive abilities. The relations between oral and written language are fundamental and reciprocal; reading and writing are initially dependent on oral language and eventually extend oral-language abilities (Flood & Lapp, 1987). Young children use their oral language skills to learn to read, while older children use their reading ability to further their language learning—they read to learn. Once children are able to decode and read words and simple sentences, their focus should shift from the decoding of learning to read to the comprehension of reading to learn. In order to read to learn, students must learn how to learn from reading; they must learn how

Acknowledgments

Information on narrative development and suggestions for narrative assessment have emerged from a project conducted by the author and Dr. Zelda Maggart and Dr. Richard Van Dongen at the University of New Mexico and Dr. Natalie Hedberg at the University of Colorado.. Many of the practical activities in this chapter have been suggested and implemented in the classroom by Linda Costlow, Cynthia Garcia, Rosario Roman, Barbara Stirbis, and numerous graduate students.

to use their language, cognitive abilities, and background knowledge to comprehend text so they can acquire new knowledge (Brown, 1982; Pearson & Fielding, 1991).

Reading to learn, or comprehending texts, requires understanding a literate language style, which involves comprehension of novel words and increasingly complex sentences; yet, more than comprehension of novel words and complex sentences is required for reading to learn. Readers must possess and acquire ever-increasing knowledge of their physical and social world, and they must know why they are reading; they must be aware of the communicative function or genre of the text (Brewer, 1980; Cope & Kalantzis, 1993). A text may be a narrative with the purpose to entertain or teach, a description with the purpose to explain how to do something, an exposition with the purpose to present an organized body of information and develop a theory, or an argument with the purpose to persuade readers to change their opinions or ideas.

If students are to read to learn, they must also expect texts to make sense. Beaugrande (1984) proposed that reading to learn is dependent on one's having a model of, or purpose for, reading and on one's capacities for building models to organize the information encountered. To develop a model for the reading act and for gaining knowledge requires metacognitive processes; that is, the self-regulatory ability of students to design and monitor their own reading comprehension processes (Brown, 1982; Pressley, Woloshyn, & Associates, 1995).

A major difference between good and poor readers is their view or model for the reading act and the way they build models for gaining knowledge during the act of reading. Good readers know that texts should make sense and that one reads to learn new information, while poor readers believe reading is sounding out words or saying the words fast, fluently, and with expression (Clay, 1973; Johns & Ellis, 1976; Myers & Paris, 1978; Reid, 1966; Weaver, 1994). If students recognize the goal or purpose of reading as comprehending text, they are more likely to be actively involved in achieving this goal by monitoring their progress toward it. Effective readers must have some awareness and control of cognitive strategies they use while reading (Baker & Brown, 1984). Poor readers exhibit less awareness and use of these strategies (Bos & Filip, 1982; Meyer, 1987; Owings, Peterson, Bransford, Morris, & Stein, 1980; Willows & Ryan, 1981; Wong, 1982).

The definition of what it means to be literate—and comprehend what one has read—has changed (Morris & Tchudi, 1996). When the United States was colonized in the seventeenth through the nineteenth centuries, being literate meant the ability to decode and encode, to say the words on a printed page, and to say what the words meant. This *basic literacy* is what has been associated with the 3Rs. Basic literacy is no longer sufficient in a technological, global economy. Persons must also have *critical literacy.* They must be able to move beyond literal meanings, to interpret texts, and to use writing not simply to record, but to interpret, analyze, synthesize, and explain. Students must be able to do more that retell the events of a story or the steps in an experiment. They must be able to determine story theme, interpret characters' motivations, and perceive interrelationships among themes in different stories; they must be able to hypothesize what will happen in an experiment and explain their observations. Even critical literacy, however, is not sufficient to meet the demands of current society. Persons must possess *dynamic literacy.* They must be able to go beyond the texts, acting on the content gained from texts and interrelating the content for problem-raising and problem-solving matters. For example, recently students in Minnesota discovered many deformed frogs on a field trip. They, and the scientists they have interested, asked why the frogs were deformed and what the significance of the deformed frogs might be to people. They must integrate information about frog DNA, frog biology, ecology, and toxicology to determine the cause or causes of the deformities. Once this knowledge is acquired, they must determine what might need to be changed and how it could be changed.

In this chapter, I will discuss how language abilities, schema knowledge, and metacognitive processing function in comprehending narrative and expository texts. The chapter will focus on assessment and remediation of deficits in these areas. Methods for assessing and facilitating a literate language style, the development of the types of schema knowledge that underlie texts, the structure of texts, and the metacognitive or self-monitoring strategies of the comprehension process will be presented.

Comprehending Narrative and Expository Texts

Information Used in Text Comprehension

If readers are to make sense of texts beyond comprehending novel words and complex syntax, they must use three kinds of information: content facts, content schemata, and text grammars (Kieras, 1985). Content facts are the simple propositions that are conveyed by the texts (e.g., facts about ants or facts about a character in a story). At this level, information does not have any superordinate organizational content. If students recognize the vocabulary words used to present the facts, they can comprehend the individual pieces of information. To gain meaning from the overall text, however, a student must have a content schema, or be able to organize a content schema from the facts presented in the text. A content schema represents a superordinate organization of a mass of possible content facts. For example, one can have a content schema for the social structure of ant or bee colonies, the metamorphosis process of caterpillars and tadpoles, or the activities at a birthday party. The speed of reading and comprehension of a text becomes easier when the reader possesses intuitive knowledge of the text grammar structure of a text (Kieras, 1985). A text grammar or macrostructure is a schema that represents a frequent organizational pattern of textual elements that is independent of specific content.

The role of schemata in text comprehension has been extensively studied (Anderson, 1994; Baker & Stein, 1981; Bartlett, 1932; Bransford, 1994; Rumelhart, 1980; Stein & Glenn, 1979; Van Dijk & Kintsch, 1983). Schemata are hierarchically organized sets of facts or information describing generalized knowledge about a text, an event, a scene, an object, or classes of objects (Mandler, 1984). (Note: Some authors use the term *script* to refer to an event schema—the stereotypical knowledge structures that people have for common routines such as going to a restaurant, taking a subway, or going to a party [Beaugrande, 1980; Bower, Black, & Turner, 1979; Nelson, 1985; Schank & Abelson, 1977]. A script can be viewed as a specific type of schema.) Our schema knowledge enables us to behave appropriately in familiar situations, and when our schema information is applied to discourse (oral or written), it enables us to make the *inferences* necessary to comprehend the text—it enables us to read between the lines. If you have an elaborated schema or script for restaurants and you read the sentence "John was hungry, so he looked in the yellow pages," you know that

John may be intending to call a restaurant for reservations or to order a pizza—you also know that he is not intending to eat the yellow pages. The ability to draw inferences is essential for critical and dynamic literacy. Although children who are poor comprehenders (despite adequate decoding skills) are less able than good readers to answer all types of questions about texts, they exhibit particular difficulty answering questions that require them to draw inferences (Oakhill & Yuill, 1996). In fact, when both good and poor comprehenders were able to refer to the text to answer questions, there was no difference between the good and poor comprehenders on literal questions. The availability of the text made little difference in the poor comprehenders ability to answer the inferential questions. This deficit in inference may be related to lack of relevant schema knowledge, to difficulty in accessing relevant schema knowledge and integrating it with the text because of processing limitations, or because they may be unaware that inferences are necessary.

Readers' schemata affect both learning and remembering of information in a text. Schemata have a variety of functions in relation to texts (Anderson, 1994):

- A schema provides a scaffold for assimilating text information. Schemata provide slots for information. For example, there is a slot for a weapon in a murder mystery and a slot for a horse in a Western. Information that fits the slots is easily learned.
- A schema facilitates selective allocation of attention. Having a schema enables readers to know what is important in a text and to devote attention to that which is most important.
- A schema enables inferences. No text is completely explicit. Readers must read between the lines. This is particularly necessary when interpreting character emotions and intentions. Consider, for example, the story *Alice Nizzy Nazzy: The Witch of Santa Fe* (Johnson, 1995). The witch is preparing a stew to keep herself young. She has put Manuela, a young child who has wandered into her home, into the cooking pot. The witch cannot find the petals from the black cactus flower to add to the pot "Suddenly she (Manuela) shouted out, "I know where the black flower is!" If students have a schema for witches, children, and cooking, they can predict that Manuela intends to trick the witch.
- A schema allows orderly searches of memory. Readers need not memorize the details of a story. For example, if the story is about a camping trip in Yellowstone Park, the reader need not focus on backpacks, tents, and sleeping bags. If the character encounters a dangerous animal, the search for the animal name is reduced—it won't be a rhinoceros or a polar bear.
- A schema facilitates editing and summarizing. Because schemata contain the criteria for importance, they are used to retrieve the information needed for a summary and to exclude irrelevant or insignificant information.
- A schema facilitates comprehension monitoring. If readers have schemas for the text content, they are more likely to recognize anomalous information in a text or attend to information that adds to or contradicts their present schema knowledge.
- A schema permits reconstruction. When readers cannot remember some components of a text, they can use what schema knowledge they have, along with the specific text information they can recall, to hypothesize about the missing information.

Activation of background schema knowledge is a fundamental aspect of comprehension, and comprehension provides a mechanism for the acquisition or construction of new schema. There are also schemata for types of discourses or texts that enable us to predict the text genre and organization of information within the text. Each type of text has its own organization. The goal of education is the development of knowledge, which is the acquisition of new schemata.

Just as there are schemata for concepts that enable us to predict the specifics of content, there are also schemata for types of discourses or texts that enable us to predict the text genre and organization of information within the text. Each type of text has its own organization or macrostructure. When readers know the macrostructure of the text they are reading, they are better able to predict what will come next and comprehend the material (Chambliss, 1995; Horowitz, 1985a,b; Meyer, 1987; Scardamelia & Bereiter, 1984; Thorndyke, 1977).

Narrative and Expository Variations in Text Grammars and Schema Content

Texts are not created equal. Bruner (1985) suggested that there are two general types of cognitive functioning—narrative and paradigmatic or logical-scientific. These modes of thought are reflected in narrative and a variety of expository texts. These texts represent different ways of knowing. Consequently, they differ in their content and overall organization (text grammar structures). Table 7-1 summarizes the differences between narrative and expository texts. Narrative texts are generally described in terms of causal event chains or story grammars. Expository texts are generally described in terms of text functions/organization such as description, procedural, comparison/contrast, problem/solution, argumentation. Because of the differences that exist between narrative and expository texts, readers must use different strategies to comprehend the texts.

Research has shown that readers make use of story grammar or schema knowledge in the comprehension of narrative texts (Pearson & Fielding, 1991). Most stories conform to a stereotypical pattern. They begin with a setting, followed by an event or perception (initiating event) to which a character reacts (emotionally, cognitively, and/or behaviorally). The initiating event motivates a character to establish a goal to cope with the event or perception. To achieve the goal, the character must implement a series of attempts that yield consequences or outcomes to which characters respond emotionally (e.g., relieved), cognitively (e.g., decided to forgive), and/or behaviorally (e.g., returned home). The reader uses knowledge of this pattern to make comprehension a very rapid and efficient process. It is not clear whether a story grammar is a content schema or a macrostructure text grammar (Mandler, 1982). Most stories follow a content schema having to do with events and goal-directed activities of characters. The text grammars specify how to take these events and activities and generate stories. Although the ordering of characters' activities may be modified to produce different stories, there is a strong relationship between the order of the story events and the order in which the events appear in the story text. The story content schemata and story text grammars or macrostructures facilitate students' abilities to recognize the gists or themes of passages. The gist or theme of a text represents the overall coherent topic of the text and its essential points. The macrostructure also facilitates readers' abilities to keep

TABLE 7-1   Text Differences

Narrative	Expository
Purpose to entertain	Purpose to inform.
Familiar schema content	Unfamiliar schema content.
Consistent text structure; all narratives have same basic organization	Variable text structures; difference genres have different structure.
Focus on character motivations, intentions, goals	Focus on factual information and abstract ideas.
Often require multiple perspective taking—understanding points of view of different characters	Expected to take the perspective of the writer of the text.
Can use pragmatic inferences, i.e., inference from similar experiences	Must use logical-deductive inferences based on information in texts.
Connective words not critical—primarily *and, then, so*	Connective words critical—wide variety of connectives, e.g., *because, before, after, when, if-then, therefore.*
Each text can stand alone	Expected to integrate information across texts.
Comprehension is generally assessed informally in discussion	Comprehension often assessed in formal, structured tests.
Can use top-down processing	Relies on bottom-up processing.

the gist or theme in mind and to use this information to construct text coherence by relating each sentence to preceding and following sentences and to the overall theme or gist. Recent literature on narrative abilities has shown that students with reading disabilities are not as knowledgeable or efficient in using story content schemata and text grammars to tell, retell, or comprehend stories. Students with reading disabilities tell shorter, less complete, less organized stories; comprehend and remember less of stories; and make fewer inferences about stories (Graybeal, 1981; Hansen, 1978; Liles, 1985, 1987; Merritt & Liles, 1987; Roth & Spekman, 1986; Weaver & Dickinson, 1979; Westby, Van Dongen, & Maggart, 1984).

As students advance in school, they are exposed to more and more expository texts (Otto & White, 1982). In early grades, the focus is on narrative texts. Even the material presented in history and science lessons is often presented in a narrative mode. By junior high and high school levels, however, narrative material usually appears only in literature/language arts courses. The information in all other classes is presented in a variety of expository formats. Students experience more difficulty understanding expository passages than they do narrative passages (Dixon, 1979; Hall, Ribovich, & Ramig, 1979; Lapp & Flood, 1978; Spiro & Taylor, 1987; Vacca, Vacca, & Grove, 1991). Compared to expository prose, narratives are read faster, are more absorbing, and are easier to comprehend and recall (Freedle & Hale, 1978; Graesser & Goodman, 1985;). Minimal research has been done exploring learning disabled students' abilities with expository text. Considering the difficulties they experience with narrative text, however, one would expect similar and likely greater difficulties with comprehension of expository texts.

Expository text usually contains content that is novel to the reader; consequently, the reader cannot readily apply content schema knowledge to aid comprehension (Kieras, 1985; Spiro & Taylor, 1987). Therefore, unlike comprehending narrative text, comprehending expository text is not primarily a matter of matching the content to a previously known pattern, but rather involves dealing with the passage content at the level of individual facts. Once readers have processed the individual facts, they may organize them into schemata. Even if a content schema is available to the reader, this schema provides no strong expectations about the text grammar form of the material. For example, there are no textual rules that state in what order one must describe the facts about ant and bee colonies. This relative independence of content facts, content schemata, and text grammars marks a major difference between expository prose and stories. Because the content schema and text grammar are generally not available to the student prior to the first reading of an expository text, processing of expository texts is much more a bottom-up process than the top-down processing used in comprehending narrative texts, where the content schema and text grammar guide the reader's comprehension (Meyer & Rice, 1984). Bottom-up processing puts more of a load on the memory and integrative processes of readers because they must hold facts in memory, organize the facts into content schema, and attempt to search for a text structure that may facilitate their processing of the content schema (Beaugrande, 1984; Britton, Glynn, & Smith, 1985). Comprehending expository texts requires that readers use the individual facts of the text to construct a content schema, a text grammar or macrostructure, and the coherence relations among the sentences of the text.

Although the structure of expository texts is not as predictable as narrative text grammars, expository texts still follow some text grammar rules that govern the placement and order of information within text. A number of expository text grammar structures have been proposed. Because the function and content of expository texts is so variable, unlike a story grammar, which can fit most content schemata, there must be different expository grammars for different types of texts. Common expository text grammars include structural organizations for comparison-contrast, problem-solution, cause-effect, temporal order, descriptive, and enumerative texts (Horowitz, 1985a, b; Meyer, 1987; Piccolo, 1987; Richgels, McGee, Lomax, & Sheard, 1987). The various expository text patterns are often signaled by headings, subheadings, and specific words (Finley & Seaton, 1987).

Narrative and expository texts differ not only in their text grammars, but also in the types of information in their content schemata. All texts can be analyzed in terms of content or idea units and relationships, which connect the content ideas (Black, 1985; Graesser, 1981; Graesser & Goodman, 1985). Content ideas are usually stated explicitly in the text and include the following:

1. Physical states: Statements that report ongoing states in the physical or social world (e.g., *The forest was cold; The king had three daughters*).
2. Physical events: Statements that report changes in the physical and social worlds (e.g., *The tornado destroyed the town; The monster killed the villagers*).

3. Internal states: Statements that describe the ongoing mental and emotional states of animate beings (e.g., *The big frog was jealous of the new baby frog*).
4. Internal events: Statements that refer to metacognitive or thought processes. (e.g., *The big frog knew he was in trouble; The lost duck forgot how to get home*).
5. Goals: Statements that refer to animate beings' attempts to attain future states and events (e.g., *The big frog wanted to get rid of the baby frog*).
6. Style: Statements that modify an action or a state (e.g., *The angry child screamed furiously; The lion crept slowly forward inch by inch*).

The following types of relationships can exist between the content ideas (the relationships between the content ideas often are not explicitly stated, but must be inferred):

1. Reason: This refers to the reasons that relate goals (e.g., *The villagers collected weapons to kill the monster*. There is a subgoal to collect weapons and a goal to kill the monster).
2. Initiate: Goals are created from somewhere. The initiate relationship links states, actions, and events to goals (e.g., in the book, *One Frog Too Many* [Mayer & Mayer, 1975], the arrival of a baby frog links to a state of jealousy in the big frog and the state of jealousy initiates the big frog's attempts to get rid of the little frog).
3. Consequence: States, events, and actions can lead to other states and events by causally driven mechanisms (e.g., the ship's sinking is a consequence of its being hit by a torpedo).
4. Property: Objects and characters have attributes. Property relations are descriptive relations that link statements about how objects or characters look or relate to other objects and characters (e.g., *The jacket was brand new. It was made of real leather*).
5. Support: Support relations link general statement ideas that make assertions (e.g., in the statements, *Spiders are not insects; they have eight legs, whereas insects have only six*).

These content ideas and the relationships among the ideas represent the types of conceptual knowledge that students must possess to comprehend texts. Narrative and expository prose differ in the types of ideas and connections represented, and, consequently, these two types of texts require differing kinds of knowledge on the part of readers. Narrative texts unfold primarily in terms of goals and the reasons for these goals, whereas expository texts have more physical state ideas linked by consequences, property, and support relationships (Black, 1985; Graesser & Goodman, 1985). In order to understand texts, one must understand the content ideas and relationships among the content ideas that underlie the text. For narrative texts one must understand human motivations and goal-seeking behavior. For expository texts one must comprehend a variety of logical relationships (Black, 1985; Bruce & Newman, 1978; Voss & Bisanz, 1985).

Narrative content can also be described in terms of *landscape of action* and *landscape of consciousness* (Bruner, 1986). In narratives with primarily a landscape of action, temporally patterned sequences of actions are reported in the third person with minimal information about the psychological states of characters. In narratives with primarily a landscape of consciousness, the story is told from the perspectives of the various characters. Most stories have aspects of both a landscape of action and a landscape of consciousness; however, some focus on one landscape more than another. Folktales and stories told by young children generally are primarily landscapes of actions. As children mature they include more aspects of the landscape of consciousness in their stories, and comprehension of stories beyond the third-grade level becomes increasing dependent upon an understanding of a landscape of consciousness. The following excerpt from *The Bunyans* (Wood, 1996) is an example of writing characteristic of the landscape of action:

> *One summer, Little Jean and Teeny wanted to go to the beach. Ma Bunyan told them to follow a river to the ocean. But all the rivers flowed west back then, so they missed the Atlantic Ocean and ended up on the other side of the country instead.*
>
> *Ma Bunyan tracked them out to the Pacific Ocean, where she found Teeny riding on the backs of two blue whales and Little Jean carving out fifty zigzag miles of the California coast.*
>
> *When Ma Bunyan saw what her son had done, she exclaimed, "What's the big idea, sir!? From that time on, the scenic area was known as Big Sur.*

In contrast, a great deal of the story *Too Many Tamales* (Soto, 1993) has a landscape of consciousness. Maria fears that she has lost her mother's ring:

> *Maria didn't dare look into Teresa's mouth. She wanted to throw herself on the floor and cry. The ring was now in her cousin's throat, or worse, his belly. How in the world could she tell her mother?*
>
> *But I have to, she thought. She could feel tears pressing to get out as she walked into the living room where the grownups were chatting.*

Interpretation of a landscape of action requires only the uses of familiar cognitive processes to explain the physical world (e.g., balls break windows, hurricane winds generate high tides, dogs chase cats). Interpretation of landscape of consciousness requires understanding of human intentionality and how humans (or animals with human characteristics) deal with the vicissitudes of life (Feldman, Bruner, Renderer, & Spitzer, 1990). This requires that readers have a theory of mind, that is, an awareness that the mind exists apart from the physical world and what the mind does. In addition, interpretation of the landscape of consciousness aspects of narratives requires interpretation of two types of linguistic phenomena: (1) mental state terms such as *remember, forget, hypothesize, think, believe,* and (2) tropes that are figures of speech such as metaphor, irony, metonym (a word used to evoke an idea through association, e.g., "He gave up the *sword*" is used to convey the idea that he left the military).

Metacognitive Processing in Text Comprehension

Metacognitive abilities are essential for comprehending texts in order to read to learn (Brown, 1982). There are two aspects to metacognition. One aspect involves self-appraisal or knowledge about cognition and conscious access to one's own cognitive operations and reflection about those of others. The other aspect of metacognition involves self-management or regulation of cognition, which involves planning, evaluating, and regulating strategies (Brown, 1987; Jacobs & Paris, 1987). Both types of metacognition are critical for reading comprehension. First and foremost, students must be able to monitor their comprehension (self-appraisal)—they must know if they are understanding what they are reading; and they must be able to take actions if they are not comprehending (self-management). The self-appraisal component requires three types of knowledge: declarative, procedural, and conditional (Paris, Lipson, & Wixson, 1983). *Declarative knowledge* is knowledge of *what*—for example, what a journal entry or summary is. *Procedural knowledge* is knowledge of *how*—for example, the steps one takes to write a journal entry or summary. *Conditional knowledge* is knowledge of *when* and *why*—for example, when and why one writes a journal entry or summary. The self-management metacognition component for planning and controlling actions is related to reading comprehension in two ways. Awareness of when and how to plan is critical for understanding characters' goal-directed behavior in narratives, and the ability to evaluate one's comprehension and plan are critical for employing comprehension repair strategies. Poor comprehenders show less evidence of metacognitive awareness and strategic behaviors. Compared to good comprehenders, they exhibit less use of spontaneous study strategies, correct fewer errors during reading, detect fewer anomalous phrases, do less self-questioning, and have less of an awareness of the goals of reading (Gardner, 1987; Paris & Myers, 1981: Yuill & Oakhill, 1991).

Not all the information necessary to comprehend texts is available in scripts and schemata. Our ability to comprehend the theme of a story requires that we be able to figure out a character's plans and goals (Black & Bower, 1980; Bruce & Newman, 1978; Schank & Abelson, 1977; Voss & Bisanz, 1985). Bruce (1980) maintained that perception of plans plays a major role in the way we structure our social reality. The research on plans and social actions in a number of fields has concluded that (1) understanding plans is a critical part of understanding actions, (2) the ability to understand plans is a very complex inferential task, and (3) children require many years to develop these skills (Kreitler, & Kreitler, 1987a,b; Miller, Galanter, & Pribram, 1960; Piaget, 1932; Schmidt, 1976; Sedlack, 1974). In discussing the work of Sacerdoti (1975), Bruce (1980) noted that in order to interpret actions as being intentional, one needs the ability to plan and to recognize actions of others in terms of goals. He stated that persons who have difficulty in recognizing plans and social actions in others will have difficulty comprehending texts that report such plans.

Reading to learn requires comprehension, and any attempt to comprehend must involve *strategic reading* and *comprehension monitoring*—which are metacognitive behaviors (Paris, Wasik, & Turner, 1991). Bruce (1980) proposed the following metacognitive behaviors as essential for reading comprehension:

1. Understanding the purpose of the reading assignment (e.g., for enjoyment, to be able to explain a principle, to compare one story to another, to complete a worksheet)
2. Identifying the important aspects and main ideas of a message
3. Focusing attention on major content rather than trivia
4. Monitoring to determine if comprehension is occurring
5. Engaging in self-questioning to determine if one's goals in reading are being achieved
6. Taking corrective action when comprehension fails

If students are using these strategies, then they will actively use information from content and text grammar schemata to facilitate comprehension by making predictions about what is to come in a text and by monitoring their comprehension to determine if their predictions are met (Meyer, 1987). For example, if you are reading a murder mystery, you are alert to clues that will lead you to discover the identity of the murderer. In expository text that begins with a topic sentence, you read to find information that supports the statement. You look for organizing words that signal sequence (*first, next, eventually*), cause-effect (*because, since, as a result of*), comparison-contrast (*similar to, however, although*), analysis (*characteristics, types, some features*), and so on. (Finley & Seaton, 1987). If readers are unfamiliar with the structure of a text, they experience difficulty in determining what is and what is not important and the interrelationships among the information presented. Consequently, comprehension of the passage is limited.

The selection, maintenance, or changing of schemata during text comprehension requires monitoring (Pearson & Spiro, 1980). When we listen or read, we are matching the present information to our schema knowledge and attempting to determine if we have a schema for what is being presented. As new information arrives, one must determine if it fits the selected schema or if another schema is needed. For example, a group of students were reading a story in which the main character, Jim, suggested that rustlers were responsible for the rocks rolling down the mountains. If the students retrieved their schema for rustlers, they should then expect some mention of cattle and perhaps a sheriff to appear as the story continued. If this is not forthcoming, then they must assume that they have selected the wrong schema and must look for other information to instantiate a different schema.

Many students with reading disabilities exhibit deficits in metacognitive abilities involving comprehension monitoring, planning of their own behavior, and, in metacognitive awareness, that planning is something that they or someone else might do (Baker, 1982; Hallahan, Kneedler & Lloyd, 1983; Wong & Wong, 1986; Yuill & Oakhill, 1991). If students lack such metacognitive abilities, then they will likely not recognize planning on the parts of characters in texts, nor will they attempt to use metacognitive strategies to interpret text and to monitor their own comprehension of the text.

Assessing Language and Cognitive Skills for Text Comprehension

The discussion in the first section of this chapter has summarized the language and cognitive skills that are essential for reading to learn—for comprehending text. They include a literate style of language, schema knowledge (including content schemata and text grammar schemata), and metacognitive processing. This section will address assessment of each of those aspects of language and cognition essential for text comprehension.

Assessing Literate Language Style

Literate language style involves more explicit language and more complex syntactic sentence structures than oral conversational speech (Horowitz & Samuels, 1987; Scott, 1994). Although there is no specific linguistic analysis system designed to identify a literate language style as opposed to an oral style, there are some systems that capture components of a literate style. In addition, there are some specific aspects of language associated with literate style that can be noted in a language sample.

Hunt's T-unit analysis has been a popular linguistic analysis system to code increasing syntactic development during the school years (Hunt, 1965). A *T-unit* is defined as a main clause plus any subordinate clauses or nonclausal structures that are attached to it. Subordinate clause structure is associated with a literate language style and has been shown to increase with a culture's exposure to literacy (Kalmar, 1985). T-unit length increases through adolescence largely as a result of increasing use of subordinate clauses.

Crystal's grammatical analysis system (LARSP) for language samples captures some of the aspects of literate language style (Crystal, 1979). This system is generally used with younger students, but it does code structures associated with a more literate style. The LARSP codes elaborations of noun phrases, coordinating conjunctions (*and, but, or, for*), subordinating conjunctions (*because, when, while, since, although*), relatives (*who, that, which*), adverbial conjuncts (which have a connective function such as *then, so, now, however, if-then, next, secondly, for a start, yet, lastly*), and adverbial disjuncts (which have a stylistic or attitudinal function such as *of course, really, probably, actually, practically, certainly*).

Pellegrini (1985) reported four aspects of children's language during play that were related to literate language style. These included temporal and causal conjunctions, elaboration of noun phrases, endophoric reference (i.e., linguistic ties between elements in the discourse, as opposed to exophoric ties, which link linguistic elements to items in the context), and verbs referring to mental processes and future events. A T-unit analysis accompanied by noting the following aspects of language occurring in each T-unit provides some sense of the degree to which a student is using a literate language style. The following sentences were written as parts of stories generated by a wordless video, *Baby Bird*, a video in the Max the Mouse series (Society for Visual Library, 1989):

1. Types of subordinate clauses, for example:
   - Dependent clauses that work as adverbs:

     While Max went to the store, the bird ate all the food in the house.

     Max fed the bird *until he had no food left*.

     After the bird was full grown, it took off with Max's house.

     Although Max fed the bird a lot of food, the bird was still crying.

     Max kept feeding the bird *because he wanted it to be quiet*.

     The bird took off into the sky *as Max stepped onto his porch*.

   - Dependent clauses that work as adjectives:

     The yellow bird *that had eaten all of Max's food* flew off with the house.

     Once there was a mouse named Max *who found a little yellow bird*.

     The bird flew to Mexico *where Max got a job making sombreros*.

- Dependent clauses that work as nouns:

  Max explained to his girlfriend Maxine *how the bird had eaten all his food.*
  Max's friends didn't know *what happened to him.*

2. Connectives: *And, then,* and *and then* are not included in the tally because it cannot be determined if they are being used in their logical sense or only to keep the conversation going. Literate connectives coded include, but are not limited to, *when, since, before, after, while, because, so, as a result, if, until, but, therefore, however, and although.*
3. Elaboration of noun phrases:
   - Modifiers: Note the words in the noun phrase immediately preceding the head noun (e.g., The *two, expensive, big, white* cockatoos).
   - Qualifiers: Note the words that follow the noun (e.g., The big white cockatoos *in the pet store window*).
4. Mental/linguistic verbs: These are verbs that denote cognitive processes (e.g., *think, know, forget, remember, consider, hypothesize*) and linguistic processes (e.g., *say, report, promise*). Also note verb tenses other than present, present progressive, and simple past.
5. Adverbs: Adverbs often code aspects of tone, attitude, and manner that in oral language would be coded through stress and intonation. Cook-Gumperz and Gumperz (1981) noted that adverbs provide information as to the necessary tone of voice to use when reading (*angrily, hotly, ominously*), and that children will recycle passages in which their previous reading intonation did not agree with the adverb.
6. Emotional words: Although not specifically associated with a literate language style, it is useful to note the use of emotional words because they reflect an awareness of landscape of consciousness.

Assessing Knowledge of Narrative Content Schemata and Text Grammar Schemata

Two general questions need to be asked with respect to students' schema knowledge in relation to reading. First, do the students have the necessary schemata and can they retrieve the relevant schema information in response to visual and language cues so they can recognize or interpret the situation or comprehend the text or discourse? Second, can the students retrieve and organize schema information to initiate and carry out a task when little or no contextualized information is provided? In a sense these two questions represent aspects of receptive and expressive schema knowledge and use.

One can evaluate students' schema for a particular situation or concept and for a particular text genre. Evaluation of a students' narrative schema crosses both knowledge of world events and situations and knowledge of the structure of stories. As children develop, they acquire increasing understanding of their physical and social world. This knowledge is first coded in narrative texts and later in exposition and other genres. As their knowledge and understanding of the world increase and change, the structure of their narrative texts changes to reflect the changing construct of their thought. Children first read to learn through narrative, and research suggests that children learn more readily through narrative than through expository text (Freedle & Hale, 1979).

Traditionally, there have been two approaches to the assessment of children's narrative schema knowledge: (1) comprehension-based measures (e.g., asking questions about settings, characters, events) and (2) productive measures that require students to generate a story. Comprehension-based measures tend to tap students' schema understanding, while productive measures tend to tap students' ability to use schema knowledge to produce a text. In the literature, all productive measures have tended to be grouped together, whether the student is retelling a story, developing an original story with no stimulus provided, or describing the story in a wordless picture book. These do not, however, place the same demands on the storyteller. Telling a story from a wordless picture book requires only that a student recognize the story content schema. It does not require that the student generate story content schema and organize it into a text grammar structure. The pictures in the book lay out the story, and if students do little more than describe the pictures, their "story" contains the story grammar elements. For this reason, stories students tell when they are provided with highly structured stimuli (wordless picture books or films) are more similar to the comprehension-based measures because they focus on students' understanding or comprehension of content schema, but not on students' abilities to use story grammars. In this chapter, the narrative assessment section has been divided into (1) assessment of recognition/comprehension of narrative content schemata and (2) assessment of ability to organize content schema and text grammar in stories.

What conceptual knowledge is needed for a student's understanding and production of narratives? A narrative relates a time-ordered sequence of events that are interrelated in some way. The speaker/ listener must, therefore, have an understanding of temporal relationships and two types of cause-effect relationships: physical and psychological. Physical cause-effect relationships obey the laws of the physical world (e.g., heavy rains cause floods or a dropped glass breaks). Psychological cause-effect relationships are the result of motivations or intentions of characters within the narrative. Behavior that is motivated or intentional is planned behavior. Understanding of planning or intentional behavior is essential for understanding story narratives because stories relate characters' plans to reach goals (Bruce, 1980; Wilensky, 1978). Recognition of the plans of characters in narratives requires (1) knowledge that people plan, (2) perspective taking (knowing what others are seeing), (3) person perception (knowing traits or attributes of others), and (4) role taking (knowing intentions, thoughts, and feelings of others).

Narratives also require that the story producer and receiver deal conjunctively with what happened in the action of the story and what the protagonists were thinking or saying. Preschool children begin to deal conjunctively with action and thought in play scripts when they alternate between describing the ongoing action and attitudes of characters in the play, taking on the roles of characters in the actual play activity, and acting as a stage manager (Wolf & Hicks, 1989). The distinction between what is intended and what is actually done is a difficult one for young children, particularly when there is a disjunction between what is said and what is done (Bruner, 1985). Trickery tales—that is, tales of deceit—involve a disjunction between action and intention. Abrams and Sutton-Smith (1977) reported that children become fully able to comprehend trickster tales between eigth and ten years of age. Appreciation of many television cartoons, such as the Roadrunner and the Pink Panther, is dependent on children's understanding of trickery. In addition to knowledge of temporal and cause-effect relationships, planning, and role taking, comprehension of trickster tales requires that the child (1) realize that deception can exist, (2) recognize that messages can be intentionally false and that the intention is more important than the content or consequence of the message, and (3) be able to detect deceit by noting visual and vocal cues that suggest that the speaker's words are not truthful and that the speaker is attempting to mask his or her true intentions (DePaulo & Jordan, 1982).

Table 7-2 presents aspects of the development of narrative structure in the first column, the development of physical and social schema knowledge about the world that underlies the narrative structure in the second column, and a narrative example in the third column.

TABLE 7-2   Narrative Development

Preschool

Narrative Structure	*Narrative Contents*	*Example Stories*
Description: Unconnected sentences; order not important	Labels/simple descriptions of objects, characters, surroundings, ongoing actions; no interrelationships among the elements mentioned	There is a ghost and a pumpkin. The witch is a woman. She flies with a broom. The witch is black. The witch chews Skol and makes cigarettes. The witch lives in California and Arizona. She does not come to Alamo.
Action sequence: Series of actions, generally with a temporal sequence; centering may be present—story may have a central character or a central theme (actions that each character does)	Characters engage in a series of actions that may be chronologically, but not causally related; characters act independently of one another	Once there was some kids. And they were going to school. A giant bird flew over and landed. Then they got a piece of rope and put in his mouth. The bird took off. And they had a good, good, good trip. They flew over the ocean and the mountain. Finally they came home.
Reactive sequence: Cause-effect sequences of events; chaining of actions	Awareness of cause-effect relationships; set of actions that automatically cause other changes, but with no planning involved (e.g., a rock rolled down the mountain and people ran)	There were two boys who went to China. And they were there. And they made friends with the bird. And so they were flying around China. And they were going over a city were the statue was. And the boys were having a nice time. But then [the eagle's] a storm came. And the eagle's wings [went started] couldn't flap. [So the] so they crash landed in the trees.

Early Elementary

Abbreviated episode: Centering and chaining present; stories have at least an initiating event (problem), response (character's reaction to problem), and consequence	Stories with goals or intentions of characters, but planning must be inferred; awareness of psychological causality for primary emotions (happy, mad, sad, surprised, disgusted, afraid); awareness of what causes emotions and what might be done in response to them; developing theory of mind (awareness that people think and feel, which allows for some perspective taking); scriptal knowledge of common characters (e.g., wolves are bad and eat pigs; princes are good and save princesses from dragons)	One day a little girl went to mail her letter. Suddenly she heard BOooooOH!. The letter-stealing, glue-licking monster wanted her letter. He wanted to lick glue from her stamp and envelope. The little girl lost her letter. Beware the letter-stealing, glue-licking monster. He may be waiting for you!

TABLE 7-2 Continued

Early Elementary

Narrative Structure	Narrative Content	Example Stories
Complete episode: Centering and chaining present; story has an initiating event, internal response, plan, attempt (carrying out plan), and consequence	Stories with goals, intentions, and plans for reaching the goals; further development of psychological causality (secondary or cognitive emotions, e.g., jealousy, guilt, shame, embarrassment); further perspective taking—awareness of character attributes with story elements of setting and events that enable child to comprehend/predict novel behaviors of characters; understanding of longer time frames (days, weeks); meta-awareness of the need to plan; understanding of need to justify plans	For a whole month there has been a real big giant that has been throwing things in the houses, and smashing homes and getting people, and throwing them. But one day there was one man that wanted to solve the problem. So he got all the men. And they started up the mountain with torches to see what they can do about it. So they were about 10 feet from him. One of the men threw a torch at him and lit the giant on fire. And the giant fell down the mountain. And they never see him again.

Later Elementary

Complex episodes: Like complete episode, but with obstacle(s) to goal and multiple attempts to reach goal	Increases in working memory permit more complex stories including overcoming obstacles through more elaborated plans and multiple attempts to reach goals and ability to take perspective of more than one character; developing ability to perceive character growth (understanding that attributes change over course of story as result of events); ability to detect deception/trickery and to deceive and trick; awareness of time cycles (seasons, years); developing awareness of multiple meanings for words and literal versus figurative meanings	Once upon a time there was a village in the mountains. And there was a gorilla that escaped from the zoo. And they went hunting for it. And it was on top of a ledge. And they started chasing it with guns and with swords. It ran up the hill. And then it fell over the edge. And then the men tried to get it, but it jumped and it wrecked their house. And then they started chasing it up the mountain again. And he started to ski down cause he found a pair of skis at the top. And then the people got skis too. So they chased him on skis. And they chase him right to the zoo. And he got back. He got caught in the zoo again. And he was there again.
Multiple sequential episodes: More than one "chapter"; chapters are arranged in chronological order; at least one episode should be abbreviated or complete	Sequence of episodes: ability to deal with extended periods of time and more complex planning	(Not included because of length)

Adolescent/Adult

Interactive episodes: two or more characters with interactive goals

Embedded episodes: one narrative structure embedded within another. (An interactive episode may be embedded). | Increase in working memory that permits holding of ideas from beginning of first episode while a second episode is introduced. Permits flashbacks and flash forwards in stories that involve understanding of time and space and comprehension of allegory that requires comprehension of multiple meanings.

Ability to engage in metanarrative discussion, i.e., discussion of narrative structure and interpretation of characterization, themes, and plots. | An old man and an old lady lived on a ranch. There was nothing to do except watch the cows. The old man got bored. He decided to drive into town to find some excitement. The old man found some friends and he played cards with them. While he was gone, an oilman came to the ranch. The oilman asked the old lady if he could drill a well. His men worked real hard and dug a deep well. They hit oil and paid the old lady a lot of money. She used the money to build a new house. Late at night the old man came home. He had lost all his money in the card game. He wondered what his wife had done all day. |

Care must be taken when evaluating the narratives of students from non-mainstream backgrounds. Narratives in different cultures vary in content, organizational structure, and style. In addition, children are socialized to telling stories in differing ways. In some cultures, children are only to listen to stories; they are not to tell stories aloud in groups until they are adolescents—and then in some instances, only males are to tell stories in public (Westby, 1994). The narrative developmental information provided in this chapter is based on the narrative development of students from mainstream backgrounds — and on the narrative expectations of the mainstream educational system. One cannot use this information to determine if students from a non-mainstream background have a disorder in narrative language skills—only whether the students possess the narrative skills expected for their grade. To be successful in school, students must be able to comprehend and produce stories with the structural organization and thematic content of mainstream texts. Children who do not exhibit the text characteristics documented for typically developing mainstream students are at risk for academic difficulties whether they lack the specified narrative skills because of cultural differences or because of intrinsic language disorders.

Assessing Recognition/Comprehension of Narrative Content Schemata

Assessing schema recognition involves evaluation of students' understanding of the information listed in the middle column of Table 7-2. A relatively quick way to evaluate students' ability to recognize and comprehend schema knowledge is to have the children tell stories from wordless picture books. Many of the wordless books by Mercer Mayer (such as *One Frog Too Many, Frog Goes to Dinner*, and *A Boy, A Dog, A Frog and A Friend*) are especially useful for this purpose. Each story has several characters. The characters encounter a number of situations that trigger feelings that in turn trigger planned actions of the characters. The artist vividly depicts the characters' emotional experiences. To understand the stories, students must recognize what the characters are doing on each page. They must realize the relationships between activities on any two adjacent pages, as well as the relationships among all the actions in the book. They must understand temporal sequence and physical and psychological cause-effect relationships and plans and reactions of characters.

Evaluation of children's schema knowledge using wordless picture books can be done in two ways. In one method, the children are given the picture book and permitted to look through it and then told to tell the story that happened in the book as they go through the book page by page. The evaluator sits across from the child so that he or she cannot see the book and tells the child, "I can't see the book so make sure to tell the story so that I will understand it. Make it the kind of story we would read in a book." Because children suspect that the evaluator does know the story in the book, the use of a classroom peer as a listener is an even better strategy.

In a second method, the clinician asks questions that focus on a variety of schema relationships using guidelines for questions proposed by Tough (1981). This method is useful for younger children, for hesitant or shy children, and for children who have difficulty organizing extended verbal responses. The questions fall into four categories:

1. Reporting: What was the boy doing here? What happened here? Tell me about this picture.

2. Projecting: What is the boy saying to the big frog? What is the frog thinking? How does the boy feel?
3. Reasoning: Why is the frog thinking that? Why does the boy feel angry? Why did the frog bite the little frog? Why did the tree fall down?
4. Predicting: What will happen next? What will the big frog do now?

The following stories exemplify students' differing schema recognition/comprehension abilities. The first story was told by a fourth-grade boy with high-average reading ability:

> Jerry Bert smiled when he found out that he had a new present. He looked at the tag and then he said, "Look, my name's on this. I'll open it up. oh my gosh, another frog." [The other] the other frog, named Sandy, frowned. [um,] Then what was his name, what was the boy's name? [Examiner: Jerry]. Jerry lifted the baby frog out the box. His dog, his pet dog, Patty, looked at it. The other frog, Sandy, was very mad. He didn't want another frog in his life. Jerry Bert said, [um um,] "Sandy, meet my new frog. His name is Bert." Then all of a sudden, Sandy bit onto Bert's leg. Bert started crying and then, [um,] I keep forgetting, Jerry saved the little frog. He told Sandy not to ever do that again. And so they went for a little hike. They pretended they were all pirates and all part of a team. So they went down to a lake. Sandy frowned as she sat onto the turtle's back. [And] and Bert smiled. Sandy kicked Bert off. Bert started crying. Then Jerry said, "Sandy don't you dare do that again." Sandy was ashamed of herself. She didn't get to ride on the boat. They all got on the boat and went for a ride. Kerplunk. Sandy jumped onto the boat. Bert was a little scared when he saw this. Nobody else noticed. All of a sudden, Sandy kicked Bert off. Bert screamed as he flew off of the boat. The turtle looked at Sandy as he was very mad. Suddenly, [um,] suddenly the turtle told Jerry. Jerry was mad. And then Jerry was surprised. He looked at Sandy and he was very very sad. So they went off looking for him. They couldn't find him anywhere, so they decided to go home. Everybody was mad at Sandy. Sandy was ashamed of herself. Jerry went home and he was very sad. He lied down on his bed and started crying. All of a sudden he heard something going "whee" in the sky. He saw something coming. It was flying toward him out of the window. It came right in and landed right on Sandy's head. Then they became friends.

Even without seeing the book, this story provides sufficient information for the listener to determine the theme and major activities of the characters. The student infers that a box with a ribbon and a tag is a present, identifies the expression on the character's faces, gives reasons for feelings, and infers the consequences of feelings. In so doing, the student is exhibiting the ability to project into the roles of the characters.

Students with a less developed schema knowledge will tell the story as a series of actions. They may realize that the book is presenting a story about several characters, but they appear unaware of the interrelationships of activities from one page to the next, and they do not recognize goal-directed behavior of the characters. Their stories consist of descriptions of the drawings, but with minimal interpretation. The following is part of the story told by a second-grade boy with an attention deficit disorder and language delay:

The boy has a present and he's opening it. And he's looking at the tag. And the dog's sitting down and the frog's sitting down. And now after he opens it, [he] he has something. [And the and the] and the frog has a frown because he thinks it doesn't look good, and the turtle is sad because he can't see it. And the dog is happy. And the frog is happy, and the boy is happy. And now the boy had a bad face. A bad face on his face cause the big frog is biting the little frog's leg. And the turtle's sad and the dog is sad. And the turtle is taking both frogs walking. And now the turtle is taking both frogs and the big frog kicks the little frog off. And now the big frog is all alone in the forest. And someone got buried. I wonder who it was. The big frog maybe. And now they're in the water and the big one is jumping on that. The turtle is sleeping and the dog is sleeping. . . .

Although the child has labeled the expressions on the characters' faces, he exhibits no awareness of the bases for the emotions.

For students in third grade and above, one can obtain a written narrative from students using short videos without dialogue such as Max the Mouse stories (Society for Visual Literacy, 1989). Each of the Max videos is about five minutes long, and the majority of them have a complete single episode structure. Some of them include two characters with conflicting goals. These are several values in collecting written samples. It is easy to collect written samples from an entire class. The video can be shown in a language arts class and all the students in the class can be asked to write the story about the video. Students who are frequently resistant to the idea of writing a story are often willing to write in response to a video. This provides the evaluator with a quick way of comparing a particular student's performance with the performance of the class in general. In addition, it provides a way to compare written and oral narrative schema recognition skills. See Chapter 9 for more about assessing written narratives.

Another approach to evaluating students' schema comprehension ability is to probe students' understanding as they read or listen to a story. At selected points in a story, questions can be asked that focus on concepts underlying the narrative, such as "How does ___ (character's name) feel?" "'Why does he feel that way?" "What can ___ (character's name) do?" (to assess awareness of planning) "What is the problem in the story?" "How was the problem solved?" (Note: *What* questions tap associative understanding—they require only that information read in a sentence be given. *Why* and *how* questions tap causal understanding and promote integrative understanding. *Why* questions expose inferences about causal antecedents and superordinate goals; how questions expose inferences about subordinate goals and actions, causal antecedents of explicit events, and outcomes [Trabasso & Magliano, 1996]). For students third grade and above, one should ask questions regarding how more than one character feels about a situation. Between 9 and 11 years of age students are developing the ability to attend to what characters think, feel, and want, and they are developing the awareness that different characters have different viewpoints on the same situation (Emery, 1996). Understanding of characters' emotions, thoughts, and beliefs are the glue that ties the action of stories together; hence, understanding of these emotional and mental states is critical for the understanding of the landscape of consciousness aspects of stories. Students often exhibit difficulty comprehending the landscape of consciousness, particularly when the consciousness of more than one character must be tracked. Students tend to have difficulty making inferences about characters for the following reasons:

- They focus on what happened instead of why it happened.
- They misinterpret character feelings because they are considering only their own perspective—they think the characters are just like them.
- They focus on only one part of the story instead of the whole.
- They focus on the perspective of only one character.

For students with language and reading difficulties at third grade and above, it is important to explore students' abilities to interpret the landscape of consciousness that is essential for making character inferences. The evaluator can ask questions that require students to focus on the why of behavior, attending to more than one character. The evaluator can read a story, such as *The Talking Eggs* (San Souci, 1989), a southern (African American or Cajun) version of the Cinderella tale, and ask questions as the story is being read. There are two sisters in the story—Rose, the older sister who was cross, mean, and not very bright, and Blanche, the younger sister who was sweet, kind, and sharp. Blanche is told to bring Rose a drink of water. When she gives it to Rose, Rose responds, "This water's so warm, it's near boilin'," shouted Rose, and she dumped the bucket out on the porch.

- Why did Rose act in this way?
- What was Blanche thinking when this occurred?
- What did Blanche want at this point?
- How is Rose feeling now?

Blanche runs into the woods. An old woman finds her and takes Blanche to her cabin. "The old woman sat down near the fireplace and took off her head."

- How did Blanche feel?
- Is that the way you would have felt?
- In what way is Blanche different from you?
- Since Blanche is different from you in this way, how do you think she felt?

Blanche is given eggs that turn into treasures. She takes all the treasures home to her sister and mother. To understand what might happen next in the story, it is essential that students understand the evil nature of the mother and Rose. They must be aware that the mother and Rose are not totally happy with the events—they are jealous and greedy.

- How did the mother and Rose feel when Blanche brought all the treasures home? (If the student replies simply, "happy," pursue with additional questions.)
- What else might Rose and her mother want? . . . be thinking? be feeling?

If the student doesn't provide further relevant information, say:

- Think about what happened so far in the story that clues us in to other feelings the characters might be having.
- What about how they treated Blanche at the beginning of the story?
- What does that tell you about what they might be thinking now?

Three groups of elementary school students, grades three through five (matched for grade, age, and sex) who differed in reading ability were asked questions regarding emotional responses of characters (Westby, Maggart, & Van Dongen, 1984). There were twelve children in each group—a group of average readers who were reading at grade level and were placed in the middle reading groups in their classrooms, and two groups of low readers, one in public school and one attending the university reading clinic. Both low reading groups were reading a year and a half below grade level, were placed in the lowest reading groups in their classrooms, were currently receiving no special-education services, and had not been identified as having any specific oral-language deficits on traditional assessment.

The students in the three groups read stories on a variety of themes (a flood, a lost horse, a robbery, a diseased forest). The children were able to read the stories with at least 95 percent word accuracy. When they completed each story, they were asked how the main character felt about the problem or what went wrong in the story. Of the average readers' responses to the feelings questions, 87 percent were correct, whereas only 48 percent of the low and 39 percent of the clinic groups' responses were correct. Many of the children in the two low reading groups refused to answer because the story did not explicitly tell them how the characters felt, or they reported what their own feelings might be in a particular situation, regardless of the information about the character. This suggests that the low and clinic readers were less competent in perspective taking. If they were unable to recognize the character's feelings or emotional responses to the events in the stories, then it is likely that they also might not understand how and why the characters dealt with the events.

Assessing Ability to Organize Narrative Schema Content and Text Grammars

If students are unable to tell a story from a wordless picture book or respond appropriately to questions asked about story content schemata, they will not be able to produce a coherent story themselves when no stimuli or stimuli with limited structure are provided (e.g., a single picture). Many students, however, are able to recognize the schematic information presented in wordless picture books and print and can comprehend questions asked about stories they have listened to or read, but are unable to retrieve and organize schema knowledge when there is minimal environmental support. Ability to generate organized schema knowledge can be assessed by having students tell stories when minimal contextual cues are available. Students can be asked to tell stories about poster pictures or can be given small figures and asked to make up a story about them. They can be asked to tell a story of a personal experience or to make up an imaginary story without any visual or toy supports. Producing stories of this type requires not only that the students have content schema knowledge of their physical and social world, but that they also have text grammar schema knowledge for the structure of narratives.

A number of story grammar analysis systems are available. Many of these systems are, like any linguistic analysis of a language sample, time-consuming in comparison to standardized tests. A more holistic approach is more practical for clinical purposes when large numbers of students must be assessed. Applebee (1978), Botvin and Sutton-Smith (1977), and Glenn and Stein (1980) have proposed hierarchies of story structures that are logically ordered from the least to the most complex. In the Glenn and Stein hierarchy, each structure includes all of the categories, functions, and relationships between categories found in the previous structures plus at least one additional one. Westby and her colleagues (1984, 1986) modified the Glenn and Stein system by including the information from Applebee and Botvin and Sutton-Smith. This modified structural hierarchy is presented in the first column of Table 7-2. Analysis of narrative level can be done quickly by following the binary decision tree in Figure 7-1 (modified from Stein & Policastro, 1984). To use this binary decision tree, read through a child's story, then ask the following questions:

1. Does the story have a temporally related sequence of events? If it does not, then the story is an isolated description.
2. If the story does have a temporally related sequence of events, then ask, "Does the story have a causally related sequence of events?" If it has a temporally related sequence of events but does not have a causally related sequence of events, then the story is an action sequence.
3. If the story does have a causally related sequence of events, then ask, "Does the story imply goal-directed behavior?" If the story has a causally related sequence of events but does not imply goal-directed behavior, then the story is a reactive sequence.
4. If the story does imply goal-directed behavior then ask, "Is planning or intentional behavior made explicit?" If the story implies goal-directed behavior but does not make the planning of this behavior explicit, then the story is an abbreviated episode.
5. If the story does make the planning or intentional behavior explicit, then ask, "Is the story elaborated by having multiple attempts or consequences, multiple sequential episodes, or embedded episodes, or is the story told from the point of view of more than one of the characters?" If the story does make intentional behavior explicit but is not elaborated, then the story is a complete episode.
6. If the story is elaborated, how is it elaborated? Is one aspect of the story elaborated? For example, is there an obstacle in the attempt path and multiple attempts? Does the story have multiple episodes—are they sequential or embedded? Is the story told from the perspective of more than one character?

This system has been used to analyze the narratives produced by the three groups of elementary school students differing in reading ability who were mentioned earlier in the comprehension section. The three reading groups were significantly different in the complexity of the stories they told in response to two poster pictures. Of the narratives told by the low readers in the reading clinic group, 62 percent were at the descriptive level, and only 8 percent were elaborate structure narratives. Fifty-four percent of the average reading group's stories were elaborated structure narratives, and none of their narratives were of the descriptive type. The low reading school group exhibited a range of narrative structures, with the majority of their narratives (73 percent) falling in the middle range of narrative

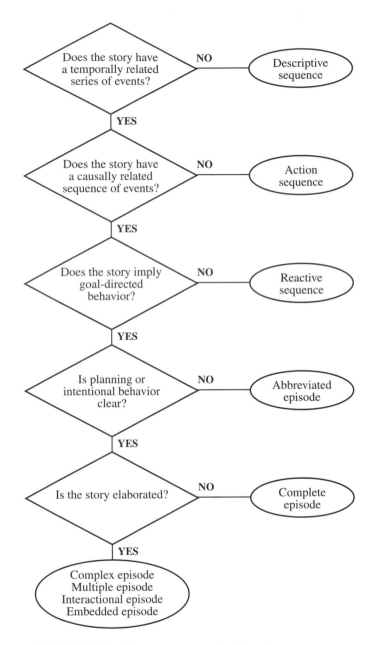

FIGURE 7-1 **Story grammar decision tree.**

structures (action sequence, reactive sequence, abbreviated episode, complete episode); 16 percent of the low reading group's narratives were descriptions, and 8 percent were elaborated structure narratives. Clearly, the low reading school group and the reading-clinic group students did not produce stories that were structurally as complex as the stories produced by the average readers. In their oral stories they made little or no reference to the intentions, plans, or goals of characters.

Assessing Metacognition

As mentioned earlier in this chapter, there are two aspects of metacognition. One aspect, self-management or regulation of cognition, involves planning and control of action. A second aspect, self-appraisal or knowledge about cognition, involves conscious access to one's own cognitive operations and reflection about those of others (Brown, 1987). If students are to recognize intentional behavior of characters in stories, they must be able to plan their own behavior (Bruce, 1980). As students read, they must monitor their comprehension and know what actions to take to facilitate comprehension when comprehension fails (Brown, 1982; Yuill & Oakhill, 1991). Evaluation of children's reading should include assessment of their metacognitive knowledge and strategies. Strategies are not the same as skills; strategies are deliberately selected means to accomplish specific goals (Paris, 1991). In strategic reading, readers know methods for figuring out new words, interpreting character behaviors and writers' intentions, and how to monitor and repair comprehension problems.

In order to assess metacognitive abilities, one needs an understanding of their development. Metacognitive processes used to regulate behavior develop early. Luria (1961), one of the first to study the development of self-regulatory language, noted that children between 2 1/2 to 4 years can use their own speech to initiate immediately following actions, but not to inhibit actions; by 4 1/2 years, children can use their own speech both to initiate and inhibit their actions. Meacham (1979) also explored the development of preschool children's use of language to guide motor activity. In a first stage, the children may accompany their motor activity with overt verbal activity, but the two activities are independent. In the second stage, children engage in verbal activity to describe the outcome of their motor activities. Language does not, however, fulfill a guiding role, either to initiate or direct motor activity, or to facilitate the remembering of anticipated goals. Consequently, there is no evaluation of the outcome of motor activity. Language follows the activity and restates the events of the activity. In the third stage, language still follows the activity, but it is used to describe the anticipated goals of motor activities rather than the actual outcome. By describing anticipated goals the child is better able to remember them, and so it becomes possible to compare the remembered thought with the actual outcome and, hence, to evaluate the outcome. In the fourth stage, language precedes activity and plays a major role in planning and guiding the course of the child's motor activities. Until children use language to plan and control their behavior, they will not develop awareness of cognitive processes.

In order to develop conscious awareness of mental processes and metacognitive strategies, children must develop a theory of mind as separate and distinct from the body. The exact time of emergence of this awareness is controversial. Bretherton and Beegly (1982) suggested that it begins in infancy. Many others dispute this. Literature is available that indicates children are developing this awareness between ages 3 and 7. Wellman

(1985) identified five different but overlapping sets of knowledge that form a person's metacognitive awareness:

1. Existence: The person must know that thoughts and internal mental states exist and that they are not the same as external acts or events.
2. Distinct processes: There are a variety of mental acts (e.g., remembering, forgetting, guessing, knowing, and daydreaming).
3. Integration: While there are distinctions among different mental acts, all mental processes are similar and related. For example, one can't remember or forget unless one first knew something. One can hope to remember, but think that one will not.
4. Variables: Any mental performance is influenced by a number of other factors or variables. For example, how much one comprehends depends on how familiar or novel the text is, the organization of the text, and the strategies used to comprehend the text.
5. Cognitive monitoring: The ability to read one's own mental states or monitor their ongoing cognitive processes. Even young children often know when they understand and when they do not, or when they are fantasizing, dreaming, or imagining.

With this metacognitive awareness, children begin to be able to talk about their planning behavior. Pea (1982) interviewed children ages 7 to 13 years to discover what they know about metacognition or planning of behavior. All the children knew that planning involves thinking about the future, and they knew when to plan, when not to plan, and why one must plan. The students reported that one must plan in order to do something and one must plan how to do something. They also stated that one must plan the specific conditions for doing something. They reported that you did not need to plan something you were just about to do, you don't plan if others plan it for you, and you don't plan if you already know what to do. You must plan because you have many actions to accomplish or because the activity won't work out if you don't plan. As indicated earlier, understanding of planning is essential in understanding the purpose or goal behind written text. If students do not plan for themselves, it is unlikely that they could interpret planning behavior of authors or characters in stories.

Kreitler and Kreitler (1987b) gathered information about children's knowledge of planning through interviews. Children exhibited a variety of developmental changes in their knowledge of and the strategies they used in planning. They gained knowledge about the components of planning behavior, the domains that can be planned, and the antecedents, purposes, and consequences of planning. Table 7-3 summarizes these developmental changes. The information reflects the changes in narrative development that have been described. Note that 5 year olds are alert to causes or triggers for plans (precursors to the development of a goal), although they do not really plan themselves. By 7 they are aware of results of plans—at least plans to get a personal need met. By 9, the age at which students comprehend and produce complete narratives, they are aware of the purpose of planning and how emotions are related to goals and plans. With this knowledge, they can interpret story characters' intentions, motivations, and goals. By 11 years of age, students can implement plans and goals for their future success. This corresponds with their ability to implement a variety of study strategies to assist themselves in comprehending texts to succeed academically.

TABLE 7-3 Development of Knowledge about Planning

Elements of Planning	5 years	7 years	9 years	11 years
Meaning dimensions	Domains that are planned and causes of plans (what triggers planning)	5 year elements + results (what follows planning or lack of planning)	5 & 7 year elements + function, purpose, role (goal of planning)	
Domains for planning	Recurrent daily actions; searching for lost items	+ manipulating adults; avoidance of obligations and punishment; performance of chores	– recurrent daily action; + relations with peers; use of instruments; fantasy & daydreams	– recurrent daily actions; planning used primarily for domains related to personal reality-bound goals (avoiding chores, entertainment, achievement) & future (studies career, marriage); domains for society at large (peace, ecology, space)
Timeframe of plan	80% immediate (few minutes to 6-7 days)	Begin to shift from immediate future to near future in planning (from 1 week to 3–4 weeks)	Begin to shift from near future to far future in planning (more than 2–3 months ahead)	21% immediate future; 38% far future
Antecedents for planning	Demand for action (e.g., take bath)	Increase in reference to special actions (e.g., alone for first time; examination)	Increased reference to emotional states	Increased reference to desire for success
Purpose and results of planning (with age increasing awareness of positive results of planning)	Perform familiar routines not year mastered	Planning in regard to knowing how to perform; get good evaluation from others	Understanding of emotional results of planning	Improvement of action in terms of correctness, precision, or speed; success in performance; aware of possible negative effects of planning

By early adolescence, students become conscious of the strategies they use to comprehend and remember information (Baker & Brown, 1984; Forrest-Pressley & Waller, 1984). They are aware of their own skills and of the ways the nature of the material to be learned (visual, linguistic, etc.), the task criteria (recognition, recall, problem solving), and the learning activities (attention, rehearsal, elaboration) will affect the strategies needed and their performance (Wong, 1985a). This level of metacognitive processing is essential for comprehension of expository texts (Meyer, 1987). Comprehension of expository texts requires students to evaluate what knowledge they have about the topic and to use a variety of strategies (rereading, outlining, underlining) to comprehend and remember the material.

Assessing Knowledge of Cognition

Awareness of mental acts must precede the development of metacognitive strategies essential for children to comprehend and remember what they read. Children must be able to know when they know and when they don't know something if they are to interact appropriately with the teacher and be able to work independently. Wellman (1985) reported that by age 7, eighty percent of children exhibit the adult pattern of understanding mental terms such as *know, remember, forget,* and *guess.* Wellman developed several tasks that are useful in determining students' understanding or appreciation of these terms.

> Task 1: Knowing-remembering condition. Children see an item hidden in one of two containers. Then, after a brief delay, the children are asked to find the item. At that point they are asked ''Did you know where the item was? Did you guess where the item was? Did you remember where it was?
>
> Task 2: Guessing condition. Children do not see where the item is hidden, and cannot know where it is, but must make a choice between the two containers.
>
> Task 3: Forgetting condition. Children watch a toy character who sees his coat put in one of two closets, and they are asked, "Does he know where his coat is? Why do you say he knows?" Later the character comes back looking for his coat and looks in the wrong closet. The children are asked "Did he know where his coat was? Did he remember? Did he forget? Why did you say he forgot?"

One can explore students' awareness of planning by asking questions such as:

> Who plans?
>
> What things are planned?
>
> Why do people plan?
>
> What happens if people plan? If they don't plan?
>
> Do you plan? Tell me about one of your plans.

We present these tasks regularly in elementary classrooms for communicatively disordered students. Initially, the majority of the children respond randomly to these tasks. If children do not know when they know or don't know, they have no basis for deciding when they need to seek assistance with a task. As a consequence, many such children are content to complete entire activities incorrectly, while others develop a pattern of learned helplessness and approach the teacher for assistance and explanation of every task, even when they have done the task in the past and should know what is expected. Frequently, it is clear that they do know (but don't know that they know), because as soon as the teacher says, "We've done that before, you know how to do it," they return to their seats and complete the work without further explanation. Any work related to metacognitive monitoring of comprehension and performance on academic tasks is based on first understanding the concepts of knowing, remembering, forgetting, and guessing. If students are to monitor their comprehension, they must *know* when they are comprehending and when they are not comprehending. They must understand that they may be expected to *remember* the material they are reading, and they must know what they can do so they won't *forget*.

Jenkins (1979) proposed a model of learning that can be used to discuss types of metacognitive processing important for comprehension monitoring:

1. The characteristics of the learner, that is, what do the learners know about themselves—about their present knowledge, what is hard and what is easy for them, what they like and what they don't like.
2. The nature of the materials to be learned. This includes the learner's awareness of the organizational structure of the texts and the types of facts and content information that will appear in the texts.
3. The criterial task; that is, what is to be the end product of the learning. For example, is the student to retell the story, complete a multiple-choice test or essay test, or teach the material to someone else.
4. Learning strategies at one's disposal, that is, can one reread, does one know how to outline or make semantic maps of the material, does one use visual imagery to remember the information, and so forth.

If students have awareness of these areas, they can use them to monitor their comprehension while reading. If students know something about themselves in relation to the topic or reading task, they can make decisions about how they will handle the task. For example, students might find history easy and know they can read and comprehend it in one reading while sitting in the cafeteria; on the other hand, they know that they find science difficult and must allow additional time to read the material and must read it in a quiet place.

If students are aware that texts can have organizational structure, they can use this knowledge to (1) identify the structural pattern of the text and (2) plan to use it strategically to identify the important aspects of the message, to focus attention on the main ideas rather than the trivia, and to predict the sequence of information in the text (Gordon & Braun, 1985).

If students are aware of the outcome requirements of the task, they can make adjustments in how they read and how well they need to comprehend. If they are reading for enjoyment or to provide a brief summary of the text to someone else, they do not need to devote a lot of attention to the task, and they do not need to comprehend everything in the text—just the main ideas. If they are to be able to write an essay about what they have read, they must understand the organization of the material and must understand the main ideas and how the other information supports the main ideas. This is clearly a task that will require more careful reading. Students who understand their own knowledge, abilities, interests, and the criterial nature of the reading task are able to choose the learning activities that will work best for them to comprehend the material at the level necessary for successful completion of the task.

One can gain insight into the comprehension monitoring strategies students use by having them read a story and stopping them periodically to ask what the story is about and to explain how they know this. Paris (1991) proposed using a think-along passage (TAP) to explore the strategies students use during reading to identify topic, predict what will happen next, monitor meaning, make inferences, and summarize. Table 7-4 shows the types of questions that can be asked about reading passages and some of the strategies reported.

With junior high students, one can sample metacognitive awareness by asking what they do to remember and how they study for tests.

- If you have to remember something, what do you do?
- What do you do if you do not understand what you are reading?
- What do you do when you are going to have a test?
- What do you do when you say you study? Do you study differently for a math test than for a history test? For an essay test than for a multiple choice test?

TABLE 7-4   Think-Along Passage Protocol for Assessing Strategic Reading

Present child with book or reading passage (Example: *Too Many Tamales* by Gary Soto).

Identifying the topic	**Possible Strategies**
1a. Look at this page. What do you think the story will be about?	Scans text Looks at title Refers to pictures
Ex: A surprise party; lots of tamales	Refers to prior knowledge Points out words Other
1b. How do you know this?	
Ex: Their eyes look like this (points)	
1c. If you don't know, how could you figure it out?	
Ex: Turn the pages; read the book	

After a significant event in the story, stop the reading (e.g., after Maria tries on her mother's ring).
Predicting

2a. What do you think will happened next?	Predicts based on prior knowledge Predicts based on text cues Rereads
Ex: Her mom'll get mad	Looks forward in the text Uses context cues Other
2b. Why do you think that?	
Ex: 'Cause she shouldn't wear her mom's ring	
2c. If you don't know, how could you find out?	
Ex: Read more of the story; look at the pictures	

TABLE 7-4   Continued

Choose a word that you think will be unfamiliar to the student.
Monitoring meaning

3a. What do you think "masa" means in
the sentence you just read?

Ex: Dough
3b. How could you tell?

Ex: From the pictures; it's in a bowl
Ex: They kneaded it. That's what you do with dough

3c. If you don't know, how could you find out?

> Uses context cues
> Substitution looks or sounds similar
> Mentions other resources
> Mentions dictionary as resource
> Relates personal experience
> Other

Select something that is not made explicit in the story.
Making inferences

4a. Why do you think they put the masa
on corn husks?

Ex: Cause they wanted to
Ex: To keep all the stuff together

4b. How did you decide this?

Ex: I just thought it
Ex: I know cause I help gramma make tamales

4c. If you don't know, how could you figure it out?

> Infers based on text cues
> Infers based on prior knowledge
> Relates personal experience
> Gives analogy
> Scans forward
> Rereads
> Other

After you or the student has finished reading the book, ask for summary.
Summarizing

5a. If you wanted to tell your friends about
this story, what would you tell them?

5b. How did you decide what things to tell
them?

5c. If you don't know, how do you think you could decide?

> Retells mostly main ideas
> Retells mostly details
> Organizes ideas in recall
> Summary is disorganized
> Expresses opinions or reactions
> Connects to personal experiences
> Uses genre structure to help recall
> Other

Based on information from: Paris, S.G. (1991). Assessment and remediation of metacognitive aspects of children's reading comprehension. *Topics in Language Disorders, 12*, 32-50.

Answering these questions is no assurance that the students actually use the strategies they say they do. Consequently, students should be observed during activities requiring strategy use (Cavenaugh & Borkowski, 1980). It is possible that the students who cannot respond to these questions may be using some unconscious comprehension and remembering strategies, but it is unlikely that they are using them effectively.

Assessing Regulation of Cognition

Awareness of planning does not ensure that students do plan. Consequently, one must also evaluate students' ability to plan. This can done in two general ways. First, one can determine if children give evidence of planning in their own behavior. For children up to 8 or 9 years of age, one can observe a child's play and interview parents and teachers to determine if the child plans. A second approach is to present children with hypothetical problem situations requiring planning for the solutions.

Garvey (1982) maintained that symbolic role-play is possible only when children conceive and plan an outcome and subsequently work toward that end (e.g., building a spaceship to travel to a distant planet where they will attack the snow monster). This outcome takes precedence over immediate sensory input, and it is the plan that guides children's response to the materials. Peers are able to join in pretend play only if they are able to recognize the others' pretend orientation and their particular plan. Sachs, Goldman, and Chaille (1984) noted that the amount of speech devoted to planning and organizing play is positively related to the content and complexity of children's narrative language. Pellegrini (1985) also reported that children with good symbolic play skills used a literate style of language and were consciously planning and organizing their fantasy play.

Observation of children's play enables us to observe planning in action. Westby (1980, 1988, 1991) developed a symbolic play scale that can be used to evaluate students' schema knowledge of their world and their manner of planning the use of this knowledge. Symbolic pretend play has a number of components. It involves (1) increasing decontextualization or decreasing reliance on concrete props and increasing reliance on verbal coding; (2) moving from representation of highly familiar themes to unfamiliar, novel themes; (3) increasing organization and preplanning of the play; and (4) increasing ability to engage in role taking. The organization category represents children's increasing ability to control and plan their behavior. The following sequence in development of organization and planning is noted:

- 17 to 19 months: The child moves quickly from one instance of pretending to another and engages in short, isolated play schemata. The child may pretend to sleep, then abruptly pretend to eat, with no links between events or elaboration of any of these schemata. Children do not announce what they are about to do or comment on what they are doing or have done.
- 19 months to 2 years: Children begin to combine objects in play; they show awareness of things that go together and will look for them. For example, a child sees a plate and then looks for a spoon to use with the plate.
- 2 years to 3 years: Children elaborate familiar schemata. For example, the 2 1/2 year old who is taking care of her baby will gather many of the items she needs. She will set the table with dishes, spoons, cups, and glasses and pull a highchair up to the table.
- 3 years to 4 years: Children produce an evolving sequence of events. At this point children will announce completed actions and actions that are to follow immediately. Now not only do they eat, but they first prepare the food, put it on the table, sit down and eat, clear the table, save the leftovers, wash the dishes, and then sit down to watch TV.

The children do not plan these events ahead of time, but as they complete one aspect of the schema they automatically move into the next aspect.

- 4 years: Children plan their play in advance, and the planning phase may take as long or longer than the actual pretend play. They announce what they are going to play.
- 5 years: Children not only plan their own behavior, but they also plan and monitor the behavior of others. In play they assign roles to other children, list what the children are to do, and during the play periodically monitor what the other children are doing.

Although normally developing children from mainstream environments have well-developed symbolic play by age 5 to 6 years, older students with language impairments exhibit deficits in many aspects of symbolic representation that develop during the preschool years. My colleagues and I have used play evaluations with children from infancy through middle school (grades six to eight). Of the four aspects of symbolic play development, students with learning disabilities usually exhibited their greatest deficits in the area of organization. Many middle school students with learning disabilities do not exhibit the sequential organization of play that is present in normal 3-year-olds' play.

The age of the students should be considered when selecting the materials used in play evaluations with school-age students. For older students collections of various building sets (Legos, Construx), battery operated vehicles, transformers, Mattel car sets (village, ore mine, service station), Fisher-Price action sets, and action figures from currently popular movies are usually appropriate. Elementary school children may also enjoy these materials, but many students have not developed the ability to represent less familiar schemata or to decontextualize and use less realistic props. Consequently, play evaluation for elementary school children with disabilities should include more realistic props and familiar materials such as household, store, and doctor materials.

One can also investigate students' planning abilities by presenting them with hypothetical problems. Goldman (1982) asked students to tell stories about how they might achieve goals such as getting out of doing chores, making friends, or wanting a dog and getting one. After the students responded to a task, such as telling a story about wanting a dog and getting one, they were asked to tell a story about wanting a dog but not being able to get one. They were asked what could stop them from getting a dog, or what could go wrong so they couldn't get one even though they wanted one. Following this response the students were asked "If that happened [child's obstacle], how could you still get a dog? How could you make that story into a story where you did get a dog?" (p. 283). Finally, they were asked if anything like this ever happened to them. Westby (1983) reported that many students with learning disabilities have marked difficulty with this task. Students who are successful with this task generally have dogs, and those who are unsuccessful do not have dogs. This result suggests that the task is ecologically valid; that is, that it is tapping a planning ability that students are using or not using in their lives.

Spivack, Platt, and Shure (1976) used somewhat similar procedures to explore the planning abilities of well-adjusted and poorly adjusted children who were identified as being impulsive, inhibited, or aggressive. They reported that well-adjusted 4- and 5-year-old children were able to give more alternative solutions to personal problems and could give more causes and consequences for the problems than poorly adjusted children. In elementary school, well-adjusted children were able to fill in the middle of problem-solving stories by giving multiple sequential steps to the solution and suggesting obstacles that might arise and ways around the obstacles. Well-adjusted adolescents were able to consider the thought processes of others in solving interpersonal problems. The Spivack, Platt, and Shure tasks can be useful in assessing the interpersonal problem-solving skills and planning that underlie narratives.

For 4- and 5-year-old students, they suggested presenting the child with the following type of problem: "Jimmy has been playing with the truck all morning and now Claire wants to play with it. What can Claire do or say to make sure she gets to play with the truck?" Or, "Manuel just broke his mom's favorite vase. What can he do or say to keep his mom from getting mad?"

At the elementary school level the student is given the beginning and end of a story and asked to complete it. For example:

> Al (Joyce) moved into the neighborhood. He (she) didn't know anyone and felt very lonely. The story ends with Al (Joyce) having many good friends and feeling at home in the neighborhood. What happens in between Al's (Joyce's) moving in and feeling lonely, and when he (she) ends up with many friends? (p. 65).

The examiner evaluates the story in terms of the number of solutions generated, obstacles to various plans that are presented, and ways around these obstacles. Westby (1983) used this task with middle-school students with RD and reported that many of them had no idea how the child could make friends.

At the adolescent level, the student is given the following type of task:

> Bill loves to go hunting, but he is not allowed to go hunting by himself. One weekend his parents go on a trip and he remains at home by himself. He has a new shotgun he received recently and a box of shells. He looks out of the window at the nearby woods and is tempted to go out hunting. (p. 95)

The student is asked to tell everything that goes on in Bill's mind and then tell what happened. This task requires not only planning abilities, but also perspective-taking abilities. Westby reported that adolescents with learning disabilities seldom deal with the conflict between what Bill wanted to do and the restrictions given by the parents. Instead, they assumed that the boy would go hunting and then they discussed problems of not finding any birds to shoot or figuring out how to hide all the dead birds.

Story comprehension can also be used to assess a student's understanding of planning. An example of how understanding of planning behavior is related to story comprehension can be shown with the story *Harry and Shellbert* (Van Woerkman, 1977). The story begins with Harry, a hare, and Shellbert, a tortoise, having lunch. Shellbert relates the original story of the race between the tortoise and the hare. When Harry hears the outcome of the race, he becomes very angry, and Shellbert challenges him to a race. Overconfident, Harry lies down to take a nap, placing a stick in the path with the long end pointing in the direction he is to run. He intends that Shellbert will trip over the stick and awaken him in time to win the race. Shellbert sees the stick, quietly passes the sleeping rabbit, and turns the stick in the other direction so that when Harry awakens, he runs the wrong way and loses the race.

The students read a portion of the story to the point at which the characters must take some action. The story is stopped at this point and the students are then asked what the character can do to accomplish his goal. For example, in the Harry and Shellbert story, after the two characters had decided to race, the students were asked, "What is something that Harry can do to make sure he will win the race?" When the students responded, they were told, "That's a good idea. What else could Harry do to make sure that he will win the race?" This was continued until the student could generate no more alternatives. The same procedure was followed with Shellbert. Student responses are scored for (1) number of plans, (2) number of steps in the plan, (3) if a justification of the plan is provided, and (4) feasibility of the plan.

This task was given to the high-average and low-average fourth-grade readers mentioned in the discussion of observing planning behavior in play. The two groups of readers did not differ in total number of plans given, but the high-average readers gave significantly more plans that were judged as feasible and gave more justifications for their plans. Low-average readers suggested activities that could not readily be associated with winning a race; for example, the turtle would wear sunglasses. The high-average readers also gave more plans that focused on activities that the character himself would do to win the race (such as running fast and not taking a nap), while the low-average readers gave more plans in which one character got rid of the other character (by hitting him over the head, tripping him, or making him fall in a hole) (Westby et al., 1986).

Facilitating Text Comprehension

Now that we know the types of linguistic and cognitive knowledge essential for text comprehension, what can be done to facilitate students' ability to comprehend what they read? Goodman (1973) proposed twelve easy ways to make reading difficult, and one difficult way to make reading easy. According to Goodman, to make reading easy for students, one must make reading easy. This can be done by providing students with interesting, comprehensible texts—texts that have a clear, higher-organizational structure, and texts that are matched to the level of the students' schema knowledge. Frameworks for facilitating comprehension instruction consider three phases of the reading process: (1) before reading, (2) during reading, and (3) after reading. Richardson and Morgan (1994) proposed an instructional framework termed PAR, which stands for Preparation, Assistance, and Reflection. The PAR acronym is associated with golf. When golfers achieve *par for the course* they have played a good game and reduced their *handicap* or overcome any disadvantages to equalize their chances of winning. The goal of using the PAR comprehension instruction framework is to reduce students' literacy handicaps. In the preparation phase, teachers need to consider the students' backgrounds and any aspects of the text that may be problematic for the students. In the Assistance phase, teachers need to provide students strategies for comprehending (such as using knowledge of text structure, how to ask questions, how to make inferences). In the Reflection phase, teachers use the material that was read to extend learning and promote critical thinking. In this phase, students may compare texts on similar themes or topics, apply information learned to different situations, or integrate information from a variety of sources in creative projects.

The focus of this section of the chapter is to demonstrate how (1) high-quality children's literature can be matched to students' present cognitive and linguistic abilities so that students can comprehend the texts and at the same time gain additional knowledge from the texts, and (2) through student-teacher interactions, professionals can facilitate the development of the metacognitive strategies students need to become independent learners.

When selecting books, one should consider not only the cognitive/linguistic aspects of the books, but also the cultural content. Children should be exposed to content that positively reflects the cultural diversity of the country and the world. Within recent years, more children's books are being published that include children and stories from diverse cultures. Such books should be used with all children, not just those from minority or nondominant cultures. There are several types of multicultural books for children. Many relate traditional stories, myths, and legends from different cultural groups. Some are culturally specific and illuminate the experience of growing up in a particular non-mainstream cultural group. Others may be termed *generically American*. These feature characters from non-mainstream groups engaged in everyday activities that contain few, if any, specific details that define them culturally. Then, there are informational books that include people from diverse cultures engaged in activities related to the topic of the book. Care must be taken in selecting multicultural books to ensure that they are authentic to the group and avoid stereotypes.

Developing a Literature Language Style

Facilitating Explicit/Descriptive Language Use

In Chapter 1, the differences between oral and written language were discussed. Compared to oral language, written literate-style language uses more specific vocabulary and more complex syntactic structures to specify the relationships among people, actions, and objects. A more literate style of language must be used any time the speaker and listener or reader and writer are not in the same time and space and do not share familiarity with the topic. In order to develop a literate language style, children must hear literate language and have the opportunity to use it in meaningful communicative contexts. Children may be exposed to a literate style in the language spoken by adults around them and in stories that are read to them.

Barrier games have been a popular means to develop explicit language. A child sits on each side of a barrier with shapes, figures, or Tinkertoys. The clinician or child makes a design or constructs a model and then must tell the student on the other side of the barrier what to do to make a design or construct the model.

Children need opportunities to hear and use literate language in conversation when minimal contextual cues are available. Show and Tell or Sharing Time serves this function in many kindergarten and first grade classrooms. These activities are often difficult for students with RD because there are no concrete clues in the environment to help trigger what they can say and because they must maintain the discourse themselves. Sharing Time can be modified to ease the transition into literate monologue by beginning with a group discussion on a topic familiar to all students. The teacher writes a number of topics on cards and then has the students draw a card for discussion. We have chosen statements such as "What would happen if you played ball in the street?" "What would happen if you invited someone home with you after school?" or 'What would happen if you got two presents that were the same?" The nature of these questions allows the teachers and children to begin by giving personal narrative examples and then to generalize to an expository form of what might generally happen in most conditions. Two adults lead the group. If no children initially respond, the adults engage in an informal discussion, for example, of a time when they invited someone home with them. If something one adult said is unclear to the other, the other adult requests clarification or further explanation. The children are permitted to interrupt at any time and add their own experience. As they do, they begin to talk about nonpresent objects and activities and must do so in a way that is understandable to others in the group. If the group discussion is about bringing a friend home after school and a child begins to talk about finding a car in the trash, an adult asks if this is related to the current topic and the child is reminded about the topic of the discussion. As the year continues, students begin to be able to ask each other questions to clarify information and, in so doing, all students become better able to talk about past experiences clearly.

Pretend play/creative dramatics activities also provide opportunities for literate language use. The decontextualization or reduction in the need for concrete props that occurs in imaginative play requires increasing use of explicit language for the play to be shared with others. Pellegrini (1985) reported that children who exhibit higher levels of symbolic pretend play also exhibit more literate language styles. They make use of more adjectives, conjunctions, words referring to metacognitive functions (I know, I think), and more endophoric reference (reference to information in the text) as opposed to exophoric reference (reference to information in the context). In sociodramatic play children must communicate effectively with each other if the play is to proceed. As props become less realistic, the need for explicit language increases. If a child puts a box on the table and intends it to be a turkey that will be carved for dinner, the child needs to make his or her intention clear to other children in the play environment.

Students also require a literate vocabulary. They need to acquire multiple words to express subtle variations of meaning. The book, *Over the Steamy Swamp* (Geraghty, 1988), provides an interesting way to introduce a variety of words referring to hunger and a variety of emotional words referring to fright. In this cumulative story, a mosquito flies across the swamp, watched by a variety of animals—a greedy dragonfly, watched by a famished frog, watched by a peckish fish, watched by a hungry heron, watched by a starving snake, watched by a craving crocodile, watched by a hostile hunter, watched by a ravenous lion. The mosquito bites the lion. As a result of the lion's roar, there is a horrified hunter, a cowering crocodile, a startled snake, a hysterical heron, a frightened fish, a dismayed dragonfly, and a flabbergasted frog. The teacher can provide dictionary definitions of the words or ask the students to find the definitions. The alliteration in the story and the detailed pictures facilitate memory for the words.

Hunger words

craving: to have an intense desire for, to beg earnestly for

greedy: wanting more than one needs

hungry: a strong desire for food

famished: extremely hungry

peckish: somewhat hungry

ravenous: wildly hungry

starving: dying from prolonged lack of food

Emotional words

cowering: shrinking as from fear

dismayed: filled with apprehension

frightened: feeling intense fear

flabbergasted: astonished, amazed

hysterical: uncontrollable emotion of fear or panic

startled: making a sudden movement in fright

For emotional words, one can construct a word web, organizing words according to mild, moderate, and strong (Figure 7-2) or by regrouping the words into a "vocabulary thermometer" (Figure 7-3) (Barton, 1996).

With students at third grade and above, we may present students with a list of vocabulary words that will appear in the text and ask them to judge the level of their knowledge (Blachowicz, 1994). For example, before reading the book, *The Fourteenth Dragon* (Seidelman & Mintonye, 1968), a descriptive poem about thirteen dragons, the teacher wrote the following words on the board and asked the students to copy them into their narrative project notebooks and to judge their knowledge of them (see Table 7-5). Then as they listened carefully to the poem being read and were shown the pictures of the dragons, there were asked to try to determine what the words meant.

Facilitating Complex Structures

Children can be introduced to the literate style of texts through familiar stories that have repetitive or cumulative organization. Listen to the language style of *The Three Billy Goats Gruff* (Asbjornsen & Moe, 1957):

> *Once on a time there were three billy goats who were to go up to the hillside to make themselves fat, and the name of all three was "Gruff." On the way up was a bridge over a river they had to cross, and under the bridge lived a great ugly troll with eyes as big as saucers and a nose as long as a poker. So first of all came the youngest Billy Goat Gruff to cross the bridge. "Trip, trap! trip, trap!" went the bridge.*

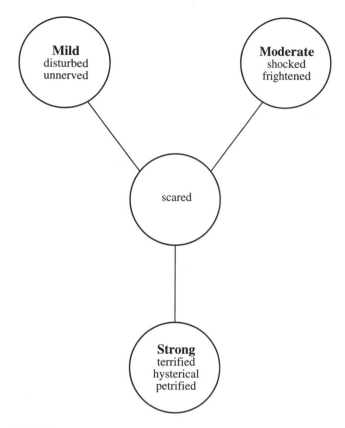

FIGURE 7-2   Emotional word web.

or from *Millions of Cats* (Gag, 1928):

> Once upon a time there was a very old man and a very old woman. They lived in a nice clean house which had flowers all around it, except where the door was. But they couldn't be happy because they were so very lonely.

The beginnings of these stories have relative clauses (introduced by *who* and *which*), literate conjunctions (*because, but, except*), inverted sentence structure (*on the way up was a bridge over the river they had to cross*), and descriptive vocabulary (*eyes as big as saucers, nose as long as a poker*).

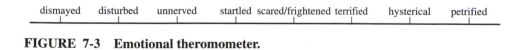

FIGURE 7-3   Emotional theromometer.

TABLE 7-5   Judging Vocabulary Knowledge

	Have never heard it	Have an idea of what it means, but not sure	Know it and use it
dismal			
disgruntled			
dastardly			
despondent			
dashing			
dainty			
drowsy			
quivering			

Some stories make considerable use of one or two aspects of literate language style. Such books can be used to highlight specific literate structures. Relative pronouns can be introduced through stories such as *There Was an Old Woman Who Swallowed a Fly* (Adams, 1973) or *The House That Jack Built* (Rogers, 1968) or its variant, *The House That Drac Built* (Sierra, 1995). In *Millions of Cats*, each cat is described by a relative clause: "a kitten which was black and very beautiful, a cat which had brown and yellow stripes like a baby tiger, another cat which was so pretty he could not bear to leave it." The repetitive nature of the first two stories facilitates role-playing by young children. The *Millions of Cats*, story can be extended by having children look through cat calendars, choose the cat they like, and describe it using relative clauses (e.g., "I like this cat that has long orange fur and a short tail.").

Many stories use complex sentence structures. It has often been assumed that complex sentences are particularly difficult to comprehend. Actually, complex sentences with certain conjunctions are sometimes easier to understand than two simple sentences, because the conjunctions signal the important relationship existing between the sentence components (Armbruster, 1984; Pearson, 1974). If-then structures are presented in books such as *If I Were a Toad* (Paterson, 1977), in which a child says what she would do if she were different animals ("If I were a fish, I would be too smart to bite the hook"), and *If I Had* (Mayer, 1968), in which a boy tells what he would do with different animals ("If I had a snake, I'd put it in my toybox. Then my sister wouldn't mess up my toys."). The teacher can reinforce the concept through role-play, asking the children to demonstrate what would they do if they were a kangaroo, a puppy, a horse, or if they had a porcupine or a lion.

A book such as *When I Was Young in the Mountains* (Rylant, 1982) can be used to introduce the temporal conjunction *when*. In this book the author reflects on the things she did when she was young and living in the mountains. This book experience can be extended by having children bring in pictures of themselves when they were younger and talking about them or making their own book of *When I Was Young*. For young children, this can be followed with *When I Get Bigger* (Mayer, 1983), in which the main character talks about all the things he will do when he is bigger.

The conjunction *but*, which is difficult to explain, can be made clear in stories. For example, in *Just for You* (Mayer, 1975), the little monster is trying to be helpful, but always ends up creating problems ("I wanted to help you carry the groceries just for you, but the bag broke."). In *One Monday Morning* (Shulevitz, 1967), the king comes to visit a little boy, but he isn't home. Each day the king and more of his retinue come to visit, but the boy isn't home. Several of Eric Carle's books emphasize the word *but*. In *The Very Quiet Cricket* (1990), a cricket encounters a number of insects. He wants to answer them. He rubs his wings together. *But nothing happened*, until he meets a female cricket. In *The Very Lonely Firefly* (1995), a firefly flies toward lights, *but it was not another firefly*, it was a lantern, cat's eyes, car headlights, and fireworks. The story, *Wombat Divine* (Fox, 1995), is particularly good for the conjunction *but* because it gives a specific reason for each *but*. Wombat wants a part in the Nativity *but* he is to heavy to be the Archangel Gabriel; too short to be a king, too sleepy to be Joseph, and so on.

In *The Gillygoofang* (Mendoza, 1982) and *Bringing the Rain to Kapiti Plain* (Aardema, 1981), explicit descriptive language is combined with relative pronouns and conjunctions:

> *The gillygoofang bewildered the giddyfish, a fish which could bounce up and down out of the water, not because it swam backward to keep water out of its eyes or changed colors to trick the bigger fish or whistled to warn the little fish or laid square eggs or slept in the weeds with one eye open, but because it couldn't bounce up and down out of the water.*

> *This is Ki-pat who watched his herd as he stood on one leg like a big stork bird; Ki-pat, whose cows were so hungry and dry, they mooed for the rain to fall from the sky; To green-up the grass, all brown and dead, that needed the rain from the cloud overhead —The big, black cloud, all heavy with rain, that shadowed the ground on Kapiti Plain.*

Developing Narrative Schema Knowledge

Skilled language users draw simultaneously on several sources of schematic knowledge in comprehending text:

1. Domain: Specific knowledge of topics, concepts, or processes for a particular subject matter.
2. General world knowledge: Understanding of social relationships, causes, and activities that are common to many specific situations and domains.
3. Knowledge of rhetorical or text grammar structures: Conventions for organizing and signaling the organization of texts (McNeil, 1987).

The conceptual knowledge underlying narrative text involves awareness of temporal action sequences, cause-effect or reactive sequences (first physical causality and later psychological causality), planning, and understanding of the concept of trickery or deception.

Family Role in Narrative Development

In order to learn to comprehend and produce narratives, children must hear a variety of well-structured narratives. Children with limited narrative abilities frequently do not enjoy listening to or reading complex stories. To ensure children's willingness to listen to or read stories, children must be provided with books that are comprehensible to them. By determining children's narrative abilities (using the guidelines presented earlier in this chapter) appropriate books can be made available. Books can be arranged according to narrative level on separate shelves in the classroom bookcase. The shelves are labeled with the names of children for whom the books would be appropriate. Children are assigned to shelves that contain books at or preferably slightly above their present narrative level. We have found that children are much more willing to listen to and read stories when they have chosen them. Narrative structure arises from understanding of conceptual relationships. Consequently, one does not teach the structure, but instead, one facilitates students' comprehension by giving them experiences with the domain-specific and world knowledge that underlie any particular structure.

The relationship between listening to stories and reading competency is explained to the students' parents. Current research shows the role that early experience with books has on children's later school success (Clark, 1976; Durkin, 1966; Wells, 1986). For example, Wells (1986) documented that the amount children were read to during the preschool years was the language variable most related to academic success at fifth grade. The teacher explains that the children will be bringing home books and that the parents are to read the books and help the child complete the book report form. Book report forms are matched to the child's level of narrative development. Table 7-6 presents the developmental sequence of questions asked on book report forms. Figure 7-4 shows a sample of a form used for an action or reactive sequence report. The book report forms provide the parents with guidelines of what they can discuss about the book with their child.

Experiences with books must also be carefully scaffolded. Storybook reading with children is not a part of all cultures, and many children come to school with no exposure to this type of activity. RD children from mainstream families also often have had limited exposure to storybook activities. Families of these children sometimes report having tried to read stories to their children, but the children were uninterested and inattentive so the family did not pursue the activity. If books are carefully matched to the child's narrative comprehension level, however, nearly every child will enjoy listening to stories.

The sequence of questions presented in the book reports is based on information regarding adult-children interaction with books and on information about narrative development. Infants' first exposure to books generally involves a labeling activity. The adult asks, "What's this?" When the child does not respond, the adult provides the label and goes on to the next page (Ninio & Bruner, 1976). Eventually, children learn to take their turn and will even initiate the game by bringing the adult a book and asking, "What's this?" Snow and Goldfield (1981) documented the following hierarchy of questions/comments that a parent used with her child between ages 2 to 4 years:

- Item levels (What's that? Who's that?)
- Item elaboration (How many pigs? What color car?)
- Event (What happened? What's ___ doing?)
- Motive/cause (Why did he want an umbrella?)
- Evaluation/reaction (How did he feel when that happened? Wasn't that a bad thing to do?)
- Real-world relevance (The pig's taking a bath. You did that this morning.)

TABLE 7-6   Book Report Sequence

Book Report 1: Description
1. Identify title either by naming or pointing to on cover.
2. Identify author either by naming or pointing to on cover.
3. Draw a picture of a favorite part of the story.
4. Describe the pictures in the book.

Book Report 2: Action Sequence
1. Identify title either by naming or pointing to on cover.
2. Identify author either by naming or pointing to on cover.
3. Name the major characters.
4. Tell the first thing that happened in the story.
5. Tell how the story ends.

Book Report 3: Action Sequence
1. Identify title either by naming or pointing to on cover.
2. Identify author either by naming or pointing to on cover.
3. Name the major characters.
4. Relate three things, in sequence, that happened in the story.
5. Retell the story using the pictures.

Book Report 4: Reactive Sequence
1. Identify title by naming.
2. Identify author by naming or pointing to on cover.
3. Respond to a why question concerning physical actions. (e.g., Why did the boy get an umbrella?)
4. Relate three things, in sequence, that happened in the story.
5. Retell the story using the pictures.

Book Report 5: Abbreviated Episode
1. Identify title by naming.
2. Identify author either by naming or by pointing to on cover.
3. Tell what the character wants.
4. Identify a feeling exhibited by one of the main characters.
5. Explain how you know a character is experiencing a particular feeling.
6. Retell the story using the pictures.

Book Report 6: Abbreviated Episode
1. Identify title by naming.
2. Identify author by naming or pointing to on cover.
3. Identify a feeling exhibited by one of the main characters.
4. Tell what the character wants.
5. Explain why the character feels as he or she does.
6. Retell the story without pictures.

Book Report 7
1. Identify title by naming.
2. Identify author by naming or pointing to on cover.
3. Tell problem in the story.
4. Tell how characters solved the problem.
5. Retell story without pictures.

Developed by Linda Costlow, Cynthia Garcia, and Carol Westby.

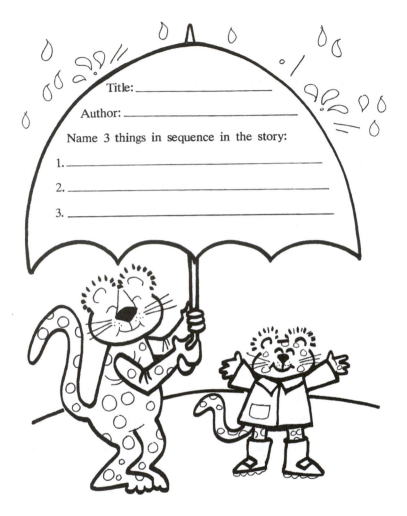

Title: _____

Author: _____

Name 3 things in sequence in the story:

1. _____

2. _____

3. _____

FIGURE 7-4   Sequence book report form.

Through this type of interactive discourse, children learn how to discuss and interpret books. Parents can also be educated to use this type of scaffolding in interacting with their children with RD when discussing personal experiences as well as when sharing books. Through such discussions, parents can facilitate children's development of a literate style oral language. At the beginning of the year, parents can be provided with a scrapbook. Periodically throughout the year, a page with a photograph of the child participating in a school activity is sent home with the child. Under the photo the teacher writes the types of questions the parent can ask to elicit a personal narrative. For young children or children with severe language handicaps, the initial questions require only labeling, such as "Who made the piñata?" Later, questions requiring event description are added, such as "What did

James do? What were you doing?" Still later, questions asking about motivation or cause are introduced, such as "Why did you make a piñata?" The photo album provides parents with information about what is happening at school and with systematic methods for facilitating their child's ability to talk about the school activities.

Developing Narrative Content Schema and Text Grammar Knowledge through Literature

Ideally, efforts should be made to involve families in facilitating students' narrative skills. Parents who are literate can be encouraged to read stories to their children and can be given guidance on how to select books and how to talk with their children about the stories. Simple book report forms can be used as a means to guide some of the interactions. Families who are not literate can be encouraged to talk with their children about pictures in books and can be encouraged to tell oral stories. Project TALES, a program to facilitate narrative and literacy skills in Native American children from pueblos without written languages has used Native storytellers to share stories with children and their families. The pueblos have had a history of rich storytelling, but with the advent of television and Nintendos, children are hearing fewer stories. Potluck dinners held after school have provided opportunities for children and parents to listen to stories from a Native storyteller and to share their own stories.

Narrative facilitation can be done in language therapy sessions and in curriculum activities in classrooms. The language arts curricula can be developed around narrative production and comprehension, and stories can be selected to supplement other academic subjects. By third grade, a meta-narrative approach can be incorporated into narrative activities. Students can be asked to identify the story elements: setting, initiating event, reaction, goal, attempts, consequences, resolution. They can also be asked to compare the elements of stories with similar themes.

Book report forms, such as in Figure 7-4, have been sent home with books that parents are to read to their children. Following the reading, the parents are to assist the children in completing the forms. The forms highlight specific aspects of narrative development. They have been kept short, so that parents and children focus on reading/listening to the story. For school-age students with RD, the purpose of their first book report is to familiarize them with the general nature of books and to play the question-answer game. In Book Report 1 in Table 7-6, children are asked to identify the title and author, describe the pictures in the book, and draw a picture of something in the book. Ability to do this results in "stories" with a descriptive structure. The books chosen for this level are those that have a central character or theme and a simple series of activities.

When children are able to describe the activities in the book, they are introduced to more concepts about the nature of a story and asked to tell how the story begins and how it ends. The children are introduced to the idea that books present a sequence of activities about a character and that one begins at the front of the book and finishes at the back of the book (Book Reports 2 and 3). Books in this category include *The Very Hungry Caterpillar* (Carle, 1969), a story about a caterpillar who eats its way through a variety of foods; *The Snowy Day* (Keats, 1962), about Peter's activities in the snow; and *Charlie Needs a Cloak* (dePaola, 1974), about the sequence of events involved in making a wool cloak for Charlie. (Note: Stories with similar content are *The Goat and the Rug* [Blood & Link, 1976], in which a goat describes how she and her Navajo friend make a rug and *Abuela's Weave* [Castaneda,

1993], a story of a how a Guatemalan child and her grandmother make and sell their weavings). To facilitate relating of a series of sequential activities, children can participate in activities similar to those in the story. For example, after reading *The Very Hungry Caterpillar*, children can sample the foods that the caterpillar ate. To extend children's experiences with *The Snowy Day*, a speech-language pathologist in Albuquerque took her ice chests to the mountain one weekend to fill them with snow so that on Monday the children in her class could make snowmen and throw snowballs. In another instance, children were studying a unit on early New Mexico. After the teacher read *Charlie Needs a Cloak*, weavers came to the classroom. They brought wool and showed the children how to spin it, then threaded a small hand loom and allowed the children to weave strips of cloth for scarves. Children can be encouraged to retell not only the stories in the books, but also to relate their own experiences. Stories of this type will result in action sequence narratives.

As children become able to deal with the beginning-to-end temporal action sequences, it is time to introduce cause-effect sequences, which give rise to stories of the reactive sequence type. In temporal sequence stories, the exact order of activities is not always critical. For example, in *The Snowy Day*, it is not important whether Peter first makes a snowball or an angel in the snow. Cause-effect (reactive sequence) stories, however, must have a set sequence of events. For example, in *Round Robin* (Kent, 1982), a small robin eats and eats until he becomes obese. When the other robins fly south for the winter, he must hop because he is too fat to fly. Because he is hopping along the snowy ground, a fox almost catches him.

Pourquoi tales that explain the origins of aspects of nature or the characteristics of certain animals are helpful to develop understanding of cause-effect because they make explicit links between actions and reactions. For example, in *Why Mosquitoes Buzz in People's Ears* (Aardema, 1975), a mosquito annoys an iguana by buzzing in his ear. The iguana puts sticks in his ears so he can't hear the mosquito. A python talks to the iguana, who cannot hear him because of the sticks in his ears. The python thinks the iguana is angry with him and runs into a rabbit hole. The rabbits run from their hole because they think the python is coming to eat them. The birds see the rabbits running and sound an alarm because they think there is danger. Hearing the alarm the monkeys swing swiftly through the trees. One of the monkeys falls on an owl's nest, causing the death of an owlet. In *Why the Sun and the Moon Live in the Sky* (Dayrell, 1968), the water refuses to visit the sun and the moon because their house is too small. The sun responds by building a bigger house. The water comes to visit; the water gets deeper and deeper, causing the sun and the moon to climb to the roof of their house and eventually causing them to flee to the sky. When reactive sequence stories are introduced, Book Report 4 can be provided. Now, in addition to being asked to relate three things in sequence that happened in the story, the students are also asked questions that focus on the physical causality or the reason for the activity. Why questions are introduced, such as, "Why couldn't the robin fly?" "Why did the rabbits run from their holes?" or "Why did sun build a bigger house?"

Repetitive or cumulative stories, which may have more complexity than action or reactive sequences, can be used to assist children in developing understanding of temporal and cause-effect sequences. Although the children may not understand all of the nuances in some of these stories, the repetitive nature of the story and chantlike nature of the language facilitates children's remembering of the words and action-reaction sequences. *Brown Bear, Brown Bear, What Do You See?* (Martin, 1983), *The Little Red Hen* (Galdone, 1973), *The Three Little Pigs* (Galdone, 1970), *Drummer Hoff* (Emberley, 1967), and *Tingo Tango Mango Tree* (Vaughn & Buchanan, 1995) are excellent examples that lend themselves to children's joining in the reading.

Development of the abbreviated and complete episode structure requires understanding of psychological causality or an understanding of motivations for behavior. Students must become aware that characters have feelings that motivate behavior or that feelings can be elicited by events. By kindergarten, children can identify and give examples of situations eliciting the emotions happy, mad, sad, and scared (Harter, 1982). Stories that explicitly label or discuss feelings, such as *Feelings* (Aliki, 1984) or *The Feeling Fun House* (Morse, Gauge, Tate, & Eickmeyer, 1985), or that elicit feelings, such as *The Quarreling Book* (Zolotow, 1963), are useful in this stage. Many of the Franklin Turtle stories and the Berenstain Bears stories deal with emotions experienced by young children. A story such as *Franklin in the Dark* (Bourgeois, 1986) is useful with young children for discussing the emotion of fear. Franklin is a young turtle who will not go into his shell because he is afraid of the dark. He visits a number of other animals who relate their fears, including a duck who wears water wings because he is afraid of deep water and a bird who wears a parachute because he is afraid of heights. In *Hetty and Harriet* (Oakley, 1981), two chickens set out to see the world. In the course of their adventures, they experience thirty-three different emotions. For older elementary school and middle school students, the popular Goosebumps books by R.L. Stein are very useful for facilitating understanding of characters' emotions. Stein frequently uses adverbs and descriptive adjectives and verbs to describe characters' behaviors and thoughts. Consider some of the following examples from *Monster Blood* (Stein, 1992):

> *"Thanks," said Evan uncertainly (p. 25).*
> *"Hi," said Andy timidly, giving the man a wave (p. 29).*
> *"Poor Evan," Andy said, half teasing, half sympathetic (p. 81).*
> *"You been in a fight?" she asked, squinting suspiciously at him (p. 86).*

Books such as these can provide children with the opportunity to discuss their own emotional experiences.

At this level, students also become alert to common scripts and character traits. To further scriptal development and awareness of character traits, a series of books having the same character or theme can be presented. Younger children will enjoy books about pigs and wolves. After children are familiar with *The Three Little Pigs* (Galdone, 1970), they can read such books as *Mr. and Mrs. Pig's Evening Out* (Rayner, 1976), in which the babysitter turns out to be a wolf, and *Garth Pig and the Ice Cream Lady* (Rayner, 1977), in which the ice cream lady is a wolf. The children can be encouraged to predict what they think will happen when they see the wolf appear at the door as the babysitter, or when Garth Pig enters the ice cream lady's truck. Older students enjoy stories about giants, trolls, and dragons. After several stories about dragons, the book *The Fourteenth Dragon* (Seidelman &

Mintonye, 1968) can be read. In this book thirteen dragons are vividly described in words and pictures. On the last page is the fourteenth dragon, the dragon that the reader of the book is to draw. Book Reports 5 and 6 are presented at this level.

The temporal sequence, physical causality, and psychological causality of the earlier stages are further elaborated in the complete episode stage. The role of planning in meeting the character's goals becomes important at this stage. Children now understand secondary emotions, such as shame, guilt, embarrassment, and pride. These emotions are dependent on higher cognitive functioning and awareness of social sanctions (Lewis & Michalson, 1983). Books that describe situations that elicit these feelings can be read and discussed. Understanding emotions should lead to a better understanding of characters' intentions and their attempts or plans to cope with their problems and emotions. The majority of stories require understanding of psychological causality and planning of characters. Some examples of such stories are described below. Internal emotion charts can be used to focus students on characters emotions, when the emotion occurred, and why it occurred. Table 7-7 shows a chart for the story *The Boy Who Lived with Seals* (Martin, 1993).

In *Chester the Worldly Pig* (Peet, 1965), Chester is dissatisfied with his life on the farm and decides to better himself by learning a skill and joining the circus. Although he succeeds in this goal, he later encounters numerous other serious threats from which he must

TABLE 7-7   Internal States Chart

The Boy Who Lived with Seals

Characters	When	Feeling	Why
parents	they discover that their son is not in camp	sad; disconsolate; despondent	because their boy is gone and may have been carried off by wild animals
parents	they learn that there is a boy living among seals	joyful	because they are sure it is their son
boy	he hears the seals calling	melancholy	because he misses his life with the seals
parents	the boy returns to live with the seals	sad but empathetic	because they didn't want to lose him but they understand his need to be with the seals
boy	he was back with the seals	joyful and grateful/ appreciative	joyful because he was back with the seals who were his family; and appreciative for the skills he learned from his human parents

escape. In *Cross-Country Cat* (Calhoun, 1979), Henry the cat is left behind at his owner's winter cabin. In order to catch up with his owners he sets out on skis and must cope with several dangers he encounters along the way. In *Fin M'Coul: The Giant of Knockmany Hill* (dePaola, 1981), Fin is being chased by a giant who is bigger and stronger than he is, and he and his wife must devise a plan to save themselves. In *Amazing Grace* (Hoffman, 1991), Grace is determined to be Peter Pan in the school play, even though classmates have told her she cannot be Peter Pan because she is a girl and she is black. Grace practices and practices; at the tryouts there is no doubt that she should be Peter Pan. Book Report 7 requires the students to identify the problem in the stories and explain how the characters solved the problems.

Between ages 10 and 12, typical students produce stories that are elaborated in a variety of ways. Early elaborations involve multiple attempts in the characters' plans or multiple minichapters or episodes. Later elaborations involve stories told from the point of view of more than one character or stories embedded within stories. Underlying these narrative structures are perception of character growth and change, awareness of deception, awareness of cyclical time, and understanding of figurative versus literal word meanings.

Beyond third grade, attention should be given to developing students' understanding of the landscape of consciousness. Not only must they be able to perceive the emotions and thoughts of the protagonists in response to events in stories, but they must also be able to perceive how other characters in stories respond to these same events. Interpretation of multiple landscapes of consciousness is critical for the story, *John Brown, Rose, and the Midnight Cat* (Wagner, 1977). Rose, a lonely and elderly woman, owns a large dog, John Brown. A black cat comes into her home. She dearly wants the cat to stay, but John Brown is jealous of the cat and sends it away. Emery (1996) suggested developing character maps to help students focus on both plot (landscape of action) and character (landscape of consciousness). Students identify the plot elements of the stories and perspectives of the various characters in the story of the events. Table 7-8 shows a character map for the story, *John Brown, Rose, and the Midnight Cat.*

Stories that rely heavily on characterization can be appreciated in the elaborated narrative stage. The book *Sarah, Plain and Tall* (MacLachlan, 1985) is an excellent introduction to this level. It contains several episodes but is short enough to be read in one long session or two short ones. This book is the story of a motherless pioneer family and the woman who answers papa's letter to come and be his wife. The changes in the emotional responses of each of the characters over the course of the story are critical to the events and outcome. Students can discuss the traits of each of the characters. For example, papa is lonely, thoughtful, industrious, sad; Sarah, the mail-order wife, is homesick, independent, optimistic, joyous, adventuresome; Caleb, the boy, is wistful, worrying, loving; and Anna, the girl, is hopeful, understanding, missing her mother. The story is told through the eyes of Anna. Students can be encouraged to retell the story through the eyes of the other characters.

By this stage, students appreciate books that require understanding of multiple meanings of words. These can be of two types: stories that involve a play on words or trickery tales. Many junior high students enjoy the books in the series *Not Quite Human* (McEvoy, 1985), which require appreciation of figurative and idiomatic expressions. In this series, a junior high teacher invents an android that can pass as a 12-year-old boy. The android's

TABLE 7-8   Character Perspective Map for *John Brown, Rose, and the Midnight Cat*

Rose's perspective	Story events	John Brown's perspective
Rose is curious and wants to see what it is.	**Initiating event:** Something moves in the garden.	John Brown does not want to look; he is hesitant and uncertain.
Rose decides there is a cat; she is lonely.	**Subsequent events:** Rose looks outside.	John Brown insists there is nobody there; he is jealous.
Rose is in bed and doesn't know what John Brown had done.	John Brown checks outside.	Feels the cat is not needed; is aggravated by its appearance.
Rose is disappointed that John Brown won't acknowledge the cat.	The next night Rose sees the cat again.	John Brown resents the cat and hopes it will go away.
Rose hopes the cat will come in and be her friend.	Rose puts out milk for the cat.	John Brown tips the milk; is irritated that the cat is around.
Rose is depressed/melancholy.	John Brown refuses to let the cat in.	John Brown is satisfied with himself that he has gotten rid of the cat.
Rose is despondent.	Rose stays in bed all day.	John Brown is concerned/ worried/alarmed about Rose.
Rose is relieved by John Brown's change of heart; is comforted by the cat.	**Resolution:** John Brown lets the cat in the house.	John Brown remains apprehensive/suspicious of the cat, but relieved that Rose is better.

"father" sends him to school. The android has been programmed with an extensive vocabulary, but his comprehension is overly literal as is illustrated in the following excerpt:

> *"My name is Chip," answered the android. "This is my first day at school."*
>
> *The man ran his hand through his thick black hair. "It's going to be your last day," he yelled, "or my name isn't Mr. Duckworth."*
>
> *"And if it isn't my last day," asked Chip, attempting to sort out the logic, "then what is your name?"*
>
> *"Your name is going to be mud if you don't tell me why you smashed my trophy case!"*
>
> *"My name will always be Chip," answered the mechanical boy. "It can't change. Although sometimes women change their names when they get married."*

The concept of deception may be introduced with trickery tales. Students must be assisted in understanding that what a person says is not necessarily what he or she intends to do. The concept can be introduced to middle school students through trickery tales from different cultures, such as the coyote tales of the Southwest Indians, Anansi the Spider tales from Africa, raven tales from the Northwest, or the Uncle Remus tales from the South, as well as trickster tales from other cultures. Because these tales come from oral histories, they include frequent repetition and lend themselves to easy role-playing. Students are given the roles of the characters in the stories, and initially the teacher takes the role of the inner thoughts of the trickster. For example, in the story, *The Crocodile's Tale* (Aruego & Aruego, 1972), a Philippino folktale, the crocodile is caught in a noose. He promises to give a boy a gold ring if he cuts him down. We know, of course, that the crocodile has no intention of giving the boy a ring, but rather intends to eat him. When a student playing the crocodile finishes saying he will give the boy a gold ring, the teacher snickers and in a loud whisper says, "I'm not really going to give him a ring. I'm just saying that. I'm really going to grab him and take him into the river and eat him." After several role-playing experiences with the teacher verbalizing the inner thoughts and actual intentions of the trickster, a student can be assigned this role. Stories of Ikotomi, the Plains Indian trickster, also provide a means of teaching the concept of trickery (e.g., *Iktomi and the Berries* [Goble, 1989]; *Iktomi and the Ducks* [Goble, 1990]). The Iktomi books use three types of discourse—the discourse of the narrator telling the story (printed in large, dark black print), the discourse of Iktomi's inner thoughts (printed in small, dark print by pictures of Iktomi), and the discourse of the narrator commenting on Iktomi's behavior and trickery (print in large, light gray print). These multiple discourses make explicit Iktomi's deceptions.

The final stage of narrative development, metaphoric, does not result in additional complexity of narrative structure. The complexity is at the content level. The entire story may be allegorical and can be read for two levels of meaning. For example, *The Phantom Tollbooth* (Juster, 1961) may be read as the story of a boy's adventures in a strange land or as a story of a boy finding beauty and purpose in life. Similarly, the Narnia stories by C.S. Lewis can be read as exciting adventures of a group of children or as a theological statement on the conflict between good and evil.

Normally developing adolescents can think of abstractions of time and space, and as a consequence will enjoy science fiction and fantasy tales that play with these concepts. Such stories frequently have multiple embedded plots that take place during different time frames. Susan Cooper's *The Dark Is Rising (1973)* (and its four sequels) and Madeleine L'Engle's *A Wrinkle in Time* (1962) (and its two sequels) are excellent examples of stories that manipulate time and space. Both move back and forth between the present situation and other times and places.

By this stage, students have a meta-awareness of narratives. They know what to expect from narratives and can compare and contrast narratives in terms of structure and theme. This ability to compare and contrast narratives can be furthered by having students read different versions of the same story or several books on a similar theme. One can begin with highly familiar stories and obvious variations. For example, *The Three Little Hawaiian Pigs and the Magic Shark* (Laird, 1981), *The Three Little Javelinas* (Lowell, 1992), *The Three Little Wolves and the Big Bad Pig* (Trivizas, 1993), and *The True Story of the Three Little Pigs* (Scieszka, 1989) are all variations of *The Three Little Pigs*. *Wili Wai Kula and the Three Mongooses* (Laird, 1983), *Somebody and the Three Blairs* (Tolhurst, 1994), and *Goldilocks and the Three Hares* (Petach, 1995) are variations of *The Three Bears*. Stories with the same goal from different cultures can be compared. For example, there are a variety of Native legends regarding how man or animals got the sun. In a Cherokee version, *Grandmother Spider Brings the Sun* (Keams, 1995); for the Northwest Indians, it is *Raven* (McDermott, 1993) who gets the sun; and in an Inuit version (*How Snowshoe Hare Rescued the Sun*, [Bernhard, 1993]) Snowshoe Hare gets the sun from the demons' cave.

Many cultures have variants of the Cinderella tale. (See the listing in Appendix A). Students can study the geography and history of regions and countries and discuss the reasons for the variations in some of these stories. Using their meta-narrative skills, students can discuss the similarities and differences in these tales in terms of story grammar components such as settings, characters, problems (initiating events), type of magic, attempts to cope with the problem, and endings. The table in the appendix summarizes the characteristics of a number of Cinderella stories.

Some story versions, such as *The True Story of the Three Little Pigs* (Scieszka, 1989), which is told from the wolf's perspective, or *The Untold Story of Cinderella* (Shorto, 1990), which is told from the stepsisters' perspective, can assist students in developing the multiple perspective taking that is a critical component of the landscape of consciousness. Some interactive CD-ROM stories also allow the child to experience stories through the eyes of different characters. For example, *The Princess and the Pea* (Softkey, 1996) allows a child to hear or read the story from the point of view of the princess, the prince, or an "objective" lion.

Narratives can be used to provide students with some of the schema knowledge they will need to comprehend expository text in science and social study lessons. For example, when beginning a unit on weather for third grade students, a teacher read the book, *The Storm in the Night* (Stolz, 1990), in which a grandfather and a grandson sit out a storm while the grandfather tells about his fear of storms as a child. Following the story, children can be encouraged to share their experiences with storms. Then the legend, *How Thunder and Lightning Came to Be* (Harrell, 1995), can be read. In this story, two birds are given the task of figuring out a way to warn people of storms. Students can be told that this is one explanation for thunder and lightning and that they will be learning other explanations for thunder and lightning and other ways to warn people of storms. The informational story book, *The Magic School Bus inside a Hurricane* (Cole, 1995), can be used to introduce students to scientific principles of weather (including a scientific explanation of thunder and lightning and methods used to predict weather) in a combined narrative-expository format. Informational story books such those represented by the popular *Magic School Bus* books by Joanna Cole have the purposes and benefits of both narrative and expository texts. They can be especially helpful in transitioning students into expository texts (Leal, 1996). Compared to narrative or expository texts, informational story books have been shown to elicit richer discussion in elementary school students in several ways: (1) Students used more of their prior knowledge along with the information gained from the text in constructing an understanding of both the story and the information; (2) they continued their discussions longer; (3) they made predictions twice as often; and (4) they exhibited a greater level of comprehension and were more likely to make extra-textual connections to interpret this text (Leal, 1994; Maria & Junge, 1994).

Facilitating Metacognition

Facilitating Metacognitive Thought and Comprehension Monitoring
Meta-awareness of cognition and emotionality is essential for the interpretation of the landscape of consciousness in narratives. Metacognitive thought is also necessary for the

monitoring of behavior and monitoring of conversation (Dollaghan & Campbell, 1987; Markman, 1981; Patterson & Roberts, 1982; Robinson, 1981). If students do not monitor their comprehension during conversation and repair conversational breakdowns, they are unlikely to monitor their comprehension during reading and engage in strategic reading practices to ensure that they comprehend texts. To engage in comprehension monitoring and strategic reading, students need declarative knowledge (e.g., what strategies one can use), procedural knowledge (e.g., how the strategies are used), and conditional knowledge (e.g., when and why the strategies are used). Although some students appear to develop strategic reading without explicit teaching, the majority of students benefit from direct teaching of specific comprehension strategies (Pressley, Woloshyn, & Associates 1995).

To encourage children to monitor what they were hearing, a teacher in an elementary classroom for students with RD intentionally gave inappropriate instructions such as "Wash these paper napkins so we can use them tomorrow," or obviously wrong or impossible suggestions such as "Hurry and put your shoes on your heads so we can go out for recess." Initially, many children attempted to respond to these instructions, but they quickly learned that they had to listen carefully to the teacher and correct her because she made mistakes. It appeared that many of the students initially assumed that teachers were always right, and consequently they never challenged anything they were told. After catching the teacher in obvious errors, they became freer to question the teacher and let her know they did not understand what was expected. Gradually, the obviousness of the inappropriate instructions was reduced so that students had to listen more carefully.

Academically successful students read for meaning (to comprehend) and read to remember (to study) (Baker & Brown, 1984). As with other aspects of learning, metacognitive comprehension monitoring must be modeled meaningfully if students are to use it. Vygotsky (1978) pointed out that verbal social interaction plays a major role in the development of higher mental (metacognitive) functions. These functions first occur on an interpersonal (social) level and later on an intrapersonal (individual) level. Gavelek and Raphael (1985) proposed that the interactive discourse that occurs in questioning introduces children to metacognitive skills. By asking appropriate questions about texts, teachers carry out the metacognitive functions that students should eventually come to exercise themselves. Comprehension monitoring requires that students learn to ask themselves the questions that previously the teacher had asked. Postman and Weingartner (1969) stated that "Once you have learned how to ask questions, relevant and appropriate and substantial questions, you have learned how to learn and no one can keep you from learning whatever you want or need to know" (p. 23).

Effective readers create meaning for a text in their own minds as they interact with passages (Tierney & Pearson, 1983). To construct a coherent meaning, readers must know what questions to formulate about a text and what questions they may be expected to answer (Fitzgerald, 1983). Comprehension monitoring can initially be practiced during a story reading time when the teacher is reading an interesting story to a group of children. By asking appropriate questions, teachers can facilitate students' retrieval of appropriate schemata, drawing inferences, and monitoring of their text comprehension to determine if they have selected the appropriate schema or if they must change their schema selection. Below, excerpts from the story *The Magic Finger* (Dahl, 1966) are used to show how this might be done. The teacher reads a passage (p. 18):

> *"We must do it," said Mr. Gregg. "We've got to have somewhere to sleep. Follow me." They flew off to a tall tree and right at the top of it Mr. Gregg chose a place for the nest. "Now we want sticks," he said. "Lots and lots of little sticks. off you go, all of you, and find them and bring them back here."*

The teacher asks the students, "What do you think this story is about?" The students are required to justify any answer from information that has been provided in the text. For example, if they respond that the story is about birds, they should refer to the fact that Mr. Gregg flew to a tree and talked about a nest. These are things that birds could do. The teacher can challenge this response by noting that Mr. Gregg talked, and birds don't talk. Students may counter with the idea that in fantasy stories, birds do sometimes talk. The teacher continues reading, stopping and questioning the students regarding what the story is about and what is happening. Later in the story, the teacher reads (p. 21):

> *"Oh, dear! Oh, dear!" said Mrs. Gregg. "They have taken over our whole house!*
>
> *We shall never get it back. And what are we going to eat?"*
>
> *"I will not eat worms," said Philip. "I would rather die."*
>
> *"Or slugs," said William.*
>
> *Mrs. Gregg took the two boys under her wings and hugged them. "Don't worry," she said. "I can mince it all up very fine and you won't even know the difference.*
>
> *Lovely slugburgers. Delicious wormburgers."*
>
> *"Oh no!" cried William.*
>
> *"Never!" said Philip.*
>
> *"Disgusting!" said Mr. Gregg. "Just because we have wings, we don't have to eat bird food. We shall eat apples instead. Our trees are full of them. Come on!"*
>
> *So they flew off to an apple tree.*
>
> *But to eat an apple without holding it in your hands is not easy. Every time you try to get your teeth into it, it just pushes away.*

The information in this part of the text should cause listeners/readers to question their choice of a bird schema for the story. The teacher stops and asks what the students now think the story is about. If they still say it is about birds, she draws their attention to parts of the text. Did Mr. and Mrs. Gregg always live in a nest? She reminds them of Mrs. Gregg's comment about not being able to get back to her house. She also notes that these birds don't like the usual bird food. Perhaps they do not like worms because they are fairy-tale birds, but she also notes that they also did not seem to know how to eat apples because they did not have hands. Even if they were fairy-tale birds, they should have been able to eat apples with their mouths.

A variant of this procedure is the Directed Reading Thinking Activity (DRTA) (Richek, 1987; Stauffer, 1969). In using the DRTA, students listen to or read a portion of a text.

Then they stop and are asked to orally predict what will happen next and to give reasons for these predictions. After this justification, they listen to or read another section of the text, noting whether or not their predictions have been confirmed. Then they report which predictions were confirmed by referring to the text for support. Students can be encouraged to make predictions about a story by using cues in the title and the picture on the book cover.

The ability to use cues is critical for comprehension of landscape of consciousness because a characters' thoughts and feelings are often implied rather than explicitly stated (Barton, 1996). The clinician or teacher can discuss the types of cues present in texts and assist students in finding the cues. Table 7-9 lists the types of cues and provides examples from the story, *Chinye* (Onyefulu, 1994), a West African version of Cinderella.

Helping students in comprehension monitoring is a worthwhile activity for all older elementary and middle school and high school students. Different types of stories and text genres provide different types of cues, and the teacher needs to demonstrate the use of these cues as he or she asks questions that focus students' attention on the cues. Modeling of comprehension monitoring and guiding students in comprehension monitoring appears to be even more essential for expository than narrative texts. Hardy (1978) has stated that narrative is a primary act of mind, and Bruner (1985) has added that narrative is a primary mode of thought. Perhaps because of this primacy of the narrative mode, less comprehension monitoring is necessary to comprehend narratives. It appears likely, however, that the unfamiliar concepts and structures of expository text require much more active metacognitive processing to be comprehended. In the section on narrative assessment, I indicated that the structure of narratives arises from the content schemata of the narratives. If one understands human goal-directed behavior, one will also understand and recognize the structure

TABLE 7-9   Clues about Characters' Emotions

Category Name	Example
Character statements	The stepmother said: "What took you so long?" she demanded, glaring.
Character actions	She stretched out a hand and touched Chinye tenderly on the cheek.
Plot events	The stepmother sends Chinye into the forest at night for water.
Text features	!(exclamation points) "My life is bad enough already, without making my stepmother angry!"
Emotional vocabulary	Nkechi's eyes gleamed greedily.
	"Look, Mother," she said proudly when she got home.
Story setting	To reach the stream, Chinye had to go through the forest. Wild animals prowled there, and even on moonlit nights the bravest villagers stayed at home.
Character thoughts	The stepmother thinks: Why couldn't it have been Adanma (her daughter) who met the old woman. . . . Maybe it was not too late!
Story mood	Note shifts in tone.
Author style	The author may use pauses or different sizes of print to convey emotions or attitudes.

of a good story. Expository texts, however, have no preordained structure. Readers must discover the text grammar structure of each expository text if they are to use it to facilitate their comprehension.

To facilitate metacognitive monitoring of expository texts, teachers can explain the functions of different types of expository texts, identify the different types of texts, the organization of the types, and the key words that students can look for (Finley & Seaton, 1987; McGee & Richgels, 1985; Piccolo, 1987). Some examples are shown in Table 7-10. The teacher can read a text aloud, modeling her or his own thought processes while doing so. The teacher can present the students with a passage, and then have them scan the passage for key words and make predictions about the structure of the paragraph.

The K-W-L procedure is a useful procedure for preparing students for the schema or content information they will encounter in expository text (Ogle, 1986). K stands for what students ***Know***—their prior knowledge before they begin to read. The teacher or clinician introduces the topic and asks students to list everything they know about the topic. W stands for what the students ***Want*** to know. This information is put in the second column. After the reading, students list what they have ***Learned*** in the third column (L) and compare this information to their prior knowledge and what they wanted to learn. The first two columns provide teachers/clinicians with an understanding of students' present schemata and what should be presented and emphasized. For example, the students who completed the information in Table 7-11 have some true information about mammals, but they may also have

TABLE 7-10   Expository Text Types and Characteristics

Text Type	Function	Key Words
Descriptive	Does the text tell me what something is?	No key words
Sequence/procedural	Does the text tell me how to do something or make something?	first . . . next . . . then; second . . . third; following this step; finally
Cause/effect	Does the text give reasons for why something happens?	because, since, reasons, then, therefore, for this reason, results, effects, consequently, so, in order, thus, then
Problem/solution	Does the text state a problem and offer solutions to the problem?	a problem is, a solution is
Comparison/contrast	Is the text showing how two things are the same or different?	different, same, alike, similar, although, however, on the other hand, but, yet, still, rather than, instead of
Enumerative	Does the text give a list of things that are related to the topic?	an example is, for instance, another, next, finally

TABLE 7-11   Learning about Mammals

What I already KNOW	What I WANT to learn	What I LEARNED
have fur	Where do they live?	
eat grass	Do they live in water?	
need to breath	What do they build their homes	
warm-blooded	out of?	
need homes	Are humans mammals?	
need shelter	What do they eat?	
give birth	Do they drink milk?	
have four legs	Do they live in salt water?	
	Where do they keep their babies	
	after birth?	

some incorrect concepts (all mammals eat grass and have four legs). The third column is a strategy that encourages students to reflect on their comprehension—an important metacognitive strategy. The teacher might want to include a fourth column—What I'd still like to know.

The ability to generate one's own questions has been shown to enhance comprehension and learning (Sternberg, 1987; Wong, 1985b). By mid-elementary school, students should be encouraged to generate and answer thought-provoking questions about the material they are reading. The questions need to go beyond memory or rote recall, requiring application, analysis, synthesis, and evaluation of the material. Teachers can provide students with generic thought-provoking questions and model examples (King, 1995). Table 7-12 shows generic, memory, and thinking questions for a unit on weather conducted in an elementary classroom.

TABLE 7-12   Generating Thought-Provoking Questions

Generic Questions	Memory Questions	Thinking Questions
Explain why (how)	What is a barometer?	Why would you use a barometer?
What is the main idea of . . . ?	What is the air pressure in	Why is the air pressure on the
How would you use . . . to . . . ?	Albuquerque? What is the air pressure	mountain top different from the air
What are the differences	on Sandia Crest (mountain top)?	pressure in Albuquerque?
between . . . and . . . ?	What is fog? What is smog?	How are fog and smog similar?
How are . . . and . . . similar?	Where do tornadoes occur? Where do	How are fog and smog different?
What would happen if . . . ?	hurricanes occur?	How are tornadoes and hurricanes
What causes . . . ? Why?		different?
How does . . . affect . . . ?		Explain what causes wind.
How is . . . related to what we		
studied earlier?		
What evidence is there to		
support your answer?		

Reciprocal peer or cooperative teaching is another helpful method to develop comprehension monitoring strategies in students (Dansereau, 1987; Palincsar & Brown, 1984). Cooperative teaching can be approached in several ways. One method that has been used with children beginning in elementary school is guided peer questioning (King, 1995). Following a teacher presentation or reading, students work together in small groups, and using the generic question types they generate two or three thoughtful questions on the material, then take turns asking and answering one another's questions. In another method, two students read the same passage. When both are finished, one student summarizes what he or she has read and the other student corrects any errors he or she has noted in the summary. In a third method, two students read different passages. Then one student summarizes the passage and the other student asks clarifying questions. Then the students switch roles. These particular cooperative teaching methods have been useful with older students in junior high and beyond who have some metacognitive monitoring skills in place.

For younger students, those with more advanced narrative abilities can be used to facilitate other students' development of narrative skills. Students who are able to comprehend and produce complete episode stories can usually work effectively with children with less developed narrative skills. The younger child may have a parent read the story, or in some instances the older peer tutor reads the story to the younger child. Then the older student asks the questions on the book report form to the younger child and judges the younger child's response.

Facilitating Regulation of Cognition or Control of Behavior

Just having the necessary language skills and content and text grammar schemas and the declarative, procedural, and conditional knowledge to engage in strategic reading does not ensure that students will comprehend. Students must be motivated to engage in strategic reading; they must be actively involved in understanding, remembering, and learning from the texts. As indicated earlier, before students can monitor their text comprehension, they must be able to plan and monitor their motoric activities. To facilitate development of regulation of cognition, children must be involved in planning many of the activities that are carried out in the classroom. To plan their behavior children must (1) determine what the task is, (2) reflect on what they know or need to know, (3) devise a plan for dealing with the task, (4) monitor progress, and (5) evaluate the outcome. Initially, the teacher models this planning behavior by thinking aloud as an activity is conducted. Meichenbaum's (1977) self-instructional training paradigm provides guidelines for what the teacher would say. For example, when the class made cheese-lion sandwiches (open-face cheese sandwiches with celery for a face and grated cheese for manes), the teacher began by defining the task or the problem ("I'm going to make a cheese-lion sandwich"). She then focused her attention on the steps in the process ("I need a piece of bread and a slice of cheese; now I need to cut some celery for his face"). Next, she verbally reinforced herself ("I cut just the right size piece of celery"), verbally corrected errors ("I didn't slice enough cheese to cover the bread—I need to cut some more"), and commented on the outcome ("This lion looks good enough to eat"). Then she talked the children through the activity step by step. As the children cut the celery and grated the cheese, she verbalized their progress toward completion of the sandwich, and finally she talked with the children about the outcome of the project—how the sandwiches looked and tasted.

As children became familiar with the process of classroom projects, they became more responsible for the planning and execution of activities. When an activity was presented, the children had to determine what was needed and how they would proceed. Ralph the Bear pictures from the Think Aloud curriculum (Camp & Bash, 1981) were enlarged and displayed in the room. In this four-poster series, Ralph models the steps in self-guiding speech by asking (1) "What is my problem" or "What am I supposed to do?" (2) "How can I do it?" or "What is my plan?" (3) "Am I using my plan?" and (4) "How did I do?" These posters helped the children remember the steps used in planning and carrying out an activity. By asking the children, "Are you following Ralph Bear's rules?" the teachers were able to reduce their overt monitoring of the children's behavior. Reduction of overt monitoring of the children's actions by the teacher is essential if children are to internalize the metacognitive monitoring process.

Symbolic play time, or creative dramatics, also provides an opportunity to plan. Elementary school children engage in play themes such as having a birthday party, going to a restaurant, visiting the doctor or hospital, going on a camping trip to the International Balloon Fiesta, or re-creating a book they have read. They must decide what roles are required for the theme, who will play each role, what events will happen, what problems might arise and how they will cope with them, what materials and props they need, and what time of day or year the event is taking place. They may also produce a play for younger children. This requires additional planning and monitoring of communication to ensure that their audience will be able to understand the story.

At the middle school level, simulation games have been used as focus units. For example, in Albuquerque, in a classroom of 24 students with RD, team-taught by two special-education teachers and a speech-language pathologist, a nine-week period in language arts was devoted to the theme of pioneers. Pioneers were described as people who chose to travel to a new unsettled area. The unit was begun by having the students view the film *Seven Alone*, the true story of the Sager children who were orphaned on the Oregon Trail in 1844. The majority of the students in the class were not originally from Albuquerque. The teacher requested that the students interview their parents and grandparents to learn where they had moved from, why they had moved, and how they had moved. In small-group discussions, the students compared their families' reasons for and manner of moving with the Sager family's. Then the students began the simulation game *Pioneers* (Wesley, 1974). *Pioneers* is a simulation that allows students to vicariously participate in situations and events similar to those experienced by pioneers who headed west in early wagon trains. The teacher and student manuals for the game provide goals that must be accomplished and situations that the travelers will experience over the course of several weeks. The 24 students were divided into three wagon teams of 8 students. Each student represented a family head. Students were assigned identities and given families and stock. The individual students had to make decisions regarding what they would take in their wagons. They were given a large selection of items to choose from, but were limited in the weight of materials they could take. Consequently, they had to make decisions regarding specific items they would take. A wrong decision, such as omission of critical supplies, could create later difficulties. The interactive CD-ROM *The Oregon Trail* (Softkey, 1996), provides a similar type of activity for individual or small groups of students. As with *Pioneers,* students select roles and must make decisions about supplies, directions, hunting, trading, resting, getting across rivers, and so on. The program gives somewhat quicker (but not immediate) feedback on their decisions.

As the simulation progressed, the wagon train groups had to make decisions, such as what to do about a lack of water, how to cross a flooded river, how to handle hostile Indians, and which trail to take. In coping with each problem that arose and arriving at a decision, the groups had to define who was involved, where the action took place, when the action took place, what the problem was, and why it was a problem. Then they had to discuss possible actions and the pros and cons of each action. Individual students and wagon trains gained points to move along the trail based on the wisdom of their decisions and by reading other books about pioneers and doing a variety of related projects, such as researching what to do in case of a snake bite, building model Conestoga wagons, and preparing a frontier meal for other class members (e.g., one class cooked buffalo meat stew). The students read from journals and diaries that were written by pioneers who had traveled on wagon trains. They also kept journals of the events they experienced during the simulation.

As the simulation progressed, students became more aware of the need to cooperate and make wise decisions. Students on one train argued heatedly and decided to split their train in two and go on separate trails. Within a few days it became clear that these two smaller trains could not survive. They did not have people with expertise in some areas; for example, one part of the train had the doctor, while the other part had the blacksmith. The smaller trains also did not have access to all of the tools or food necessary, and the students on the smaller trains could not read enough or do enough individual projects to collect sufficient points to move the train ahead quickly. The simulation activity provided students with consequential feedback on their planning and decision making.

Summary

Comprehending text is essential if students are to become independent learners. There are many tests available to measure text comprehension, but only recently are attempts truly being made to teach comprehension. We cannot teach comprehension unless we understand what cognitive and linguistic abilities underlie the comprehension process. For many years it was assumed that if students were able to decode rapidly, comprehension would automatically follow. Although this does indeed appear to be the case for many normally developing students, it is not the case for students with RD.

In this chapter, procedures to assess and facilitate text comprehension were described. Adequate assessment should include evaluation of students' (1) literate language style, (2) physical and social world knowledge, (3) ability to organize this conceptual knowledge into coherent texts such as stories, and (4) ability to monitor their own motoric activities and their text comprehension.

In order to assist students with RD in developing their reading comprehension abilities, we must first facilitate their understanding of the linguistic and cognitive concepts that occur in texts. To do this, texts must be presented that are interesting and comprehensible to the students. We must then assist the students in developing the metacognitive monitoring strategies that will enable them to be strategic readers and to learn from text without the support of a teacher. Effective intervention to develop students with comprehension skills that enable them to develop critical and dynamic literacy should (Paris, Wasik, & Turner, 1991):

- Develop in students a sense of ownership about the information they read
- Be developmentally appropriate to the students' language learning and metacognitive levels
- Call attention to the structure of texts and tasks
- Promote collaboration among peers and teachers
- Transfer control of instruction to the students so that they take responsibility for their own self-regulated learning

References

Abrams, D., & Sutton-Smith, B. (1987). The development of the trickster in children's narrative. *Journal of American Folklore*, *90*, 29–47.

Anderson, R. (1994). Role of the reader's schemata in comprehension, learning and memory. In R.B. Ruddell, M. Rapp, & H. Singer (Eds.), *Theoretical models and processes of reading* (pp. 469–482) (4th ed.). Newark, DE: International Reading Association.

Applebee, A. (1978). *The child's concept of story*. Chicago: Chicago University Press.

Armbruster, B. (1984). The problem of ''inconsiderate text.'' In G. Duffy, L. Roehler, & J. Mason (Eds.), *Comprehension instruction* (pp. 202–217). New York: Longman.

Baker, L. (1982). An evaluation of the role of metacognitive deficits in learning disabilities. *Topics in Learning and Learning Disabilities*, *2*, 27–35.

Baker, L., & Brown, A. (1984). Metacognitive skills and reading. In P. Pearson (Ed.), *Handbook of reading research* (pp. 353–394). New York: Longman.

Baker, L., & Stein, N. (1981). The development of prose comprehension skills. In C. Santa & B. Hayes (Eds.), *Children's prose comprehension*. Newark, DE: International Reading Association.

Bartlett, F. (1932). *Remembering: A study in experimental social psychology*. Cambridge: Cambridge University Press.

Barton, J. (1996). Interpreting character emotions for literature comprehension. *Journal of Adolescent & Adult Literacy, 40*:1, 22–28.

Beaugrande, R. (1980). *Text, discourse, and process.* Norwood, NJ: Ablex

Beaugrande, R. (1984). Learning to read versus reading to learn: A discourse-processing approach. In H. Mandl, N. Stein, & T. Trabasso (Eds.), *Learning and comprehension of text* (pp. 159–191). Hillsdale, NJ: Erlbaum.

Blachowicz, C.L.Z. (1994). Problem-solving strategies for academic success. In G. Wallach & K. Butler (Eds.), *Language learning disabilities in school-age children and adolescents* (pp. 304–322). New York: Merrill.

Black, J. (1985). An exposition on understanding expository text. In B. Britton & J. Black (Eds.), *Understanding expository text* (pp. 249-267). Hillsdale, NJ: Erlbaum.

Black, J., & Bower, G. (1980). Story understanding and problem solving. *Poetics, 9*, 223–250.

Bos, C., & Filip, D. (1982). Comprehension monitoring skills in learning disabled and average readers. *Topics in Learning and Learning Disabilities, 2*, 79–85.

Botvin, G., & Sutton-Smith, B. (1977). The development of structural complexity in children's fantasy narratives. *Developmental Psychology, 13*, 377–388.

Bower, G., Black, J., & Turner, J. (1979). Scripts in memory for texts. *Cognitive Psychology, 11*, 177–220.

Bransford, J.D. (1994). Schemata activation and schema acquisition: Comments on Richard C. Anderson's remarks. In R.B. Ruddell, M. Rapp, & H. Singer (Eds.), *Theoretical models and processes of reading.* (pp. 483–495) (4th ed.). Newark, DE: International Reading Association.

Bretherton, I., & Beegly, M. (1982). Talking about internal states: The acquisition of a theory of mind. *Developmental Psychology, 18*, 906–921.

Brewer, W. (1980). Literary theory, rhetoric, and stylistics: Implications for psychology. In R. Spiro, B. Bruce, & W. Brewer (Eds.), *Theoretical issues in reading comprehension* (pp. 221–239). Hillsdale, NJ: Erlbaum.

Britton, B., Glynn, S., & Smith, J. (1985). Cognitive demands of processing expository text: A cognitive workbench model. In B. Bruce & J. Black (Eds.), *Understanding expository text* (pp. 227–248). Hillsdale, NJ: Erlbaum.

Brown, A. (1982). Learning how to learn from reading. In J. Langer & M. Smith-Burke (Eds.), *Reader meets author: Bridging the gap* (pp. 26–54). Newark, DE: International Reading Association.

Brown, A. (1987). Metacognition, executive control, self-regulation, and other more mysterious mechanisms. In F. Weinert & R. Kluwe (Eds.), *Metacognition, motivation, and understanding*. Hillsdale, NJ: Erlbaum.

Bruce, B. (1980). Plans and social action. In R. Spiro, B. Bruce, & W. Brewer (Eds.), *Theoretical issues in reading comprehension* (pp. 367–384). Hillsdale, NJ: Erlbaum.

Bruce, B., & Newman, D. (1978). Interacting plans. *Cognitive Science, 2*, 195–233.

Bruner, J. (1985). Narrative and paradigmatic modes of thought. In E. Eisner (Ed.), *Learning and teaching the ways of knowing* (pp. 97–115). Chicago: University of Chicago Press.

Bruner, J. (1986). *Actual minds, possible worlds*. Cambridge, MA: Harvard University Press.

Camp, B., & Bash, M. (1981). *Think aloud: Increasing social and cognitive skills—A problem-solving approach*. Champaign, IL: Research Press.

Chafe, W. (1982). Integration and involvement in speaking, writing, and oral literature. In D. Tannen (Ed.), *Spoken and written language*. Norwood, NJ: Ablex.

Chambliss, M. (1995). Text cues and strategies readers use to construct the gist of lengthy written arguments. *Reading Research Quarterly, 30*:4, 778–807.

Clark, M. (1976). *Young fluent readers*. London: Heinemann.

Clay, M. (1973). *Reading: The patterning of complex behavior*. Portsmouth, NH: Heinemann.

Cook-Gumperz, J., & Gumperz, J. (1981). From oral to written culture: The transition to literacy. In M. F. Whiteman (Ed.), *Variation in writing: Functional and linguistic differences* (pp. 90–109). Hillsdale, NJ: Erlbaum.

Cope, B., & Kalantzis, M. (1993). *The powers of literacy*. Pittsburgh: University of Pittsburgh Press.

Crystal, D. (1979). *Working with LARSP*. New York: Elsevier.

Dansereau, D. (1987). Transfer from cooperative to individual studying. *Journal of Reading, 30*, 614–619.

DePaulo, B., & Jordan, A. (1982). Age changes in deceiving and detecting deceit. In R. Feldman (Ed.), *Development of nonverbal behavior in children* (pp. 140–180). New York: Springer-Verlag.

Dixon, C. (1979). Text type and children's recall. In M. Kamil & A. Moe (Eds.), *Reading research: Studies and applications*. Clemson, SC: National Reading Conference.

Dollaghan, C. & Campbell, T. (1987). Comprehension monitoring in normal and language-impaired children. *Topics in Language Disorders, 7*, 45–60.

Durkin, D. (1966). *Children who read early*. New York: Teachers College Press.

Feagans, L., & Short, E. (1984). Developmental differences in the comprehension and production of narratives by reading disabled and normally achieving children. *Child Development, 55*, 1727–1736.

Emery, D.W. (1996). Helping readers comprehend stories from the characters' perspective. *The Reading Teacher, 49*, 534–541.

Feldman, C.F., Bruner, J., Renderer, B. & Spitzer, S. (1990). Narrative comprehension. In B.K. Britton & A.D. Pelligrini (Eds.), *Narrative thought and narrative language* (pp. 1–78). Hillsdale, NJ: Erlbaum.

Fillion, B., & Brause, R. (1987). Research into classroom practices: What have we learned and where are we going? In J. Squire (Ed.), *The dynamics of language learning* (pp. 291–225). Urbana, IL: ERIC.

Finley, C., & Seaton, M. (1987). Using text patterns and question prediction to study for tests. *Journal of Reading, 32*, 124–142.

Fitzgerald, J. (1983). Helping readers gain self-control over reading comprehension. *The Reading Teacher, 37,* 249–253.

Flood, J., & Lapp, D. (1987). Reading and writing relations: Assumptions and directions. In J. Squire (Ed.), *The dynamics of language learning* (pp. 9–26). Urbana, IL: ERIC.

Forrest-Pressley, D., & Waller, T. (1984). *Cognition, metacognition, and reading.* New York: Springer-Verlag.

Freedle, R., & Hale, G. (1979). Acquisition of new comprehension schemata for expository prose by transfer of a narrative schema. In R. Freedle (Ed.), *New directions in discourse processing* (pp. 121–134). Norwood, NJ: Ablex.

Gardner, R. (1987). *Metacognition and reading comprehension.* Norwood, NJ: Ablex.

Garvey, C. (1982). Communication and the development of social role play. *New Directions in Child Development, 18,* 81–101.

Gavelek, J., & Raphael, T. (1985). Metacognition, instruction, and the role of questioning activities. In D. Forrest-Pressley, G. MacKinnon, & T. Waller (Eds.), *Metacognition, cognition, and human performance* (pp. 103–136). Orlando: Academic Press.

Glenn, C., & Stein, N. (1980). Syntactic structures and real-world themes in stories generated by children. (Tech. Report). Urbana: University of Illinois.

Goldman, S. (1982). Knowledge systems for realistic goals. *Discourse Processes, 5,* 279–303.

Goodman, K. (1973). On the psycholinguistic method of teaching reading. In F. Smith (Ed.), *Psycholinguistics and reading.* New York: Holt, Rinehart, and Winston.

Gordon, C., & Braun, C. (1985). Metacognitive processes: Reading and writing narrative discourse. In D. Forrest-Pressley, G. MacKinnon, & T. Waller (Eds.), *Metacognition, cognition, and human performance* (pp. 1–75). Orlando: Academic Press.

Graesser, A. (1981). *Prose comprehension beyond the word.* New York: Springer-Verlag.

Graesser, A., & Goodman, S. (1985). Implicit knowledge, question answering and the representation of expository text. In B. Britton & J. Black (Eds.), *Understanding expository text* (pp. 109–171). Hillsdale, NJ: Erlbaum.

Graybeal, C. (1981). Memory for stories in language impaired children. *Applied Psycholinguistics, 2,* 269–283.

Hall, M., Ribovich, J., & Ramig, C. (1979). *Reading and the elementary school child.* New York: Van Nostrand.

Hallahan, D., Kneedler, R., & Lloyd, J. (1983). Cognitive behavior modification techniques for learning disabled children: Self-instruction and self-monitoring. In J. McKinney & L. Feagans (Eds.), *Current topics in learning disabilities* (pp. 207–244). Norwood, NJ: Ablex.

Hansen, C. (1978). Story retelling used with average and learning disabled readers as a measure of reading comprehension. *Learning Disability Quarterly, 1,* 62–69.

Hardy, B. (1978). Narrative as a primary act of mind. In M. Meek, A. Warlow, & G. Barton (Eds.), *The cool web* (pp. 12–23). New York: Atheneum.

Harter, S. (1982). Children's understanding of multiple emotions: A cognitive developmental approach. In W. Overton (Ed.), *The relationship between social and cognitive development* (pp. 147–194). Hillsdale, NJ: Erlbaum.

Horowitz, R. (1985a). Text patterns: Part 1. *Journal of Reading, 28,* 448–454.

Horowitz, R. (1985b). Text patterns: Part ll. *Journal of Reading, 28,* pp. 534–541.

Horowitz, S., & Samuels, S.J. (1987). Comprehending oral and written language: Critical contrasts for literacy and schooling. In R. Horowitz & S.J. Samuels (Eds.), *Comprehending oral and written language* (pp. 1–52). San Diego: Academic Press.

Hunt, K. (1973). *Grammatical structures written at three grade levels.* Champaign, IL: NCTE Research Report 3.

Jacobs, J.E., & Paris, S.G. (1987). Children's metacognition about reading: Issues in definition, measurement, and instruction. *Educational Psychologist, 22,* 255–278.

Jenkins, J. (1979). Four points to remember: A tetrahedral model and memory experiments. In L. Cermak & F. Craik (Eds.), *Levels and processing in human memory.* Hillsdale, NJ: Erlbaum.

Johns, J., & Ellis, D. (1976). Reading: Children tell it like it is. *Reading World, 16:2,* 115–128.

Kalmar, I. (1985). Are there really no primitive languages? In D. Olson, N. Torrance, & A. Hildyard (Eds.), *Literacy, language, and learning.* New York: Cambridge University Press.

Kieras, D. (1985). Thematic processes in the comprehension of expository prose. In B. Britton & J.

Black (Eds.), *Understanding expository text* (pp. 89–107). Hillsdale, NJ: Erlbaum.

King, A. (1995). Cognitive strategies for learning from direct teaching. In E. Wood, V.E. Woloshyn, & T. Willoughby (Eds.), *Cognitive strategy instruction for middle and high school students* (pp. 18–65). Cambridge, MA: Brookline Books.

Kreitler, S., & Kreitler, H. (1987a). Plans and planning: Their motivational and cognitive antecedents. In S.L. Friedman, E.K. Scholnick, & R.R. Cocking (Eds.), *Blueprints for thinking* (pp. 110–178). Cambridge: Cambridge University Press.

Kreitler, S., & Kreitler, H. (1987b). Conceptions and processes of planning: The developmental perspective. In S.L. Friedman, E.K. Scholnick, & R.R. Cocking (Eds.), *Blueprints for thinking* (pp. 205–272). Cambridge: Cambridge University Press.

Lapp, D., & Flood, J. (1978). *Teaching reading to every child*. New York: Macmillan .

Leal, D.J. (1994). A comparison of third-grade children's listening comprehension of scientific information using an information book and an information storybook. In C.K. Kinzer & D.J. Leu (Eds.), *Multidimensional aspects of literacy research, theory, and practice* (pp. 137–145). Chicago: The National Reading Conference.

Leal, D.J. (1996). Transforming grand conversations into grand creations: Using different types of texts to influence student discussion. In L.B. Gambrell & J.F. Almasi (Eds.), *Lively discussions!* (pp. 149–168). Newark, DE: International Reading Association.

Lewis, M., & Michalson, L. (1983). *Children's emotions and moods*. New York: Plenum.

Liles, B. (1985). Cohesion in the narratives of normal and language disordered children. *Journal of Speech and Hearing Research, 28*, 123–133.

Liles, B. (1987). Episode organization and cohesive conjunctives in narratives of children with and without language disorder. *Journal of Speech and Hearing Research, 30*, 185–196.

Luria, A. (1961). *The role of speech in the regulation of normal and abnormal behavior*. New York: Liveright.

Mandler, J. (1982). Some uses and abuses of a story grammar. *Discourse Processes, 5*, 305–318.

Mandler, J. (1984). *Stories, scripts, and scenes: Aspects of schema theory*. Hillsdale, NJ: Erlbaum.

Maria, K., & Junge, K. (1994). A comparison of fifth graders' comprehension and retention of scientific information using a science textbook and an informational storybook. In C.K. Kinzer & D.J. Leu (Eds.), *Multidimensional aspects of literacy research, theory, and practice* (pp. 146–152). Chicago: The National Reading Conference.

Markman, E. (1981). Comprehension monitoring. In W. Dickson (Ed.), *Children's oral communication skills* (pp. 61–84). New York: Academic Press.

Max in Motion/Adventuresome Max (1989). Chicago: Society for Visual Education.

McGee, L., & Richgels, D. (1985). Teaching expository text structure to elementary students. *The Reading Teacher, 38*, 739–748.

McNeil, J. (1987). *Reading comprehension: New directions for classroom practice*. Glenview, IL: Scott, Foresman.

Meacham, J. (1979). The role of verbal activity in remembering the goals of actions. In G. Zivin (Ed.), *The development of self-regulation through private speech* (pp. 237–263). New York: Wiley.

Meichenbaum, D. (1977). *Cognitive-behavior modification: An integrative approach*. New York: Plenum.

Merritt, D., & Liles, B. (1987). Story grammar ability in children with and without language disorder: Story generation, story retelling, and story comprehension. *Journal of Speech and Hearing Research, 30*, 539–552.

Meyer, B. (1987). Following the author's top-level organization: An important skill for reading comprehension. In R. Tierney, P. Anders, & J. Mitchell (Eds.), *Understanding readers' understanding* (pp. 59–76). Hillsdale, NJ: Erlbaum.

Meyer, B., & Rice, G. (1984). The structure of text. In P. Pearson (Ed.), *Handbook of reading research* (pp. 319–351). New York: Longman.

Miller, G., Galanter, E., & Pribram, K. (1960). *Plans and the structure of behavior*. New York: Holt, Rinehart, and Winston.

Morris, P.J., & Tchudi, S. (1996). *The new literacy: Moving beyond the 3Rs*. San Francisco: Jossey-Bass.

Myers, M. (1987). The shared structure of oral and written language and the implications for teaching writing, reading, and literature. In J. Squire (Ed.), *The dynamics of language learning* (pp. 121–146). Urbana, IL: ERIC.

Myers, M., & Paris, S. (1978). Children's metacognitive knowledge about reading. *Journal of Educational Psychology, 70,* 680–690

Nelson, K. (1985). *Making sense: The acquisition of shared meaning.* Orlando: Academic Press.

Ninio, A., & Bruner, J. (1976). The achievement and antecedents of labeling. *Journal of Chad Language, 5,* 1–15.

Ogle, D. (1986). A teaching model that develops active reading for expository text. *The Reading Teacher, 39,* 564–570.

Oakhill, J., & Yuill, N. (1996). Higher order factors in comprehension disability: Processes and remediation. In C. Cornoldi & J. Oakhill (Eds.), *Reading comprehension difficulties: Processes and intervention* (pp. 69–92). Mahwah, NJ: Erlbaum.

Otto, W., & White, S. (Eds.) (1982). *Reading expository material.* New York: Academic Press.

Owings, R., Peterson, G., Bransford, J., Morris, C., & Stein, B. (1980). Spontaneous monitoring and regulation of learning: A comparison of successful and less successful fifth graders. *Journal of Educational Psychology, 72,* 250–256.

Palincsar, A., & Brown, A. (1984). Reciprocal teaching of comprehension fostering and comprehension-monitoring activities. *Cognition and Instruction, 1,* 117–175.

Paris, S.G. (1991). Assessment and remediation of metacognitive aspects of children's reading comprehension. *Topics in Language Disorders, 12,* 32–50.

Paris, S.G., Lipson, M., & Wixson, K. (1983). Becoming a strategic reader. *Contemporary Educational Psychology, 8,* 293–316.

Paris, S.G., & Myers, M. (1981). Comprehension monitoring, memory, and study strategies of good and poor readers. *Journal of Reading Behavior, 13,* 5–22.

Paris, S.G., Wasik, B.A., & Turner, J.A. (1991). The development of strategic readers. In R. Barr, M.L. Kamil, P. Mosenthal, & P.D. Pearson (Eds.), *Handbook of reading research, Vol. II* (pp. 609–640).

Patterson, C., & Roberts, R. (1982). Planning and the development of communication skills. *New Directions in Child Development, 18,* 29–46.

Pea, R. (1982). What is planning development the development of? In D. Forbes & M. Greenberg (Eds.), *Children's planning strategies.* San Francisco: Jossey-Bass.

Pearson, P. (1974). The effects of grammatical complexity on children's comprehension, recall, and conception of certain semantic relations. *Reading Research Quarterly, 10,* 155–192.

Pearson, P.D., & Fielding, L. (1991). Comprehension instruction. In R. Barr, M.L. Kamil, P. Mosenthal, & P.D Pearson (Eds.), *Handbook of reading research, Vol. II* (pp. 815–860). White Plains, NY: Longman.

Pearson, P., and Spiro, R. (1980). Toward a theory of reading comprehension instruction. *Topics in Language Disorders, 1,* 71–88.

Pellegrini, A. (1985). Relations between preschool children's symbolic play and literate behavior. In L. Galda & A. Pellegrini (Eds.), *Play, language, and stories.* Norwood, NJ: Ablex.

Piaget, J. (1932). *The moral judgment of the child.* London: Kegan Paul.

Piccolo, J. (1987). Expository text structure: Teaching and learning strategies. *The Reading Teacher, 40,* 838–847.

Postman, N., & Weingartner, C. (1969). *Teaching as a subversive activity.* New York: Delacorte Press.

Pressley, M., Woloshyn, V., & Associates (1995). *Cognitive strategy instruction that really improves children's academic performance.* Cambridge, MA: Brookline Books.

Reid, J. (1966). Learning to think about reading. *Educational Research, 9,* 56–62.

Richardson, J.S., & Morgan, R.F. (1994). *Reading to learn in the content areas.* Belmont, CA: Wadsworth Publishing.

Richek, M. (1987). DRTA: 5 variations that facilitate independence in reading narratives. *Journal of Reading, 30,* 632–636.

Richgels, D., McGee, L., Lomax, R., & Sheard, C. (1987). Awareness of four text structures: Effects on recall of expository text. *Reading Research Quarterly, 22,* 177–197.

Robinson, E. (1981). The child's understanding of inadequate messages and communication failure: A problem of ignorance or egocentrism. In W. Dickson (Ed.), *Children's oral communication skills* (pp. 167–185). New York: Academic Press.

Roth, F., & Spekman, N. (1986). Narrative discourse: Spontaneously generated stories of learning disabled and normally achieving students. *Journal of Speech and Hearing Disorders, 51,* 8–23.

Rumelhart, D. (1980). Schemata: The building blocks of cognition. In R. Spiro, B. Bruce, & W. Brewer (Eds.), *Theoretical issues in reading comprehension* (pp. 33–58). Hillsdale, NJ: Erlbaum.

Sacerdoti, E. (1975). Nonlinear nature of plans. Proceedings of the Fourth International Joint Conference on Artificial Intelligence. Tbilisi, Georgia, U.S.S.R.

Sachs, J., Goldman, J., & Chaille, C. (1984). Planning in pretend play: Using language to coordinate narrative development. In A. Pellegrini & T. Yawkey (Eds.), *The development of oral and written language in social contexts*. Norwood, NJ: Ablex.

Scardamelia, M., & Bereiter, C. (1984). Development of strategies in text processing. In H. Mandl, N. Stein, & T. Trabasso (Eds.), *Learning and comprehension of text* (pp. 379–406). Hillsdale, NJ: Erlbaum.

Schank, R. (1982). *Reading and understanding*. Hillsdale, NJ: Erlbaum.

Schank, R., & Abelson, R. (1977). *Scripts, plans, goals, and understanding*. Hillsdale, NJ: Erlbaum.

Schmidt, C. (1976). Understanding human action: Recognizing the plans and motives of other persons. In J. Carroll & J. Payne (Eds.), *Cognition and social behavior*. Hillsdale, NJ: Erlbaum.

Scott, C. (1994). A discourse continuum for school-age students. In G. Wallach & K. Butler (Eds.), *Language learning disabilities in school-age children and adolescents* (pp. 219–252). New York: Merrill.

Sedlak, A. (1974). An investigation of the development of the child's understanding and evaluation of the actions of others. (Tech. Report No. NIH-CBM-TR-28). New Brunswick, NJ: Department of Computer Science, Rutgers University.

Snow, C., & Goldfield, B. (1981). Building stories: The emergence of information structures from conversation. In D. Tannen (Ed.), *Analyzing discourse: Text and talk* (pp. 127–141). Washington, D.C.: Georgetown University Press.

Spiro, R., & Taylor, B. (1987). On investigating children's transition from narrative to expository discourse: The multidimensional nature of psychological text classification. In R. Tierney, P. Anders, & J. Michell (Eds.), *Understanding readers' understanding* (pp. 77–93). Hillsdale, NJ: Erlbaum.

Spivack, G., Platt, J., & Shure, M. (1976). *The problem-solving approach to adjustment*. San Francisco: Jossey-Bass.

Stauffer, R. (1969). *Teaching reading as a thinking process*. New York: Harper and Row.

Stein, N., & Glenn, C. (1979). An analysis of story comprehension in elementary school children. In R. Freedle (Ed.), *New directions in discourse processing, Vol. II* (pp. 53–120). Norwood, NJ: Ablex.

Stein, N., & Policastro, M. (1984). The concept of story: A comparison between children's and teacher's viewpoints. In H. Mandl, N. Stein, & T. Trabasso (Eds.), *Learning and comprehension of text* (pp. 113–155). Hillsdale, NJ: Erlbaum.

Sternberg, R. (1987). Questioning and intelligence. *Questioning Exchange, 1*, 11–13.

Thorndyke, P. (1977). Cognitive structures in comprehension and memory of narrative discourse. *Cognitive Psychology, 9*, 77–110.

Tierney, R., & Pearson, P. (1983). Toward a composing model of reading. *Language Arts, 60*, 568–580.

Tough, J. (1981). *Talk for teaching and learning*. Portsmouth, NH: Heinemann.

Trabasso, T., & Magliano, J.P. (1996). How do children understand what they read and what can we do to help them. In M.F. Graves, P.v.d. Broek, & B.M. Taylor (Eds.), *The first r: Every child's right to read* (pp. 160–188). Newark, NE: International Reading Association.

Vacca, J.A., Vacca, R.T., & Grove, M.K. (1991). *Reading and learning to read*. New York: Harper Collins.

van Dijk, T., & Kintsch, W. (1983). *Strategies of discourse comprehension*. New York: Academic Press.

Voss, J., & Bisanz, G. (1985). Knowledge and the processing of narrative and expository text: Some methodological issues. In B. Britton & J. Black (Eds.), *Understanding expository text* (pp. 385–391). Hillsdale, NJ: Erlbaum.

Vygotsky, L.S. (1978). *Mind in society*. Cambridge, MA: Harvard University Press.

Weaver, C. (1994). *Reading process and practice: From socio-psycholinguistics to whole language*. Portsmouth, NH: Heinemann.

Weaver, P., & Dickinson, D. (1979). Story comprehension and recall in dyslexic students. *Bulletin of Orton Society, 28*, 157–171.

Wellman, H. (1985). The origins of metacognition. In D. Forrest-Pressley, G. MacKinnon, & T. Waller

(Eds.), *Metacognition, cognition, and human performance* (pp. 1–31). Orlando: Academic Press.

Wells, G. (1986). *The meaning makers*. Portsmouth, NH: Heinemann.

Wesley, J. (1974). *Pioneers*. Lakeside, CA: Interact.

Westby, C. (1980). Assessment of cognitive and language abilities through play. *Language, Speech and Hearing Services in Schools, 11*, 154–168.

Westby, C. (1983). *Language in planning and problem solving*. Paper presented at the American Speech-Language-Hearing Association Convention, Cincinnati, OH.

Westby, C. (1988). Children's play: Reflections of social competence. *Seminars in Speech and Language, 9*:1, 1–14.

Westby, C. (1991). A scale for assessing pretend play. In C. Schaefer, K Gitlin, & A. Sandgrund (Eds.), *Play diagnosis and assessment* (pp. 131–161). New York: Wiley.

Westby, C. (1994). The effects of culture on genre, structure, and style of oral and written texts. In G. Wallach & K. Butler (Eds.), *Language learning disabilities in school-age children and adolescents* (pp. 120–218). New York: Merrill.

Westby, C., Maggart, Z., & Van Dongen, R. (1984). Oral narratives of students varying in reading ability. Paper presented at the Third International Congress for the Study of Child Language, Austin, TX.

Westby, C., Van Dongen, R., & Maggart, Z. (1986). The concept of trickery: Its development and role in culture and reading. Paper presented at the International Reading Association Convention, Philadelphia, PA.

Westby, C., Van Dongen, R., & Maggart, Z. (1989). Assessing narrative competence. *Seminars in Speech and Language, 10*, 63–76.

Wilensky, R. (1978). Why John married Mary: Understanding stories involving recurring goals. *Cognitive Science, 2*, 235–266.

Willows, D., & Ryan, E. (1981). Differential utilization of syntactic and semantic information by skilled and less skilled readers in the intermediate grades. *Journal of Educational Psychology, 73*, 607–615.

Wolf, D., & Hicks, D. (1989). The voices of narratives: The development of intertextuality in young children's stories. *Discourse Processes, 12*, 329–351.

Wong, B. (1982). Strategic behaviors in selecting retrieval cues in gifted, normal achieving, and learning disabled children. *Journal of Learning Disabilities, 15*, 33–37.

Wong, B. (1985a). Metacognition and learning disabilities. In D. Forrest-Pressley, G. MacKinnon, & T. Waller (Eds.), *Metacognition, cognition, and human performance* (pp. 137–180). Orlando, FL: Academic Press.

Wong, B. (1985b). Self-questioning instructional research: A review. *Review of Educational Research, 55*, 227–268.

Wong, B., & Wong, R. (1986). Study behavior as a function of metacognitive knowledge about critical task variables: An investigation of above average, average, and learning disabled readers. *Learning Disabilities Research, 1*, 101–111.

Yuill, N., & Oakhill, J. (1991). *Children's problems in text comprehension: An experimental investigation*. New York: Cambridge University Press.

Children's Materials

Aardema, V. (1975). *Why mosquitoes buzz in people's ears*. New York: Dial.

Aardema, V. (1981). *Bringing the rain to Kapiti plain*. New York: Dial.

Adams, P. (1973). *There was an old woman who swallowed a fly*. Wilts, England: Child's Play.

Aliki (1984). *Feelings*. New York: Greenwillow.

Aruego, J., & Aruego, A. (1972). *The crocodile's tale*. New York: Scholastic.

Asbjornsen, P., & Moe, J. (1957). *The three billy goats gruff*. New York: Harcourt Brace Jovanovich.

Bernhard, E. (1993). *How snowshoe hare rescued the sun: A tale from the Arctic*. New York: Holiday House.

Blood, C., & Link, M. (1976). *The goat in the rug*. New York: Aladdin Books.

Bourgeois, P. (1986). *Franklin in the dark*. New York: Scholastic.

Calhoun, M. (1979). *Cross-country cat*. New York: Mulberry Books.

Carle, E. (1969). *The very hungry caterpillar*. New York: Philomel.

Carle, E. (1990). *The very quiet cricket*. New York: Putnam.

Carle, E. (1995). *The very lonely firefly*. New York: Putnam.

Castaneda, O. (1993). *Abuela's weave*. New York: Lee & Low Books.

Cole, J. (1995). *The magic school bus inside a hurricane*. New York: Scholastic.

Cooper, S. (1973). *The dark is rising*. New York: Atheneum.

Dahl, R. (1966). *The magic finger*. New York: Harper and Row.

Dayrell, E. (1968). *Why the sun and the moon live in the sky*. New York: Houghton Mifflin.

dePaola, T. (1974). *Charlie needs a cloak*. Englewood Cliffs, NJ: Prentice-Hall.

dePaola, T. (1981). *Fin M'Coul: The giant of Knockmany Hill*. New York: Holiday House.

Ehrlich, A. (1985). *Cinderella*. New York: Dial.

Emberley, B. (1967). *Drummer Hoff*. Englewood Cliffs, NJ: Prentice-Hall.

Fox, M. (1995). *Wombat divine*. New York: Scholastic.

Gag, W. (1928). *Millions of cats*. New York: Coward, McCann, and Georhegan.

Galdone, P. (1973). *The little red hen*. New York: Scholastic.

Galdone, P. (1970). *The three little pigs*. New York: Clarion Books.

Geraghty, V. (1988). *Over the steamy swamp*. San Diego: Harcourt Brace.

Goble, P. (1989). *Iktomi and the berries*. New York: Orchard.

Goble, P. (1990). *Iktomi and the ducks*. New York: Orchard.

Grimm (1978). *Cinderella*. New York: Larousse.

Harrell, B. (1995). *How thunder and lightning came to be*. New York: Dial.

Hoffman, M. (1991). *Amazing Grace*. New York: Dial.

Johnson, T. (1995). *Aunt Nizzy Nazzy: The witch of Santa Fe*. New York: Putnam.

Juster, N. (1961). *The phantom tollbooth*. New York: Random House.

Keams, G. (1995). *Grandmother spider brings the sun*. Flagstaff, AZ: Northland.

Keats, E. (1962). *The snowy day*. New York: Viking.

Kent, J. (1982). *Round robin*. Englewood Cliffs, NJ: Prentice-Hall.

Laird, D. (1981). *The three little Hawaiian pigs and the magic shark*. Honolulu: Barnaby Books.

Laird, D. (1983). *Wili Wai Kula and the three mongooses*. Honolulu: Barnaby Books.

L'Engle, M. (1962). *A wrinkle in time*. New York: Dell.

Louie, A. (1982). *Yeh-Shen*. New York: Philomel.

Lowell, S. (1992). *The three little javelinas*. Flagstaff, AZ: Northland Publishing.

MacLachlan, P. (1985). *Sarah, plain and tall*. New York: Harper and Row.

Martin, B. (1983). *Brown bear, brown bear, what do you see?* New York: Holt, Rinehart, and Winston.

Martin, R. (1993). *The boy who lived with the seals*. New York: G.P. Putnam.

Mayer, M. (1968). *If I had*. New York: Dial.

Mayer, M. (1974). *Frog goes to dinner*. New York: Dial.

Mayer, M. (1983). *When I get bigger*. Racine, Wl: Western Publishing Co.

Mayer, M. (1975). *Just for you*. Racine, WI: Western Publishing Co.

Mayer, M., & Mayer, M. (1971). *A boy, a dog, a frog, and a friend*. New York: Dial.

Mayer, M., & Mayer, M. (1975). *One frog too many.* New York: Dial.

McDermott, G. (1993). *Raven: A trickster tale from the Pacific Northwest.* San Diego: Harcourt Brace.

McEvoy, S. (1985). *Not quite human: Batteries not included.* New York: Archway.

Mendoza, G. (1982). *The gillygoofang.* New York: Dial.

Morse, J., Gouge, B., Tate, D., & Eickmeyer, J. (1985). *The feeling fun house.* Dallas: Family Skills, Inc.

Oakley, G. (1981). *Hetty and Harriet.* New York: Atheneum.

Onyefulu, O. (1994). *Chinye: A West African folktale.* New York: Viking.

Paterson, D. (1977). *If I were a toad.* New York: Dial.

Peet, B. (1965). *Chester the worldly pig.* Boston: Houghton Mifflin.

Petach, B. (1995). *Goldilocks and the three hares.* New York: Grosset & Dunlap.

Rayner, M. (1976). *Mr. and Mrs. Pig's evening out.* New York: Atheneum.

Rayner, M. (1977). *Garth Pig and the ice cream lady.* New York: Atheneum.

Rogers, J. (1968). *The house that Jack built.* New York: Lothrop, Lee, and Shepard.

Rylant, C. (1982). *When I was young in the mountains.* New York: E. P. Dutton.

San Souci, R.D. (1989). *The talking eggs.* New York: Scholastic

Scieszka, J. (199). *The true story of the three little pigs.* New York: Puffin.

Seidelman, J., & Mintonye, G. (1968). *The fourteenth dragon.* New York: Harlin Quist.

Shorto, R. (1990). *The untold story of Cinderella.* New York: Citadel Press.

Shulevitz, U. (1967). *One Monday morning.* New York: Scribners.

Sierra, J. (1995). *The house that Dave built.* New York: Gulliver Books.

Society for Visual Literacy. (1989). *Max in motion/ Adventuresome Max.* Chicago.

Softkey. (1996). *The princess and the pea.*

Soto, G. (1993). *Too many tamales.* New York: Putnam & Grosset.

Stein, R.L. (1992). *Monster blood.* New York: Scholastic.

Stolz, M. (1990). *Storm in the night.* New York: Harper & Row.

Tolhurst, M. (1994). *Somebody and the three Blairs.* New York: Orchard.

Trivizas, E. (1993). *The three little wolves and the big bad pig.* New York: Simon & Schuster.

Van Woerkman, D. (1977). *Harry and Shellbert.* New York: Macmillan.

Vaughn, M. & Buchanan, Y. (1995). *Tingo tango mango tree.* Morristown, NJ: Silver Burdett.

Wagner, J. (1977). *John Brown, Rose, and the midnight cat.* Scarsdale: Bradbury Press.

Wood, A. (1996). *The Bunyans.* New York: The Blue Sky Press.

Zolotow, C. (1963). *The quarreling book.* New York: Harper and Row.

Appendix A: Cinderella Variants

Analyzing Cinderella

Version/Country	Setting/Cinder's Job	Other Characters	Problem	What Solves the Problem	Transportation	Where Going	Ending
French	housework	stepmother 3 stepsisters	needs clothes for ball	fairy godmother	pumpkin	ball	marries prince
Italian	Venice; maid	stepmother 2 stepsisters	needs clothes for ball	fairy mother	gondola	ball	marries duke
Korean	cooking, cleaning, hulling rice	stepmother stepsister	must weed rice paddy before going to festival	frog, birds, ox	—	festival	marries magistrate
Egyptian	slave (stolen by pirates)	servant girls master	falcon takes shoe		—	Memphis to see Pharaoh	marries Pharaoh
Chinese	cooking, cleaning	stepmother stepsister	must watch fruit; has only rags	fish	—	feast	marries king; stepmother and step sister live in cave and are crushed to death by stones
Magic Eggs (Southern)	iron, chop cotton	mother older sister	poor	old woman	—	old woman's house	moves to the city
Mufaro's Beautiful Daughters (African)	African countryside	father sister	to be judged worthy by king	girls' character, snake, boy, old woman	—	king's city	becomes queen; sister a servant
Turkey Girl (Zuni)	caring for turkeys	orphan; no other characters	needs clothes	turkeys	—	Dance of the Sacred bird	doesn't keep word; loses clothes and friends
Turkey Girl (Santo Domingo)	caring for turkeys	no other major characters	needs clothes	turkeys	—	powwow	enters mountain with turkeys
Cinderlad (Irish) (boy with big feet)	cowherd	father (peddler) stepmother stepsister, giant	runs away from home	ox	—	—	saves princess from dragon and marries her
Golden Slippers (Vietnamese)	worked in rice fields	stepmother stepsister	finishing her work; clothes	fish, ricebirds	horse	autumn festival	marries prince
Cinder Edna (modern)	housework lawn mowing clean bird cages	stepmother stepsisters	money for the ball	earns her own money	takes the bus	ball	marries prince's brother; studied waste disposal engineering
Cinder-Elly (rap)	New York City	mom, dad, 2 older sisters	no money for clothes	godmother	bicycle	basketball game	dates basketball player named Prince
Baba Yaga and Vasilisa the Brave (Russian)	Russian woods	stepmother 2 stepsisters witch	needs candle	doll	walk	Baba Yaga's	stepmother, sisters burned to death; weaves cloth; marries tzar

Cinderella Stories

Brown, M. (1954). *Cinderella*. New York: Macmillan. (French version of Cinderella)

Bernhard, E., & Bernhard, D. (1994). *The girl who wanted to hunt: A Siberian tale*. New York: Holiday House. (A young girl uses her skills as a hunter to avenge her father's death and to escape her evil stepmother).

Climo, S. (1989). *The Egyptian Cinderella*. New York: Harper Collins Publishers. (In this version of Cinderella set in Egypt in the sixth century B.C., Rhodopis, a slave girl, eventually comes to be chosen by Pharaoh to be his queen.)

Climo, S. (1993). *The Korean Cinderella*. New York: HarperCollins.

Climo, S. (1996). *The Irish Cinderlad*. New York, HarperCollins. (An Irish version with a boy instead of a girl. Boy belittled by stepmother and stepsisters rescues a princess after meeting a magical bull.)

Delamare, D. (1993). *Cinderella*. New York: Simon & Schuster. (Italian version)

Ehrlich, A. (1985). *Cinderella*. New York: Dial. (French)

Han, O.S. (1996). *Kongi and Potgi: A Cinderella story from Korea*. New York: Dial.

Jackson, E. (1994). *Cinder Edna*. New York: Lothrop, Lee & Shepard. (Modern day version of Cinderella)

Lewis, S. (1994). *Cinderella: Lamb Chop's play along*. New York: Bantam Doubleday Dell.

Louie, A. (1982). *Yeh-Shen: A Cinderella story from China*. New York: Philomel.

Lum, D. (1994). *The golden slipper*. New York: Troll Associates. (Vietnamese Cinderella)

Martin, R. (1992). *The rough-face girl*. New York: G.P. Putnam's Sons. (In this Algonquin Indian version of the Cinderella story, the rough face girl and her two beautiful but heartless sisters compete for the affections of the invisible being.)

Mayer, M. (1994). *Baba Yaga and Vasilisa the brave*. New York: Morrow Junior Books. (Russian Cinderella. Beautiful Vasilisa uses the help of her doll to escape from the clutches of the witch Baba Yaga, who sets in motion the events that lead to the once ill-treated girl's marrying the tzar.)

Minters, F. (1994). *Cinder-Elly*. New York: Viking. (An inner-city rap version of Cinderella)

Onyefulu, O. (1994). *Chinye: A West African folk tale*. New York: Viking.

Perlman, J. (1992). *Cinderella penguin*. New York: Puffin.

San Souci, R. D. (1898). *The talking eggs*. New York: Scholastic. (Southern [Cajun or Gulluh] Cinderella story)

Shorto, R. (1990). *The untold story of Cinderella*. New York: Citadel Press. (Told from the perspective of Cinderella's stepsisters)

Steptoe, J. (1987). *Mufaro's beautiful daughters*. New York: Scholastic. (African Cinderella)

Velarde, P. (1989). *Old father story teller*. Santa Fe: Clear Light. (A collection of tribal legends from Santa Clara Pueblo, including Turkey Girl, a version of Cinderella)

Wegman, W. (1993). *Cinderella*. New York: Hyperion Books. (Dog version of Cinderella)

Chapter 8

Learning to Write

CHERYL M. SCOTT

In the book *Reading Disabilities* (Kamhi & Catts, 1989), several chapters were devoted to the topic of writing development and writing problems of children with developmental language-based reading disabilities. I pointed out that writing is an area of great difficulty for a majority of these children and one that frequently persists into adulthood, affecting personal, academic, and vocational domains (Blalock & Johnson, 1987). Several other reasons were cited for including information about writing in a book on reading. Research in emergent literacy had documented close connections between writing and reading (Dobson, 1988), and young children's "invented" spelling was thought to reflect a broader facility in phonological awareness so important to reading (Read, 1985, 1986). I emphasized that throughout school, writing and reading are inextricably connected. Kindergartners are asked to "read" what they "write." High school students read to find out what to write and write to demonstrate that they understand what they read.

Writing is a formidable topic of great interest to scholars in many disciplines, to regular and special educators and language clinicians, and even to politicians. It is a form of communication with roots in early childhood and a lifelong learning curve. Any discussion of developmental writing problems must be grounded in a knowledge base about the development of writing. Both topics in turn require a framework for talking about writing—the purposes served by writing, the contexts where it takes place, the cognitive processes involved when we write, and the linguistic forms writing can take. This was the strategy followed for the material on writing in Kamhi and Catts's *Reading Disabilities* (1989) and remains a viable strategy for this chapter.

Several perspectives about writing and its development in children are important to emphasize at the start. First is the point that *writing is always an act of writing a particular text*. A child (or adult for that matter) who is adept at story writing may or may not be able to pen a convincing argument. The two types of writing call on very different cognitive abilities, employ different sentence and text level forms, and appear at different times in different ways in school curricula. Two children may have very different experiences and exposure to different types of writing, depending on their sociocultural and educational circumstances. A second perspective is the *fine line between "normal" and "disordered" writing*. As the title of this chapter implies, learning to write is a task for all children. Although information about the writing of children with language and reading disabilities is included, the title does not single out "writing disorders," "writing disabilities," or some other label for children with these problems. Writing is not easily reduced to a dichotomous standard of acceptable/unacceptable. More often, writing difficulties are a matter of degree rather than outright difference.

The present chapter is organized into three major sections: a framework for considering the topic of writing, the development of writing in children and adolescents, and problems in writing encountered by children with language and reading disabilities. This chapter lays the groundwork for the consideration of writing assessment and intervention, as addressed by Westby in Chapter 9.

A Framework for Writing

What kind of activity is writing? If this question were put to a variety of people, most likely there would be a variety of answers, depending on the individual's age, education, cultural background, and work history. The answer of some might reveal that they consider writing to be a *transcription process*—the physical act of transforming spoken language into written language, much like an ancient scribe or modern-day court stenographer. This view actually reflects the thinking of a prominent linguist of the first half-century, Leonard Bloomfield, who dismissed writing as "merely a way of recording language by means of visible marks" (Bloomfield, 1933, p. 21). Other answers might highlight the *form of writing*— for example, spelling words or making correct sentences, paragraphs, or even an entire five-paragraph essay. In fact, elementary school children, particularly those with language and reading disabilities, are likely to say that writing is "making the words right," or "making good sentences." High school and college students see writing mainly as a *demonstration of knowledge*, done for the purpose of giving teachers what they want and making a good grade (Evans, 1993). Young and older students alike realize that they will be judged through their writing, for either their form or content or both. Hopefully some who answered the question would concentrate on the function of writing as a *type of communication*—for example, writing a story to entertain, writing a letter to the editor to persuade, or writing an E-mail message to keep in touch with a friend. A last group of answers could conceivably highlight writing as a *tool*—one that can be used as a memory aid or a means of personal reflection and growth (e.g., the minutes of a meeting, or a private journal). Writing is also a *learning tool*. By writing about a topic, we come to understand the topic in a different or deeper way (Bereiter & Scardamalia, 1987). Writing, of course, is all of these things. Writing serves a variety of communicative and cognitive purposes, takes on a variety of linguistic forms consistent with those purposes, and requires the coordination of highly complex mental processes to produce. It is the "final common pathway" of cognition and language— making simultaneous statements about linguistic knowledge as well as world knowledge and social cognition.

Context and Purpose: Where, for Whom, and Why?

A hypothetical list of distinctive types of writing, each with its unique purpose and unique form, would presumably be limited only by our patience. We could discuss writing according to the place where it is done—writing done at home, in school, in the workplace, in community and government institutions. Such broad contextual categories suggest some obvious categories of writing. A teenager's self-sponsored home writing might consist of letters and/or a diary while school-sponsored writing would include book reports, essay test questions, science lab reports, and so forth. Writing can be a solitary activity, with absolute silence from start to finish, or for a first grade child it could be a social activity, done in the context of talking, playing, and drawing with classmates. Something is written to be read by an audience. The audience may be the writer (e.g., a locked personal journal), only one other person (a report for a teacher), a group of known people (the minutes of a faculty meeting), or a group of unknown people. Mature writers "write to an audience"; as they write they are inside the mind of the eventual reader, constructing the reader's response and adjusting their writing accordingly. In addition to the obvious communicative purposes of writing, texts also store and preserve information. A newspaper article about a family member is cut out for a scrapbook; a difficult article is put aside for later re-reading. Writing is all of these variations and many more. The contexts and purposes for writing change dramatically over the course of elementary and secondary schooling and beyond.

Linguistic Form

For purposes of this chapter, text is defined broadly as a piece of writing done for a particular purpose. For a young child, a text might be a few words that accompany a drawing. For the tenth grader, the five-paragraph theme supporting a point of view is a text. A written genre is a distinctive type of text—for example, narrative text, persuasive text, factual text, and so forth. To write in a particular genre is to conform to a particular set of linguistic constraints at the text level (e.g., narratives start with a setting) and also at the sentence level (e.g., narratives usually employ simple past tense forms of verbs). Conveniently, then, writers do not have to invent a new form each time the same situation arises. Genre acquisition cannot be reduced to learning a specified set of skills; however, writers must gain at least some control over major formal features of genre (Popken, 1996). Text and sentence-level features of narrative and expository (informational, factual)[1] genres important in school writing have been described elsewhere by Scott (1988, 1994, 1995) and Westby (1994).

In addition to linguistic constraints imposed by genre, written sentences have distinctive grammatical properties that arise from *modality*—the fact that they are written rather than spoken (Perera, 1984, 1986; Scott, 1988, 1994, 1995). Without direct teaching, children's writing takes on this distinctive "written" grammatical flavor at an early age.

Writing requires other types of linguistic knowledge; words must be spelled and sentences must be punctuated. Whereas spelling and punctuation are frequently described as lower level "mechanical" activities, learning how to spell and punctuate are more recently seen as cognitive-linguistic activities of considerable dimension. For example, punctuation

---

[1]The terms *expository, informational,* and *factual* text will be used interchangeably.

used by novice writers is said to reveal much about children's developing metasyntactic and metatextual knowledge (Kress, 1982; Simone, 1996). Recent information about the development of punctuation is included in the chapter. Any adequate treatment of the development of spelling would require a chapter in its own right; therefore, the topic is not addressed here.

The Process of Writing

Among those who model the writing process, there seems to be unanimous agreement that it is a complex mental process (Bereiter & Scardamalia, 1987). Compared to speaking, writing requires a high level of abstraction, elaboration, conscious reflection (Gombert, 1992), and self-regulation (Graham & Harris, 1994). Models of the writing process are not concerned with very casual sorts of writing, for example, dashing off a note to a friend or a quick reminder memo. Rather, models of writing attempt to explain the *composition* process—how we would proceed to write an essay, or a report, or a story of some length. Another term for this type of writing is *epistemic* writing—the type that both advances the writer's knowledge of a topic and is credible to the reader (Bryson & Scardamalia, 1991). One well-known model conceives of writing as a problem-solving activity with three overlapping and even recursive stages[2] (Hayes & Flower, 1980, 1987). A model based on this work is portrayed schematically in Figure 8-1. Writers first develop an internal representation of the problem and establish goals (e.g., "write a paper that effectively describes deforestation of the American Northwest, is at least five pages, and earns an A from the teacher"). In the *planning* phase, writers select information from their knowledge base and organize that information for an effective presentation. Subprocesses of planning include (1) generating relevant information by retrieving it from long-term memory, (2) organizing the retrieved information, (3) setting goals for the text and criteria for its evaluation, and (4) developing "en route" strategies for completing the paper (Black, 1981; Graham & Harris, 1993). Mature writers draw on their knowledge of text structure during the planning stage (e.g., "I need to follow a point-counterpoint structure for each of the three points"). Topic knowledge alone does not necessarily ensure clear writing.

In the *generation* phase, pen is put to paper and text is produced. Writers must now choose the words and structures that encode the meanings they wish to convey. Hayes and Flower (1987) reported that ideas in an outline are expanded by mature writers on the average by a factor of eight as text is actually generated. Writers work by producing a part of a sentence, pausing, generating the next part, pausing, all in a left-to-right manner. By studying the types of errors writers make, researchers have gained insight into the nature of the text generation process (e.g., Daiute, 1984).

Revising is the final phase of the composition model. In an attempt to improve the text, writers make changes that range from changing a word, adding a comma, to reorganizing

---

[2]Hayes and Flower (1980, 1987) emphasized the recursive nature of operations in their model—a characteristic that distinguishes the model from previous sequential stage models of writing and underscores the constructivist problem-solving nature of writing (Fitzgerald, 1992). Planning and revision operations may occur at any point in the composing process and may cycle back to earlier portions of the text.

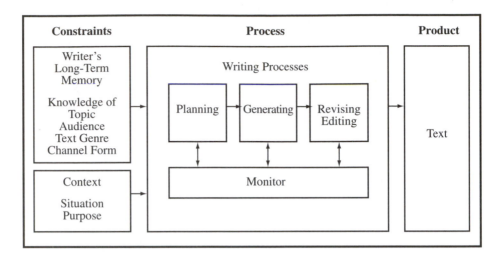

FIGURE 8-1   A simplified schematic of the writing process, based on the
Hayes and Flower (1980, 1987) model.

or adding/deleting major portions. Research challenges the view of revision as an end-stage process, stressing instead the recursive nature of revising (Witte, 1983). Older writers and expert writers devote proportionally more time to revising and make changes involving larger stretches of discourse and text meaning. Revisions of younger writers and novice writers are more frequently devoted to the word or sentence level and are less apt to change the meaning.

This three-stage model of writing was devised in response to *protocol analysis*, a research paradigm in which writers are asked to *think aloud* (Hayes & Flower, 1980, 1987) as they write. Verbatim transcripts of what writers say, along with observations of what they do (e.g., analyses of pause behavior), make inherently private cognitive processes more accessible for study. Recently, think-alouds have been used to study how writing processes change with development and whether different processes are used by children with learning disabilities.

Whereas the Hayes and Flower model was designed as a model of mature, or expert writing, Bereiter and Scardamalia (1987) distinguish between novice and mature writing in their work. The novice writer uses a *knowledge-telling model* to generate a text. Like the expert writer, the novice writer sees composition as a problem to be solved, but a different kind of problem—namely one of accessing enough relevant information to satisfy length and genre requirements for the writing assignment or task. Bryson and Scardamalia (1991, p. 45) illustrated this model for the hypothetical writing assignment "Is television a good influence on children?" Two types of cues are used to generate text: topic identifiers such as "television shows" and "children," and discourse knowledge (e.g., "say what you think and then give reasons"). These cues are the entree to long-term memory where information is called up and transcribed in "think-say" cycles. The composition moves forward in an linear, sometimes associative, manner in which the mention of one point can trigger the mention of an associated point (e.g., "It's good for children to watch comedy shows. My favorite comedy show is . . . .").

Expert writing, on the other hand, is described in a *knowledge-transforming model* (Bereiter & Scardamalia, 1987). This writer is guided by a "discover what I know" rather than a "tell what I know" mandate. Presumably, the discoveries would not have come about without the act of writing. Differences between the novice and expert models are evident in longer start-up times and more extensive note-taking. Think-aloud analysis reveals an active "dialectic" between content (what the writer knows and believes) and rhetorical issues (how the writer should best say it); in the course of this internal conversation, thinking can evolve in new directions (Bryson & Scardamalia, 1991). The knowledge-transforming model is stressed increasingly in current writing pedagogy literature, particularly in response to what some perceive as an overemphasis of "vacuous" writing process instruction (Writing and Thinking, Interview with Leif Fearn, 1996). Some writers continue to use a knowledge-telling model throughout their school years and beyond.

Two additional views of the nature of writing have surfaced in recent years. First, the social-interactive model of writing (Nystrand, 1989) sees writing as fundamentally an interaction of minds—that of the writer and the hypothesized or real reader. Writing is an act of thinking as the reader would think and making text adjustments that result in a better communication. Whereas problem-solving models focus on cognitive processes of the writer, the social-interaction model emphasizes two sets of cognitive processes (the writer and the reader) and their interaction. The details of the social-interaction model are beyond the scope of this overview, but adopting the model does have implications for descriptions of writing development and for writing pedagogy (Fitzgerald, 1992). A second trend is to view writing within a broader framework of theories of self-regulated learning (e.g., Zimmerman, 1989). Basically, these models categorize a variety of strategies and feedback mechanisms whereby writers move forward in the composing process. For example, a writer could impose a minimum number of words that must be written before something less taxing (e.g., going to the movies) is done. Or, it might be necessary to rearrange the environment (e.g., move the computer to another room). Zimmerman (1989) stressed three strategies in particular—self-observation, self-judgment, and self-reaction—as critical in writing and learning. Graham and Harris (1994) have drawn extensively on self-regulation models in designing intervention approaches for poor writers.

Writing in the Future

It is not uncommon to hear questions about writing and its uses in the future. We hear and read that the electronic/technological age, with its thirst for speed in the delivery of information, will turn us into information consumers with no patience for writing, which, by nature, takes more time. Perhaps voice recognition technology in computers will impact writing. When Donald Graves was asked recently about the future of writing (Writing Process: In Retrospect, 1996), he predicted an increase in the volume of writing:

> Computers and writing are a perfect match. I see greater opportunities for publishing and getting your work out. Certainly the mechanical aspects are much easier than ever before, so I see the computer as a wonderful friend. (p. 6)

Stephen and Susan Tchudi (Why Write?, 1995) share Graves's optimism. They point out that E-mail, for instance, has actually revived interest in print literacy. Whereas letter writing declined when long distance telephoning became affordable, many people who once corresponded by phone are once again writing their messages on E-mail and actually prefer this method to the phone. In an age of information bombardment, perhaps people will write more, not less, because writing provides an opportunity to slow down, reflect, and process information more thoroughly. Technology may actually "increase the need to think critically about reading *and writing* [italics added] as interpretive, critical acts" (Why Write, 1995, p. 5). The Tchudis also responded to a question about whether writing is really necessary for success in the world of work. They responded that although there are a few truly successful people who can't write, this is the exception rather than the rule.

Learning to Write

In the last twenty years, students of writing development have turned their attention from the products of writing to the process of writing as well as the contexts in which writing occurs. The research focus on written products required that children be writing somewhat fluently at the text level; thus, the youngest children studied were at the mid-elementary level. The specific focus was sentence-level grammatical maturity (e.g., Harrell, 1957; Hunt, 1965, 1970; Loban, 1976; O'Donnell, Griffin, & Norris, 1967). More recently, interest in the earliest stages of print literacy, along with social constructivist views of young children (Vygotsky, 1978), led researchers to study the emergence of writing in naturalistic contexts—at home, and in preschool and early elementary classrooms. The results of this inquiry have been dramatic. Whereas writing had been viewed as a relatively late-developing linguistic skill, built on a foundation of reading competence through explicit instruction, the developmental map of writing has essentially been rewritten (Jensen, 1993, citing a communication from Thomas Newkirk). Recently a group of prominent researchers in writing development were asked what was the most important thing learned in the last several decades (Jensen, 1993). Their responses could be summarized as four major points:

Writing is a gateway to literacy: Children learn to write very early and feel a sense of control and ownership of the written word earlier in writing than in reading.

All children can be writers: The view of what constitutes writing has been expanded so that many more children are seen as writers and see themselves that way.

Writing is a complex process with psychological, cultural, linguistic, and social influences: At every level, writing is embedded in social and cultural contexts and cannot really be understood apart from these.

Children write to say something important: Writing comes from the desire to know what we think, communicate that to others, and feel closer to others as a result.

Emergent Writing, Age 4 to 6 Years

Researchers have used two basic approaches in studying the beginning of writing. One approach is as unobtrusive, passive observer, exemplified in the work of Dyson (1989,

1993a). Such approaches yield rich descriptions of early writing in its social context and tentative interpretations about the individual psychological and larger sociocultural processes at work. In a second approach, researchers interact more directly with children around instances of writing. For example, they might ask the children questions about what they are doing or what something "says" (e.g., Ferreiro, 1984), or even why they (and people in general) write (e.g., Merenda, 1996). Another more active approach is to ask children to "write" something "their own way" (e.g., Sulzby, Branz, & Buhle, 1993) or to dictate a story for an adult to write down (Zuccermaglio & Scheuer, 1996). Interactive paradigms like these provide valuable insights into how children analyze the forms and functions of writing.

Types of Writing

One of the main contexts for writing in this period is drawing, as shown by Dyson (1993b) in an extensive observational study of an urban San Francisco K-1 classroom. She described draw-write instances as "multimedia productions" (p. 12) in which children talk, draw, write, and sometimes dramatize the stories they are communicating. At first, the writing may be only a small part of the production, for instance a few letters, or letter-like forms, or words. Eventually, proportions shift so that a longer text is accompanied by smaller pictures that may be added after the text is finished. Many children continue to draw small pictures on their written work even beyond the mid-elementary years.

Gundlach (1982) observed that the processes served by writing and drawing combinations are not well understood. Dyson's observations (1993b), however, may shed some light on this activity. She observed that children began to talk playfully (and critically) about each others' writing as a separate object from the drawing. Gradually, children begin to differentiate the type of information conveyed in print versus picture, with writing conveying more of the narrative action and drawing illustrating key ideas. Writing also became more integrated into the children's social worlds; friends became characters in their writing, and the children would write specific words that they knew would amuse their friends. Dyson's tentative conclusion is that children's writing changes from a type of social prop to a social mediator:

> A major developmental change may be from young children's use of writing as a kind of prop, an interesting object to be used in various kinds of social and often playful activities, to the deliberate manipulation of written language as a mediator through which social activity occurs . . . (1993b, p. 28)

Other contexts and purposes besides draw-write combinations have been observed. As early as 5 years, and often by age 6, some children write messages for others, labels, and lists to help them remember or organize information. Messages may have clear-cut and sometimes even urgent purposes. Consider the now-classic RUDF (*are you deaf?*) message presented by 5-year-old Paul Bissex to his mother when more conventional ways of getting her attention had failed (Bissex, 1980).

Knowledge about Writing

In addition to describing types of spontaneous emergent writing and their social contexts, researchers have been interested in the types of knowledge (albeit tacit knowledge) children may have about the forms of writing. How do children come to realize that letters stand for speech sounds (the alphabetic principle), or that written sentences have a distinctive grammar? Can young children talk about writing as an object, for example, why they wrote something a particular way, or why people write at all? Answers to these types of questions require researchers to interact with emergent writers in a more direct manner.

The classic study of the young children's discovery of the alphabetic nature of writing is Ferreiro's work with young Mexican children aged 3 to 5 (Ferreiro, 1984; Ferreiro & Teberosky, 1982). Using a Piagetian interview strategy, Ferreiro asked children questions about their drawing and writing. At first, children view *letters as objects* that have names. The question "What does it say" is meaningless because letters are not viewed as symbols. There is no discernable relationship between placement of letters and drawings on the page; letters may even appear inside the drawn object. Eventually children come to view *letters as substitute objects* that "name" something. One sign of the change is the contrastive use of definite articles for the picture of an object (e.g., *a chair*) but omission of the article for the printed word "chair." Although letters represent other objects, they do not yet represent the sound pattern of that object (and the child does not yet use a consistent set of letters for the object). Additionally, the child is much more likely to symbolize (write) objects than events. At this stage, writing is still a first-order symbol system (Donaldson, 1984). For writing to become a second-order symbol system, one equally suited to objects and events, the child must realize that written symbols designate speech sound symbols— that writing, in essence, "draws" speech (*letters as sounds*).

An appreciation of the alphabetic nature of writing may be gradual. Sulzby (1986) observed that the same child may use different types of graphic systems (e.g., scribbling, letter-like forms, and invented spelling) at the same developmental point, although perhaps for different tasks and in different settings. Some children adopt a quantity strategy, distinguishing objects by the number of "letters" they write. Later, a syllabic hypothesis might be used in which number of letters equal the number of syllables, even though a consistent letter-sound correspondence is still lacking. Eventually, consistent letter-sound associations are made.

Sulzby and her colleagues have been interested in the question of what children know about literate language patterns before they are conventionally literate. Her research paradigm is to ask children to "read" favorite storybooks and also to "write a story" and then to "read me your story," with the rationale "to see if it is just the way you want it to be" (Sulzby, 1996, p. 39). Sulzby's research documents children's ability to use *written-like language* in both tasks (e.g., *once there was a bug . . .*); in addition, children use *oral-like language* (quoted speech) in both activities. Sulzby's work is interesting because it demonstrates that spoken and written forms are potentially separable from the medium of delivery, or modality. Not only are preliterate children able to talk like a book, they are also beginning to write like they talk. The ability to speak in a literate style while at the same time writing in a spoken style (if the need arises) has been touted as the highest level of literary style (e.g., Kroll, 1981). Sulzby's work indicates that the seeds for this literacy agility may be sown very early.

As a final observation about emergent writing, we can ask whether children can talk on a metalinguistic level about writing—their own and writing in general. To illustrate the potential of this type of inquiry, Goodman (1996) related her conversation with a first grade child (first week of the school year) over the child's drawing-writing piece, a stick-figure person standing under a rainbow with a tree to the side. Above the drawing, there were the neatly written capital letters OOSOORB OB and underneath SOT. When asked to read her writing in the picture, the child read "I am outside, under a rainbow and beside a tree." Her teacher saw little association between the speech and letters and asked the child to tell her about the "Os". The child responded that they weren't Os, they were circles. When asked why she put circles in the middle of her writing, she said:

> Because. See, I couldn't tell what letters make those sounds so I just put circles for what goes there because something goes there only I don't know what. I can't tell what letter makes that sound, so I just put circles. (Goodman, 1996, p. 349).

After that explanation, it was obvious the child had correctly written S for *side*, RB for *rainbow*, BS for *beside*, and T for *tree*. The child used a placeholder, which she was quite aware of and able to explain when asked. Merenda (1996, p. 12-13) also talked with preschool and kindergarten children about writing. She asked them, simply, "tell me why you write." Among the answers were:

> to tell a story
>
> if you're little, you write things . . . if you're big, you write homework
>
> because we don't want anybody to touch it (referring to a plant)

These emergent writers had varied but accurate ideas about why people write.

Conventional Writing: The Early School Years

Sulzby (1996) defined conventional writing as "connected discourse that another conventionally literate person can read without too much difficulty and that the child can read conventionally" (p. 27). By that standard, most children become conventional writers by the end of the first grade (Chapman, 1994). To be a conventional writer, the child must have some understanding of (1) sound-symbol relationships, (2) words as stable, "memorable" units, and (3) text as a stable, memorable object (Sulzby, 1996, p. 27). Furthermore, children who are conventional writers in fact believe that they can write. Emergent writers, when asked to "write" (by a teacher or researcher) may say that they can't write even though they can usually be persuaded to "write" something.

The writing of children aged 6 and older has most often been studied in the context of the classroom. Writing activities in the first several years of elementary school today are very different from those of twenty years ago. Previously children were engaged in activities designed to help them learn the *writing system*—spelling, punctuation, and layout. Children copied spelling words and sentences from the board, wrote sentences that used certain words, and practiced forming letters and later, penmanship. Today a paradigm shift spurred by whole language, literature-based, and writing process approaches has resulted in classroom contexts designed to help children learn the *written language*—to write in the genres characteristic of schools and the broader community (Pontecorvo & Orsolini,

1996). Children may still copy words from the board, but in most classrooms children are also provided with opportunities to write at the text level (e.g., stories), both teacher-assigned and self-chosen pieces. The latter type of writing is discussed in this section. This provides for developmental continuity with the previous overview of emergent writing, which was also frequently self-sponsored (e.g., writing and drawing together).

Chapman (1994) studied the *emergence of genre* in the writing of six first grade children. She defined genre as a "typified form of discourse or way of organizing or structuring discourse, shaped by and in response to recurring situational contexts" (p. 352). In her study the recurring context was the "Writing Workshop"—a time when children could write and draw about things of interest to them. This daily period followed interactive reading and writing activities such as "Morning News" and shared reading of "big books." As the children wrote, the teacher circulated among them, talking about their writing if they wished. Chapman constructed a genre typology and chronology of change in the production of fifteen identified genres over the course of the school year. Moreover, writing similarities and differences between children described by their teacher as advanced, average, and delayed in their overall development were of interest. The raw data were all texts produced by the children throughout the school year (724 texts in all). The year was divided into three periods: beginning (September through November), middle (December through February), and end of year (March through June).

The texts were first categorized as either *chronological* (action/event oriented) or *nonchronological* (object-oriented). Chronological texts were based on the children's own experiences, either past or planned for the future, or imaginative. Distinctive forms in chronological texts included action verbs in past tense or future time, temporal connectives (e.g., *then, next*), and temporal adverbials (e.g., *yesterday, at Christmas*). There were two distinct strands of nonchronological texts. Descriptive texts provided information about a picture; interactive texts had as their goal some form of social action (e.g., a written question-answer dialogue between two children). Distinctive forms in nonchronological genres were verbs of attribution (e.g., *are, have, got*) or attitude (e.g., *like, want*) that took generalized present tense form.

Over the course of the year, there were dramatic changes in the children's writing. One major change was the gradual disassociation of drawing and writing. At the beginning of the year, almost all writing was associated with picture drawing (99%); in the last third of the school year, this association had declined (67%, range 45% to 98%) so that free-standing texts of several clauses were common. In addition, major changes occurred in both quantity (i.e., genre repertoire) and quality of genre writing. The children produced eight different genres in the first three months, adding an additional six in the next three-month period. Labels (a nonchronological type of writing) accounted for half of all texts (49%) at first, but were negligible (1%) in the last period. Basic records (chronological) declined from 18 percent to 1 percent, but expanded records increased from 6 percent to 31 percent. Attribute series (nonchronological, e.g., *This is an army base. I like it.*) increased from <1 percent to 24 percent. Texts were usually single clauses (e.g., the label text *this is a soccer game*) at the start of the year (69%, range 44% to 86%), but texts of two or more clauses, rare at first, comprised 95 percent of all texts in the last period. In fact, at the end of the year, the average number of clauses per text ranged from 3.15 to 5.52. Chapman (1994, p.

368) provided the following example from one of her subjects to illustrate the increase in text length between September and March:

At Windsor Park I played soccer with my brother. (September)

Last Saturday and Sunday my brother went to soccer tournaments. There was two tournaments a day. His team was in third place. At the end every team got a trophy even though the team might not have won. And everyone got a popsicle. Last Saturday and Sunday I was sick. (March)

There were individual differences in genre frequency and distribution among the six children. However, in spite of "arriving by different routes" (Chapman, 1994, p. 371), there were many common features in the children's texts at the end of the first grade. There were also plateaus and sudden leaps. But all six children, even those who were identified as delayed in language development by their teachers, wrote texts that could stand alone, without pictures, by the end of the year.

Similar to Sulzby's (1996) observation for emergent writers, Chapman's conventional writers also had *oral-like* and *written-like* features in their texts. The attribute series genre, for example, is similar to children's oral commentary (e.g., *this is a haunted castle. I like it. It's neat*) (p. 372). The children wrote speech more directly in "speech balloons." Book language, on the other hand, was also evident in the use of phrases such as *far, far away in another land* (p. 370).

Where do these genres come from? Perhaps they are "invented" by the children, much like invented spelling (a cognitive constructivist position), or alternatively, they are "appropriated" from the environment (a social constructivist position). Chapman's (1994, 1995) observations of the larger classroom context for her subjects led her to believe that both origins contribute and interact. All children clearly used language experiences in the classroom as resources for their writing; however, they were individuals when it came to their genre preferences and unique styles.

Newkirk (1987) also studied self-sponsored school writing of young elementary school children, but restricted his sample to non-narrative writing (one text from 100 different children in grades 1 through 3). Like Chapman's much smaller group, children in Newkirk's study were in classrooms with teachers trained in the writing process approach and wrote regularly on self-chosen topics. The nonchronological genres identified by Chapman (1994) for first grade were also evident in texts examined by Newkirk, but were seen in a more developed form in older children. For example, whereas lists in Chapman's study were usually single words, a third grade writer made a list of sentences describing *10 Bad Things About My Brother* (Newkirk, 1987, p. 131). The general trend uncovered by Newkirk was one of redistribution. Several genres frequent in the texts of younger children were less frequent by the third grade, and vice versa. Figure 8-2 shows an example of a nonchronological text written by a second grade child describing a bearded seal (from the present author's files). This text would be classified as an attribute series text in both the Chapman and Newkirk investigations. In this genre, facts are stated about a topic, but they are in no particular order and could be rearranged without affecting text coherence. Attribute series texts were frequent in the first and second grade texts examined by Newkirk (21% and

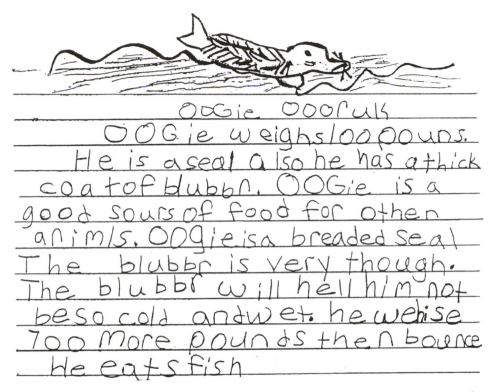

OOGie OOOruK
OOGie weighs 100 pounds.
He is a seal also he has a thick
coat of blubbn. OOGie is a
good sours of food for othen
animls. OOGie isa breaded seal
The blubbr is very though.
The blubbr will hell him not
beso cold andwet. he wehise
700 more pounds then bounce
He eats fish

FIGURE 8-2   An example of nonchronological (factual) text written by a second grade child (author's files).

26% of all nonchronological writing, respectively), but accounted for only 6 percent of third grade texts. There were substantial increases in the length of texts: Only 15 percent of first grade texts were more than one paragraph, but 49 percent of third grade texts exceeded one paragraph. Newkirk interpreted his findings as support for the idea that young elementary children can write in genres that lay a foundation for later expository writing. The young child's labels, lists, and attribute texts are the tools of informational texts to come.

While research reviewed thus far reveals that young elementary children write in both narrative (chronological) and expository (nonchronological) genres in school at times when they can choose their topics, writing assignments (*school-sponsored writing*) favor narrative writing, according to Christie (1986) and Martin (1989). This is a trend that continues into the mid-elementary years, as shown in the following section.

Learning the Genres of School Writing

Learning to write means learning new ways of making meaning. Although in theory one can speak or write the same information, in practice discourse genres tend to be delivered in one or another medium but not both. Consequently, learning to write, particularly learning to write expository and argument (persuasion) genres, opens new avenues of making meaning for children. There are three major requirements involved in learning genre writing:

Generating the right content and enough of it.

Organizing the content to conform to an appropriate global text structure (e.g., narrative, persuasive, factual, etc).

Calling up the right structures and words that accomplish text-level goals (e.g., cohesion markers, foregrounding/backgrounding structures, temporal connectives in narratives, universal present tense in factual writing).

Typically growth in all three domains occurs concurrently, but developmental asynchronies can also occur. For example, a child may know a great deal about the solar system (i.e., the child can generate enough content), but still be unable to organize that information in an effective written text. It is not always possible to isolate these three domains in the developmental literature, particularly when children's texts are rated holistically. This is due to the fact that a rating may contain features from several domains (e.g., a rating of 5 means "elaborated content clearly organized according to content expectations").

The question of how children and adolescents learn to write in these new genres is also complicated by the difficulty of separating intrinsic cognitive and linguistic developmental factors from the filter effects of school curricula and writing instruction. Thus, if a child writes a poor persuasive piece, is it because persuasion is too demanding cognitively and/or linguistically, or is it due to a lack of exposure to persuasive text and little or no instruction in the genre? The curricular/instruction explanation has gathered a vocal and growing number of proponents in recent years (e.g., Christie, 1986; Martin, 1989), with many calling for expanding the scope of genre teaching in schools and lowering the age for teaching the non-narrative genres (Perera, 1992).

School-Sponsored Genres

A variety of classification schemes of typical school writing genres have been proposed. Two examples, one by Scott (1988) and another by Martin (1989), are shown in Table 8-1. Most classification schemes distinguish between narrative (chronologically based text) and expository (factual, nonchronological, or logically based text). It is then common to distinguish several kinds of narrative text and several subtypes of expository text. School writing done within any one curricular subject could call for several different genres. For example, science writing could be a procedure (steps in an experiment), a report (what bats are like), or an explanation (why the theory of relativity is plausible).

It needs to be pointed out that the portrayal of writing genres characteristic of schools, and the discussion to follow on writing development within this context, is representative of U.S. mainstream and European-based education systems. Gee (1994) refers to this as "essay-text literacy" and points out that it is only "one cultural way of making sense among many . . ." (p. 179). This form of literacy values textual explicitness and an impersonal stance. Depending on a child's social and cultural background, the essay-text literacy mode, with all its many "unspoken ground rules" (see Sheeran & Barnes, 1991) will be more or less transparent. Cazden (1993) contends that the canonical report genre (e.g., *A cat is a*

TABLE 8-1   Classification Schemes of Typical School Writing Genres

	Scott (1988)	
	Chronological	Nonchronological (logical)

Personal	Narratives
	    personal experience
	    biographical
	    fictional
	    historical
	Personal journals
	Letters	

	Procedures	Persuasion
		Reports
		Composition
		    generalization
		    speculation

Impersonal		argument

	Martin (1989)	
	Narrative (what happened)	Factual (the way things are)
	Recount	Procedural (how something is done) Descriptions (what some particular thing is like) Reports (what an entire class of things are like) Explanation (a reason why a judgment has been made) Exposition (arguments why a thesis has been proposed) Persuading *that* (analytic) Persuading *to* (horatory)

feline mammal. Also it is warm-blooded. Cats can be wild or domestic. Domestic means . . .) of the essay-text literacy tradition raises several dilemmas for genre development and teaching for children from mainstream and minority cultural backgrounds (see also Scott & Rogers, 1996).

Several studies of elementary school writing curricula confirm the domination of narrative writing, followed by informational writing, with persuasive writing addressed least frequently, if at all. Martin (1989) examined writing in an Australian suburban infants' and primary school in years 1 through 6. Only 15 percent of the texts were factual (13% reports, 2% procedural, and 0.5% explanations and expositions).[3] According to Burkhalter (1995),

---

[3]Unfortunately, Martin (1989) does not clarify whether the texts were all school-sponsored, or whether some were self-chosen.

the same situation exists in U.S. schools. She speculates that the rationale for the neglect of informational and persuasive texts is adherence to a Piagetian developmental model that reserves formal operational reasoning abilities until age 11. In practice, however, persuasive writing is further delayed until late secondary school or even college (Applebee, Langer, & Mullis, 1986; McCann, 1989).

The most extensive recent data on school writing curricula for older students was gathered in 1992 as part of the National Assessment for Educational Progress (NAEP). The 1992 NAEP was administered nationally to a representative sample of fourth, eighth, and twelfth grade students who wrote open-ended text-level responses to prompts in three genres: narrative, informative, and persuasive. Part of the 1992 assessment included an examination of school writing instructional practices. Students, teachers and school administrators completed questionnaires that asked about the type and length of writing assignments among other things. The survey choices for types of writing assignments were log/journal, story or narrative (personal or imagined experience), report or summary, essay or theme in which you analyze or interpret, and persuasive essay or letter. Frequency of writing was noted only as "at least monthly" or "never or hardly ever." Unfortunately, the only types queried for fourth graders were log/journal and story or report (which were not separated). Results generally confirm smaller-scale study results and anecdotal observations. Log/journal writing decreased (62% of the fourth graders but only 45% of the twelfth graders reported at least monthly writing), as did narrative writing (75% of eighth graders and 62% of twelfth graders). At grades 8 and 12, the majority of students said they wrote monthly reports/summaries (78% and 82%), essays or themes requiring analysis or interpretation (66% and 84%), and persuasive essays or letters (57% and 54%). For the most part, however, these assignments were short. Two-thirds of the grade 8 and 12 students reported writing one- or two-paragraph papers weekly, and one- or two-page papers at least once a month (81% and 87% respectively). The frequency for longer assignments (three or more pages) decreased for both groups; 52 percent of eighth grade students and 37 percent of the twelfth grade students said they never wrote papers of three or more pages. When compared with the previous 1988 NAEP results, however, more students are writing longer texts.

Learning to Write School-Sponsored Genres

Researchers have studied children's writing development in single-genre and cross-genre designs. Cross-genre designs compare children's ability to write in at least two genres (e.g., narrative writing is compared to expository writing). Evidence suggests that students first gain proficiency in narrative writing, followed by informative writing, with persuasive writing last (e.g., Crowhurst, 1987; Langer, 1985; McCutchen & Perfetti, 1982)—a sequence that matches the timing of genre work in school writing curricula, as discussed previously. Proficiency has been measured in a variety of ways, including overall text length, types and frequency of cohesion markers, local and remote connections between sentences, and analyses of text structure. Scott's (1994) review of cross-genre research showed that children write longer narrative texts and use more advanced systems of cohesion in narrative versus other types of texts. There is anecdotal evidence that children rely on narrative formats when other types of discourse are called for (Crowhurst & Piche, 1979). Likewise, Applebee (1984) found that adolescents beginning to write analytic texts sometimes start by embedding narrative stretches within a global analytic framework.

Within any one genre, fine-grained analyses reveal content and form developments across the school years. McCutheon and Perfetti (1982), for example, found that cohesion developed in essay writing in texts written at second, fourth, sixth, and eighth grades. Freedman's (1987) analysis of narratives written by fifth, eighth, and twelfth grade students revealed continuing change in text structure. Several investigators have been interested recently in the development of persuasive writing. In a cross-sectional design, Knudson (1994) traced the development of persuasive writing in third, fifth, tenth, and twelfth grade students. Students were asked to write a letter to the school principal arguing that a school rule either should or should not be changed; types of arguments offered were categorized. Simple statements without supporting evidence decreased over time. The major developmental growth trend was a significant increase in the use of compromise. Whereas third grade children never offered a compromise, 11 percent of the twelfth grade arguments were compromises. A similar developmental increment was found by Golder and Coirier (1994). They reasoned that the two most important processes in argumentative text writing are the supporting process (stating reasons to back a claim) and the negotiation process (convincing the reader to accept those reasons). Negotiation markers included (1) counterarguments (e.g., *even if, however*), (2) obligation and judgment (e.g., *one should, it's good . . .*), (3) degree of certainty (*maybe, surely*), and (4) writer endorsement and accountability (*in my opinion*). Significant increase in the frequency of negotiation markers occurred between the ages of 10 and 16. Furthermore, for the oldest subjects, there was a strong association between negotiation in writing and the ability to judge the "argumentativity" of texts based on weak-strong argumentative text structure. Results were interpreted as lending support to the importance of text structure schema in genre writing. Golder and Coirier's study is particularly interesting because they presented subjects with several different tasks in an effort to explain as well as describe argumentative writing.

Durst, Laine, Schultz, and Vilter (1990) looked at factors that contributed the most to holistic scores of persuasive writing of high school seniors. Of the seven linguistic and rhetorical variables studied, four contributed the most: the use of logical appeals, the number of total words, and degree of coherence (defined as "explicit interconnectedness of the various parts of the essay" including transitional sentences, cohesive ties, overall structure made explicit with an introduction, conclusion, and so on [p. 236]), and the use of the five-paragraph structure. There was no relationship between ratings and number of fragments, punctuation errors, agreement errors, and spelling errors.

A final overview of genre writing can be found in the results of the 1992 NAEP (Applebee, Langer, Mullis, Latham, & Gentile, 1994). Major findings have been reproduced in Table 8-2 and provide comparisons of narrative, informative, and persuasive writing as well as performance within each text type.[4] Texts were rated by trained readers who scored each piece on a 5-point scale as *response to topic* (the lowest rating), *undeveloped, minimally developed, developed,* or *elaborated* (the highest rating). The most general summary statement of the NAEP results is that the majority of students are capable of writing developed

---

[4]It should be noted that the informative text prompt to fourth graders (only) asked them to tell about a favorite story that they had read, heard, or seen at the movies. It could be argued that this is really a narrative genre. The narrative prompt asked them for an imaginative story.

TABLE 8-2   Major Findings for Writing, 1992 National Assessment of Educational Progress

For Informative Writing

About three–fourths (or more) of the students at all three grades provided at least minimally developed responses to the informative tasks. However, minimally developed responses were brief, vague, or somewhat confusing.

About one–third of the fourth graders (32 to 39%) provided developed or better responses to the informative tasks, while very few (6–11%) provided elaborated or better responses. Responses rated as developed were typically uneven but contained the elements necessary for successful completion of the task. In contrast, elaborated responses were well developed and detailed.

At grades 8 and 12, the results were more varied across tasks. Students had the least difficulty discussing a school problem—27 percent at grade 8 and 46 percent at grade 12 wrote elaborated or better responses. They had the most difficulty with the challenging task of describing an invention—4 to 6 percent provided elaborated or better responses for both grades.

For Persuasive Writing

Fewer than half the fourth graders (36 to 47%) and from 59 to 76 percent of the eighth and twelfth graders wrote at least minimally developed papers.

All students, even at grade 12, had considerable difficulty moving beyond the minimally developed level. Across all three grades, from 7 to 25 percent of the students wrote developed or better responses to the persuasive tasks and very few (0 to 3%) wrote elaborated or better responses.

For Narrative Writing

Approximately one-fourth of the students at grade 4 (20 to 29%) wrote narratives rated as developed or better, but only small percentages (2 to 4%) wrote narratives rated as elaborated or better.

At grades 8 and 12, there was considerable variation in narrative writing. Across both grades, from 33 to 59 percent of the students provided developed or better responses to the narrative tasks and from 4 to 16 percent provided elaborated or better responses.

Most students showed some grasp of the narrative form. At least 55 percent and often 80 percent or so across the grades provided at least minimally developed or better narrative responses.

narratives and informational texts at the end of high school, but continue to have difficulty with persuasive test. Elaborated texts were not characteristic of any genre or any age group.

Interpreting Genre Research

As indicated previously, genre research results may reflect experiential rather than intrinsic cognitive/linguistic limitations. Children simply are not exposed to, taught, or expected to write in informational and persuasive genres to the extent necessary for writing competence. Some critics see political overtones in the relative lack of factual and persuasive writing—the idea being that such writing confers power that is more properly reserved for adults in general and mainstream groups in particular (viz., Martin, 1989). Others see the reason as an overemphasis of Piagetian cognitive theory at the expense of Vygotskian social constructivist theory (e.g., Burkhalter, 1995). Still others have attempted to empirically test the experiential versus developmental explanations. If the explanations for shortcomings in children's genre writing result from cognitive limitations, children's writing should not improve following explicit instruction in the genre. Both Burkhalter (1995) and

Crowhurst (1991) have demonstrated significant improvement in persuasive writing in children as young as fourth grade, for example, following explicit instruction.

A final argument for curriculum changes that would introduce factual writing earlier can be found in the emergent literacy research. When Pappas (1991) asked four kindergarten children to "pretend read" information books (a paradigm usually reserved for storybooks), she found that all four children, from both middle SES and lower SES homes), expressed textual properties of information books. Moreover, the children's renditions were "constructive" and went beyond mere memorization of facts from the books. Duthie (1994, p. 588) asked first grade children directly "What is nonfiction?" Among the answers were:

> It gives information about things around us.
>
> If you have a sick cat and you can't call a vet, you could look in nonfiction.
>
> It can teach you about fruits and vegetables.

After Duthie devoted a segment of her usual reading and writing workshop time to nonfiction, her students showed more confidence and comfort writing nonfiction and, for some, it became their favorite form of writing. Following the experience with nonfiction writing, when she asked the same question again, the children's answers reflected the writer's perspective (Duthie, 1994, p. 594):

> You can teach people what you know about stuff.
>
> You use a good title and lead in nonfiction just like fiction because you have to get the reader interested or they won't read it.

It remains to be seen whether the developmental sequence for genre writing from narrative to factual and persuasive writing will stand in future years if school curricula do in fact change. Ironically, Donald Graves, whose writing process approach (Graves, 1983) is sometimes equated with a perceived overemphasis on narrative writing in the early years, clearly believes children are capable of writing in a variety of informational genres; his book *Investigative Nonfiction* (Graves, 1989) suggests ways to encourage such writing in kindergarten, first, and second grade classrooms.

Learning the Grammar of Writing

The Effects of Modality

Children learning to write face several new grammatical challenges. Some challenges stem from the requirements of genre and others from the nature of the medium (the written *modality*), as discussed previously. Projects comparing written and spoken text provide insight into the development of a specifically "written" grammar.[5] Several large-N investigations

---

[5]It is important to remember that emergent and young conventional writers have some tacit knowledge about the special characteristics of writing, as shown by comparisons of telling, dictating, and writing (e.g., Sulzby, 1986). The topic considered here, however, is when texts reflect more explicit control over such grammatical and textual features

of speaking and writing grammar have tracked syntactic changes throughout the school years (Harrell, 1957; Loban, 1976; O'Donnell, Griffin, & Norris, 1967). The focus of other investigations has been more limited in terms of age range or specific research questions (De Temple, Wu, & Snow, 1991; Golub & Frederick, 1971; Pelligrini, Galda, & Rubin, 1984; Scott & Klutsenbaker, 1989). With one exception (Loban, 1976), these studies have compared written and spoken samples of the same genre, usually narrative (e.g., spoken and written versions of a film, two films in the same series, or similar pictures, and so on). As a result, the structures identified in writing can be assumed to reflect the influence of modality alone. The large-N studies in particular demonstrate that between mid-elementary through high school years, children's writing shows increasing frequency of later developing syntactic forms such as relative clauses, expanded noun phrases, and nonfinite adverbial clauses (e.g., *looking out the window* he could see they were in trouble). Reviews of this literature are available in Perera (1986) and Scott (1988).

Kroll (1981) proposed four periods in the evolution of spoken/written form relationships. During a *preparation* phase in the early period of conventional writing, texts may not be up to the standard of spoken language. Sentences are shorter and grammatical errors, usually omissions, occur that would be unusual in speech. Presumably spelling, punctuation, and layout decisions, being far from automatic at this early age, take up a large amount of the child's resources and attention. In a *consolidation* phase, writing more closely resembles speech. At the age of 9 or 10, many children enter a *differentiation* phase in which a more "written" grammar emerges, as shown by: (1) absence of distinctly oral structures (e.g., *well, you know*), (2) fewer coordinated main clauses with *and* and more subordinate clauses, and (3) structures more often found in written language such as passives and nonfinite verb forms. Further, patterns of written text organization appear such as moving adverbial elements to the front of the sentence. Perera (1984) noted that this can be a somewhat awkward period; at times "spoken" and "written" grammar are mixed in the same text. The text in Figure 8-3, written at school by a third grade child (age 7;8) provides an example. The text is an imaginative narrative, written in the first person. There are several structures characteristic of mature writing including: (1) a series construction (lines 8-11) and (2) adverbial fronting, *there stood a little tiger cub* (line 13, also lines 1, 2, 6, 16, and 22). At the same time, the child writes the spoken form *well* (line 19). Finally, in Kroll's (1981) last phase, the *integration* phase, writers move easily between oral and written form, adapting structure to fit the needs of a variety of text types. Using Sulzby's (1996) terminology for emergent literacy, the writer can now write *oral-like* if necessary (and is also able to speak *written-like*). Some writers may never reach an integration phase (Perera, 1984: Rubin, 1987).

One question of interest is whether written grammar is, in some sense, more complex than spoken grammar and, if so, when this is evident in development. When average sentence length (in words) is used as a metric of overall complexity, writing eventually overtakes speaking in late elementary or early secondary years, although studies differ in the exact point of crossover. The actual differences are small, however (e.g., 9.34 words for writing compared with 8.90 words for speaking by fifth graders in the 1967 O'Donnell et al. project). Whether this represents a true complexity difference is open to interpretation. Drawing on the work of Halliday (1985, 1987) and Biber (1986, 1992), Scott discussed the notion of whether speaking and writing differ in some global sense of syntactic complexity (1994, 1995). She concluded, along with Halliday and Biber, that mature writing and

TIGERCUB

One hot Summer I was walking in the field
Just me, privace at last, feeling
proud of myself I sat down with
a little sac lunch I had made.
I opend my thermas and set out
my blanket. as I ate my lunch
I planned what I was going to do.
I was going to: pick some wild
flowers, swim in the field lake,
and biuld things in the fields
sandpile I heard this little
new new. I looked behind me
there stood a little tiger cub.
he sat down beside me. mew
mew he said. I stroked his soft
tiger fur After I hat done
my three tasks I noticed
the tiger cub had follod me.
Well I did the thing most
children would do I decied to
ask my folks if I could have him.
When I got home I asked
my dad why he was mewing?
My dad studeyd his mewing
for a minuit

..... **story continues**

FIGURE 8-3 **An example of narrative (imaginative) writing by a third grade child (author's files). The text illustrates several "written" grammatical features as well as developing punctuation.**

speaking are both complex but differ in terms of the *types* of complexity favored in each (i.e., particular syntactic structures and operations).

A study of oral and written form in a picture description task (De Temple et al., 1991) provides a caveat to the interpretation of modality effects on children's grammar. Even though the stimulus was the same (scenes of people and animals from storybooks), children's written versions contained many more structural features associated with narrativity; for example, non-present-tense verb forms and clauses describing events that "went beyond" the picture (e.g., *later they will eat dinner*). The children (second through fifth grade) apparently interpreted the task somewhat differently depending on whether they were asked to say or write their description. Genre and modality may be totally separable, therefore, in theory only.

The Effects of Genre

Cross-genre studies of children's writing show that type of writing has an impact on syntactic complexity, summarized by Rubin (1984) as follows:

> First, discourse function exerts a profound effect on syntactic complexity. Within-age style shifts are of a magnitude equal to or exceeding between-age contrasts. Second there is a strong tendency for style-shifting in writing to increase with age. That is, more mature writers are sensitive to the differential sytlistic demands of the various functions to a greater degree than younger writers. (p. 220)

When children are asked to write in several genres, narratives show the least amount of syntactic complexity, followed by reports, and finally persuasion (Langer, 1985; Rubin, 1984). Persuasion brings about the highest degree of syntactic complexity because of the interdependence of subordination operations and the expression of logical relationships (Rubin, 1984). Syntactic complexity in cross-modal studies has usually been measured in terms of sentence length and/or subordination ratio (subordinate/main clauses). These effects are not usually obvious before the late elementary or early secondary years, however, when children have sufficient fluency in factual as well as narrative writing. Kress (1982, pp. 100-101) published two texts written by a 7-year-old that illustrate this point quite well. An imaginative story written at home was thirty-one sentences with an average sentence length of 9.90 words; a factual piece from school, written at the same age, was eight sentences with an average sentence length of 7.00 words.

Learning about Punctuation

Another interesting question about the development of written form is how children learn to punctuate. Far from being a trivial "mechanical" skill, punctuation reveals children's "theories" about grammar and text in an explicit way. Research on the development of punctuation is sparse and complicated by the lack of "normativity" for the placement of most markers. With a few exceptions (paragraph-end periods followed by capital letter, and commas in a series of nouns), punctuation is a matter of choice (Simone, 1996). In addition, punctuation has evolved from marking "places to breathe" to serving many syntactic, semantic, emphatic, and organizational functions, sometimes concurrently. Indeed, punctuation remains difficult even for mature writers.

It is not surprising, then, to find that it takes a long time for children to make inroads into the punctuation system. Ferreiro and Zucchermaglio (1996), in a study of Spanish-speaking second and third grade children in Mexico and Argentina, analyzed punctuation in written versions of *Little Red Riding Hood*. Some texts (12%) had no punctuation at all, and some had only text-boundary markers, an initial capital and final period (27%). When punctuation was used within the text, it was common for children to use just one marker (e.g., one or more instances of a period and no other markers). Commas and periods accounted for 38 percent and 29 percent of all punctuation marks found in the texts and were also the most multifunctional markers, being used in several nonconventional as well as conventional ways. Of interest was the finding that children were more likely to use punctuation within quoted speech portions of the text.

Periods have received the most attention in developmental writing research. Cordeiro (1988) found that third grade children were not much more accurate than first graders in using periods at sentence boundaries (46% and 53% respectively). In the same two years, however, there was significant change in the children's use of incorrect periods from a seemingly random placement to more syntactically motivated placement at phrase or clause boundaries. The third grade author of the *Tiger Cub* text (Figure 8-3) marks sentence boundaries two-thirds of the time, but sometimes uses a comma rather than a period. This child uses three markers in addition to periods—commas, a question mark (line 24), and even a colon in line 8 to mark the beginning of a series construction. Although this child appears to be well on her way to conventional punctuation, another imaginative story written a few months later revealed periods at only 45 percent of end-sentence boundaries. Given the complexity of punctuation, it is not surprising that the developmental course appears to be a long one with variability along the way.

Learning the Process of Writing

The development of writing process has been studied from several vantage points. Some studies have simply observed writers—for example, recording the time spent in initial planning or, once writing starts, the amount of time actually writing as opposed to pausing (see reviews in Faigley, Cherry, Joliffe, & Skinner, 1985). Other investigators have intervened at various points in the writing process. As an example of this type of paradigm, an experimenter might provide a model of planning before children begin to write or provide suggestions for revisions.

The seminal developmental work on processes involved in writing remains the work of Bereiter and Scardamalia, much of it summarized in their 1987 book *The Psychology of Written Composition*. Children between the ages of 10 and 14, students in the fourth, sixth, and eighth grades, were asked to generate factual text from information in a matrix; they also wrote an opinion piece in response to the prompt "Should students be able to choose what things they study in school?" In a study of planning, Bereiter and Scardamalia (1987) provided specific planning instructions prior to writing the opinion text. In general, 14-year-olds were able to able to utilize planning prompts about audience and purpose, whereas the younger children used their planning time in a more constrained way to merely generate content. One analysis centered on a comparison of notes made before writing and the actual finished text. Whereas the 14-year-olds' written notes listed "gists" of ideas that were expanded into complete ideas in the text, the notes of the 10-year-olds were already complete sentences, which then recurred practically unchanged in the text. The product of planning for the younger children was the text itself, not an intermediate plan. As another indication of planning productivity, an analysis of think-aloud protocols from the planning period revealed that the number of idea units doubled between the ages of 10 and 13. Another sign of developmental change in planning was evident in the children's ability to recognize when planning, as modeled by an adult, took place. With age, then, there is an increasing differentiation of planning from text production. Even though considerable planning development occurred by the age of 14, college undergraduates, by comparison, were more skillful planners (Burtis, Bereiter, Scardamalia, & Tetroe, 1983). Bereiter and Scardamalia stressed that more mature planning "consists of thinking *about* the composition rather than planning that consists of mentally rehearsing or creating the composition" (p. 210).

One explanation of younger children's difficulty in planning is that they are still in a state of "cognitive overload" when they write (Gombert, 1992, p. 169). Specifically, energies devoted to spelling, grammar, and punctuation are thought to interfere with planning efforts. Perhaps it is no coincidence, then, that planning begins to show developmental change at about the same time that these competing subprocesses are becoming more automatic. MacArthur (1996) cited evidence that by late elementary years, the superiority factor for dictated stories compared to written stories has disappeared. Although dictated stories may still be longer, they are not qualitatively better. Because dictation eliminates on-line transcription (spelling) requirements, improved writing via dictation is thought to indicate that an inordinate amount of resources are being allocated to transcription.

Hayes and Flower (1987) reviewed developmental literature on the revision phase of writing. They noted that adult and more expert writers devote proportionally more time to revising. Adults also view revising from a more global perspective, as a way of "molding the argument." On the other hand, high school and even some college students devote little time to revision, and when they do revise, changes are largely limited to the sentence level (correcting/changing grammar and punctuation), in other words "fixing up" the current version. Sometimes the changes are harmful rather than helpful. More recent studies confirm that high school and some college students avoid making major organizational and content changes in their texts, perhaps because major problems are not detected (e.g., Beason, 1993; Yagelski, 1995).

Being able to revise one's writing subsumes some type of an internal standard of comparison. Internal standards for writing are also shown in evaluations of others' writing. According to McCormick, Busching, and Potter (1992), the evaluation of a particular text involves "the conversion of multiple kinds of knowledge into specific criteria" (p. 314). A beginning literature on the development of internal standards of writing as revealed in evaluations of others' texts indicates that children between second and sixth grade frequently justify their evaluations with personal affective responses (e.g., *I didn't like it 'cause I'm scared of snakes*) (McCormick et al., 1992). Towards the end of elementary school years, development is seen in the move from affective to objective responses and from simple to multiple criteria. McCormick and colleagues (1992) sought to provide a more detailed account of children's evaluation of writing. They studied 27 fifth grade children identified as either high or low achievers, with follow-up one year later. The children were asked to rank order four of their own pieces of writing and another four "peer" texts that were actually written by the researchers to capture degrees of topic interest and craft. The children's comments were assigned to one of five criteria categories (p. 320-324):

> <u>Text-based</u>   Refers to characteristics, qualities, and content of the text itself (e.g., *that just isn't a good story to me; it's all right but it's not my favorite one; they don't tell when they seen the big creature and everything; it's just dull, . . . you don't think The pencil's all mine!; it sounds like a little kid wrote it*)
>
> <u>Non-text association</u>   Evaluations based on events and ideas from student's own experience (e.g., *'cause I love my dog . . . like to help my dog and he likes to help me*)
>
> <u>Surface qualities</u>   Refers to mechanics, spelling, or another aspect of linguistic correctness or image (e.g., *well I made a lot of obvious mistakes in that one; and it's neat and everything*)
>
> <u>Process</u>   Refers to processes of creating and sharing/publishing text (e.g., *I just kind of threw it down so that's why I put it last*)
>
> <u>Not interpretable</u>

Within each of these categories, further subcategories were created by the authors for a total of thirty-one distinct types of criteria.

Most fifth grade students used at least three (of the 31) criteria to justify their rankings, and 70 percent were <u>text-based</u> in nature. For example, the students commented on features of the text that created (or failed to create) interest, or they commented on whether the text was easy or hard to understand. Interestingly, and at odds with some previous research, only 5 percent of the children's comments, on average, referred to <u>surface qualities</u> (however, low achievers cited surface qualities more often than high achievers). There was considerable variation among children, with many struggling to articulate any criteria, some merely repeating parts of the text they liked, and others resorting to personal associations. High-achieving students voiced a mixture of personal and objective reactions, were able to state multiple criteria, and seemed to have a growing sense of awareness of the craft of writing. However, they did not use a "teacher's grid" (the same set of criteria) for each story; rather, each story was treated separately according to a unique template. In sum, the study showed that older elementary children are beginning to develop a meta-evaluative stance toward writing. An association between highly developed internal standards of writing and the ability to write well would be expected and has been demonstrated recently for college freshman (Johnson, Linton, & Madigan, 1994).

Writing Problems of Children and Adolescents with Reading Disabilities

The publication of *Reading Disabilities* (Kamhi & Catts, 1989) occurred at a turning point in research on the writing of children with RD.[6] Prior to that time, investigators concen-

---

[6]The studies reviewed in this section typically have involved children classified as learning disabled. However, because most of these children received this classification on the basis of their reading disabilities, they are referred to here as children with reading disabilities. This is also in keeping with the terminology used throughout this book.

trated on describing written texts (*products*) of such writers. The general design was to compare children with RD to typically developing students on a variety of product measures at word, sentence, and text levels (e.g., number of words, sentence complexity, grammatical errors, text organization, cohesion, etc.). As expected, when such comparisons were made, texts written by children with RD were almost always inferior. I reviewed available studies, most of them on written products in the 1989 volume (Scott, 1989). As discussed by Graham and colleagues (Graham, Harris, MacArthur, & Schwartz, 1991), the product approach has limitations: (1) little insight is gained into *processes* used in producing these inferior texts, (2) product measures are situation specific, precluding the development of general models; and (3) quality writing is difficult to define and measure. As a remedy, Graham and colleagues (1991) recommended studies designed to answer questions about

> what students with LD know about the act of composing (what writing means to them), what processes they employ when producing text, how these processes interact either to enhance or impede performance, how different conditions for producing text influence what and how they write, and how competence in writing is acquired. (p. 90)

In fact, studies of writing processes employed by students with RD have increased in the last decade. This last section of the chapter provides an overview of research that could be called product-oriented and then reviews more recent findings with a process orientation.

Product-Oriented Research

At the text level, for both narrative and expository genres, one of the most consistent findings for problem writers across a wide age range is the *production of shorter texts*, whether the measure is total number of words or total number of sentences (Anderson, 1982; Blalock & Johnson, 1987; Houck & Billingsley, 1989; Morris & Stick, 1985; Scott & Klutzenbaker, 1989). Underscoring the importance of this simple measure, text length is a consistently good predictor of holistic quality ratings of writing (Durst et al., 1990; Freedman, 1987; McFadden & Gillam, 1996). Because short texts do not present the same opportunities for text structure development as longer texts, the findings for productivity and genre inadequacies (e.g., missing components of stories) should be seen as related. An obvious process explanation for the lack of fluency and productivity of students with RD is their inability to sustain a topic or use self-directed memory search strategies (Thomas, Englert, & Gregg, 1987).

Narratives written by children and adults with RD have been examined in some detail. Although many have acquired some basic knowledge of *narrative text structure* schema, and some can write good stories, a majority of students with RD have difficulty with at least some text-level dimensions of the narrative genre. These include: (1) pronominal referencing in texts with several characters, particularly same-gender characters (Bartlett, 1984), (2) narrator stance—shifting inappropriately between first and third person (Anderson, 1982), and (3) omission of critical story grammar components, especially those relating characters' internal responses, plans, and motivations (Barenbaum, Newcomer, & Nodine, 1987; Newcomer & Barenbaum, 1991). When narratives are rated for overall quality, those written by RD children receive lower ratings than age-matched controls (e.g., McFadden &

Gillam, 1996). Difficulty with *expository texts* has also been documented. Specific characteristics of expository writing include (1) fewer lexical and grammatical cohesive ties
(Morris & Stick, 1985), (2) fewer logical adverbial clauses per sentence (Scott & Klutsenbaker, 1989), (3) overuse of sentence-initial *and* (Scott & Klutsenbaker, 1989) and (4) less
developed text structures including redundancies and abrupt termination (Thomas et al.,
1987). Of the several types of expository text structures, sequencing is easiest for students
with RD, and compare/contrast and explanation texts are more difficult (Thomas et al.,
1987).

The most common metric for investigating sentence-level writing competence is *average sentence length*, where texts are usually segmented as T-units (Hunt, 1965). A measure
of overall syntactic complexity, the T-unit has not reliably shown deficiencies in children
with RD. Whereas shorter T-units characterized low-achieving subjects (Hunt, 1970) and low
language-ability students (Loban, 1976) in earlier large-N studies, more recent work with
RD students has failed to find differences in T-unit length (e.g., Houck & Billingsley, 1989;
Morris & Crump, 1982). The sensitivity of the T-unit as a measure of complexity, plus its
susceptibility to task and genre, have been addressed by Scott (1988). Finer grained methods of analysis seem to be called for in studies of sentence-level syntax of poor writers. As
an example, when researchers have looked at *lexical and syntactic variety*, poor writers are
shown to have a more limited repertoire of complex syntactic structures (Loban, 1976; Scott
& Klutsenbaker, 1989).[7] *Grammatical and punctuation errors* also characterize the writing
of RD students (Anderson, 1982; Gregg, 1983; Morris & Stick, 1985). Omissions of
inflectional suffixes, which may create subject-verb agreement or tense problems, are typical (Rubin, Patterson, & Kantor, 1991). A frequent punctuation error is the lack of capitalization. Sentence fragments can also be created by problems with sentence-end punctuation.
However, it is unclear whether RD students make more of these errors than control subjects (Houck & Billingsley, 1989).

Cross-genre and cross-modality studies also shed light on the nature of writing problems. Evidence suggests that students with RD are not insensitive to genre influence. In a
study of sixth, eighth, and tenth grade students with RD, Blair and Crump (1984) found
that *argument* texts were structurally more complex than *descriptive* texts. Scott and Klutsenbaker (1989) compared persuasive, narrative, and expository summary writing in three
students with RD (fifth and eighth grade) and also found that argument texts exceeded
descriptive writing in terms of structural complexity; for these writers, however, narrative
writing was also more complex than expository writing, indicating a relative lack of development in informational text. Although students with RD make some adjustments in text
depending on genre requirements, they appear to have inordinate difficulty with expository
writing. Given that younger typically developing children usually write longer and more
complex narrative than factual texts (Kress, 1982), this finding for older RD children is not
unexpected.

---

[7]A child who uses a small number of complex structures over and over again could produce a text
with the same average number of words per T-unit as another child who uses a larger variety of complex structures. This may explain, in part, the inability of average T–unit length measures to detect
syntactic differences.

In a *cross-modal* investigation, Gillam and Johnston (1992) explored narrative speaking and writing in children with spoken language disorders. Compared to age- and language-matched subjects, children with language disorders used fewer complex sentences in spoken and written narratives, and group differences were even more pronounced in writing. In fact, there was a complete reversal of modality effects. Whereas age- and language-matched subjects used more complexity when they wrote, children with language impairments used more complexity when they spoke. Placed in the context of Kroll's stages discussed earlier, these students appeared to be "stuck" in the preparation phase, when spoken sentence complexity exceeds what the child is capable of writing. The findings of Scott and Klutsenbaker (1989) corroborate those of Gillam and Johnston (1992); a fifth grade student with RD produced more subordination in spoken narrative, persuasive, and expository summaries compared with written versions, but the opposite was true for the age-matched control subject.

Process-Oriented Research

Students with RD have difficulty with all parts of the writing process, from beginning to end. Hallenbeck (1996) described the problem faced by the RD student writing a paper as akin to "building a house without a blueprint; they don't know where they're going or how to begin" (p. 107). The metaphor aptly describes research on *planning* phases of writing. Research suggests that RD students are less likely to think about the readers' needs during initial and ongoing planning or in revision—as if readers are supposed to "just know" what they think (Gombert, 1992). Further, the analysis of think-aloud protocols indicates that students with RD do not think of genre-specific text structure schemes (Englert, Raphael, Fear, & Anderson, 1988). Without a picture of "the whole," which text structure facilitates, there is little conscious thought about what to include and what to omit. These students also have difficulty generating ideas (Graham, et al., 1991). As a general strategy, students with RD are said to use a *knowledge-telling* strategy (Bryson & Scardamalia, 1991; Thomas et al., 1987), but they have difficulty sustaining even that effort, and produce shorter texts as a result. Graham (1990) learned that students with RD do respond well to "contentless" props to "write more," producing texts on average two to four times as long as the original, although some of the added material was not useful (40% of all added statements). This finding underscores the major role played by the these students' difficulties with *self-regulation* of cognitive processes.

Revision behavior and knowledge has also been a focus for process-oriented research on the writing of students with RD. MacArthur, Graham, and Schwartz (1991) asked seventh and eighth grade students with RD about the types of changes they would make to improve a paper. They were also invited to make suggestions for improvements on another student's paper, and they wrote and revised both narrative and expository papers of their own. Only one-fourth of the students made any suggestions based on content (e.g., add more information); all other revisions mentioned dealt with surface features such as spelling, neatness, and so on. Revisions to their own texts were similar—just 19 percent changed the original meaning in any way. And only half of all revisions, either surface or content-related, were rated by the researchers as real improvements to the text. Interestingly, when placed in the role of editor of another's paper, however, the students did a better job. Three-fourths of their suggestions in this case dealt with meaning; most frequently they suggested adding information and changing the beginning of the paper. These findings correspond well with results from a later study of knowledge and attitude about writing (Graham, Schwartz, & MacArthur, 1993). In this project, normally achieving fourth, fifth, seventh, and eighth grade students were more likely than students with RD to mention substantive activities when describing "what good writers do"; they were also more likely to mention substantive solutions (e.g., "study or look for more information") rather than surface solutions (e.g., "write bigger") to writing problems. The one area where there were no differences, however, was in the students' beliefs about themselves as writers (termed *self-efficacy* by Graham et al., 1993). To measure self-efficacy, students responded on a 5-point scale to statements such as "when writing a paper it is easy for me to get ideas", or "it is hard for me to keep the paper going." The tendency of students with RD to overestimate their writing competence may explain, in part, the difference in their ability to revise their own versus others' papers.

As a final perspective on writing processes of RD students, we can ask how different writing "mediums" affect writing processes and text quality. MacArthur and Graham (1987) studied the effects of three methods of writing stories—by hand, on the computer, and by dictation, in fifth and sixth grade children with RD. The students had used computers regularly for two years prior to the study. There was no effect of method on planning time, which was less than a minute in each case, even though the children were prompted to plan before starting to write. Composing was actually slower on the computer (an average of 30.6 letters per minute on the computer vs. 54.9 handwritten letters). Also, computer-produced writing had more errors (7.3 per 100 letters compared with 2.5 errors by hand). The hand-written and word-processed stories did not differ on any product measures (length, story structure, grammatical errors, average T-unit length). Likewise, the number and type of revisions were similar for handwritten and word-processed stories, even though the time when the revisions were made differed. When composing on the computer, revisions were interspersed throughout; revisions were made at the end of the handwritten text. Major differences occurred for dictated stories, however. Produced nine times faster than handwriting and twenty times faster than word processing, the dictated stories were also of higher quality. MacArthur and Graham (1987) concluded that the difficulties RD children have getting "language onto paper" (the children misspelled 12% of the words they wrote and made numerous capitalization and punctuation errors) got in the way of text planning and generating processes. Students were so slow writing by hand and at the computer that they may have actually forgotten plans already made or disrupted plans being made on-line. In a later study, Graham (1990) designed a task to isolate the effects of on-line transcription (spelling words, etc.) from rate. In a slow dictation condition, students dictated their compositions to an examiner who then transcribed it at a much slower rate (actually the student's usual writing rate was used). The texts produced from slow dictation were generally as good as normal-rate dictation texts, thus indicating that transcription rather than slow rate is the actual distractor for RD students. When students had more time to think on-line (as the examiner finished transcribing each sentence), they used that time to plan better texts.

To summarize, Graham and Harris (1993) categorized the wide array of processing difficulties of students with RD into three basic types: (1) lack of proficiency in text production skills (spelling, punctuation, etc.), (2) lack of knowledge central to the process of writing, including knowledge about the topic, retrieving what they know, text structure schemas, and recognizing what strategies are needed, and (3) difficulty planning and revising. Furthermore, these difficulties interrelate (MacArthur, Graham, Schwartz, & Schafer, 1995). To illustrate, difficulties with basic text production skills may lead the writer to think of good writing as a matter of form rather than substance, which in turn leads to ineffective revision.

Summary

We have seen that writing in its earliest period is usually a self-chosen activity—almost a prop among others like drawing—within a social context of peers and talk. These short texts comment on both events and objects; thus the seeds of both narrative and factual writing are sown early. Gradually writing must accommodate school curricula; children become composers responding to writing assignments with a paragraph to several pages in narrative, factual, and persuasive genres. Planning and revising of texts as well as automaticity in transcribing (e.g., spelling words) are all expected. New linguistic skills deriving from the need to be explicit and make longer stretches of text cohere are called for. The knowledge base for written content increasingly draws on new "encyclopedic" knowledge rather than older, experiential knowledge. The ability to write is not something learned "once and for all." Research shows that the writing of college students benefits significantly from a variety of instructional programs (Charney & Carlson, 1995; Cheng & Steffensen, 1996).

Some children will become good writers capable of producing *integrative* text (Kroll, 1981) and using writing for *knowledge-transforming* purposes (Bereiter & Scardamalia, 1987). Many will apparently grow to like writing less and less (Evans, 1993; Harris & Graham, 1992). Still others—children with RD—will have difficulties of such a magnitude that academic survival is threatened and later vocational plans are altered. The texts produced by students with RD are shorter, more poorly organized from the standpoint of genre-specific text structure, with fewer grammatical markers of genre and modality. Spelling and punctuation errors abound. Furthermore, the process of composing for such students differs at all levels and in all domains. Students with RD are unable to marshall the conscious monitoring and regulating strategies that would result in better writing. Writing is a permanent record of such difficulties. Its visibility makes it a "tangible threat" (Hallenbeck, 1996, p. 107) to children and consequently a high priority for assessment and intervention attention, as addressed in the following chapter.

References

Anderson, P. (1982). A preliminary study of syntax in the written expression of learning disabled children. *Journal of Learning Disabilities, 15,* 359–362.

Applebee, A. (1984). *Contexts for learning to write.* Norwood, NJ: Ablex.

Applebee, A., Langer, J., & Mullis, I. (1986). *The writing report card: Writing achievement in American Schools.* Princeton, NJ: Educational Testing Services.

Applebee, A., Langer, J., Mullis, I, Latham, A., & Gentile, C. (1994). *NAEP 1992 writing report card.*

Report No. 23-W01. Washington, DC: Office of Educational Research Improvement, U.S. Department of Education.

Barenbaum, E., Newcomer, P., & Nodine, B. (1987). Children's ability to write stories as a function of variation in task, age, and developmental level. *Learning Disability Quarterly, 10,* 175–188.

Bartlett, E. (1984). Anaphoric reference in written narratives of good and poor elementary school writers. *Journal of Verbal Learning and Verbal Behavior, 23,* 540–552.

Beason, L. (1993). Feedback and revision in writing across the curriculum classes. *Research in the Teaching of English, 27,* 395–422.

Bereiter, C., & Scardamalia, M. (1987). *The psychology of written composition.* Hillsdale, NJ: Erlbaum.

Biber, D. (1986). Spoken and written textual dimensions in English: Resolving the contradictory findings. *Language, 62,* 383–414.

Biber, D. (1992). On the complexity of discourse complexity: A multidimensional analysis. *Discourse Processes, 15,* 133–163.

Bissex, G. (1980). *GYNS AT WRK: A child learns to write and read.* Cambridge, MA: Harvard University Press.

Black, J. (1981). Psycholinguistic processes in writing. In C. Frederiksen, M. Whiteman, & J. Dominic (Eds.), *Writing: The nature, development, and teaching of written communication* (pp. 199–216). Hillsdale, NJ: Erlbaum.

Blair, T., & Crump, W. (1984). Effects of discourse mode on the syntactic complexity of learning disabled student's written expression. *Learning Disability Quarterly, 7,* 19–29.

Blalock, J., & Johnson, D. (Eds.) (1987). *Adults with learning disabilities: Clinical studies.* New York: Grune and Stratton.

Bloomfield, L. (1933). *Language.* New York: Holt, Rinehart, & Winston.

Bryson, M., & Scardamalia, M. (1991). Teaching writing to students at risk for academic failure (Report No. UD 028 249) In *Teaching advanced skills to educationally disadvantaged students* (ERIC Document Reproduction Service No. ED 338 725).

Burkhalter, N. (1995). A Vygotsky-based curriculum for teaching persuasive writing in the elementary grades. *Language Arts, 72,* 192–199.

Burtis, J., Bereiter, C., Scardamalia, M., & Tetroe, J. (1983). The development of planning in writing.

In B. Kroll & G. Wells (Eds.). *Exploration in the development of writing* (pp. 153–176). New York: John Wiley.

Cazden, C. (1993). *A report on reports: Two dilemmas of genre teaching* (ERIC Document Reproduction Service No. ED 363 593).

Chapman, M. (1994). The emergence of genres: Some findings from an examination of first-grade writing. *Written Communication, 11,* 348–380.

Chapman, M. (1995). The sociolinguistic construction of written genres in the first grade. *Research in the Teaching of English, 29*(2), 164–192.

Charney, D., & Carlson, R. (1995). Learning to write in a genre: What student writers take from model texts. *Research in the Teaching of English, 29,* 88–125

Cheng, X., & Steffensen, M. (1996). Metadiscourse: A technique for improving student writing. *Research in the Teaching of English, 30*(2), 149–181.

Christie, F. (1986). Writing in the infants grades. In C. Painter & J. Martin (Eds.). *Writing to mean: Teaching genres across the curriculum* (pp. 118–135). Melbourne, Australia: Applied Linguistics Association of Australia, Occasional Papers, No. 9.

Cordeiro, P. (1988). Children's punctuation: An analysis of errors in period placement. *Research in the Teaching of English, 22,* 62–75.

Crowhurst, M. (1987). Cohesion in argument and narration at three grade levels. *Research in the Teaching of English, 21,* 185–201.

Crowhurst, M. (1991). Interrelationships between reading and writing persuasive discourse. *Research in the Teaching of English, 25*(3), 314–338.

Crowhurst, M., & Piche, G. (1979). Audience and mode of discourse effects on syntactic complexity in writing at two grade levels. *Research in the Teaching of English, 13,* 101–109.

Daiute, C. (1984). Performance limits on writers. In R. Beach & L. Bridwell (Eds.), *New directions in composing research* (pp. 205–224). New York: Guilford Press.

De Temple, J.M., Wu, H-F., & Snow, C. (1991). Papa pig just left for pigtown: Children's oral and written picture descriptions under varying instructions. *Discourse Processes, 14,* 469–495.

Dobson, L. (1988). *Connections in learning to write and read: A study of children's development through kindergarten and grade one.* Urbana, IL: Center for the Study of Reading. Technical Report No. 418.

Donaldson, M. (1984). Speech and writing and modes of learning. In H. Goelman, A. Oberg, & F. Smith (Eds.). *Awakening to literacy* (pp. 174–184). London: Heinemann.

Durst, R., Laine, C., Shultz, L., & Vilter, W. (1990). Appealing texts: The persuasive writing of high school students. *Written Communication, 7*(2), 232–255.

Duthie, C. (1994). Nonfiction: A genre study for the primary classroom. *Language Arts, 71*, 588–595.

Dyson, A. (1989). *Multiple worlds of child writers: Friends learning to write*. New York: Teachers College Press.

Dyson, A. (1993a). *Social worlds of children learning to write in an urban primary school*. New York: Teachers College Press.

Dyson, A. (1993b). A sociocultural perspective on symbolic development in primary grade classrooms. In C. Daiute (Ed.), *The development of literacy through social interaction* (pp. 25–40). San Francisco: Jossey-Bass Publishers.

Englert, C., Raphael, T., Fear, K., & Anderson, L. (1988). Students' metacognitive knowledge about how to write information test. *Learning Disability Quarterly, 11*, 18–46.

Evans, R. (1993). Learning "schooled literacy": The literate life histories of mainstream student readers and writers. *Discourse Processes, 16*, 312–340.

Faigley, L., Cherry, R., Joliffe, D., & Skinner, A. (1985). *Assessing writers' knowledge and processes of composing*. Norwood, NJ: Ablex.

Ferreiro, E. (1984). The underlying logic of literacy development. In H. Goelman, A. Oberg, & F. Smith (Eds.), *Awakening to literacy* (pp. 154–173). London: Heinemann.

Ferreiro, E., & Teberosky, A. (1982). *Literacy before schooling*. Exeter, NH: Heinemann.

Ferreiro, E., & Zucchermaglio, C. (1996). Children's use of punctuation marks: The case of quoted speech. In C. Pontecorvo, M. Orsolini, B. Burge, & L. B. Resnick (Eds.). *Children's early text construction* (pp. 177–205). Mahway, NJ: Erlbaum.

Fitzgerald, J. (1992). Variant views about good thinking during composing: Focus on revision. In M. Pressley, K. Harris, & J. Guthrie (Eds.), *Promoting academic competence and literacy in school* (pp. 337–358). San Diego, CA: Academic Press.

Freedman, A. (1987). Development in story writing. *Applied Psycholinguistics, 8*, 153–170.

Gee, J. (1994). Orality and literacy: From *The savage mind* to *ways with words*. in J. Maybins (Ed.), *Language and literacy in social practice* (pp. 168–192). England: Multilingual Matters, LTD.

Gillam, R., & Johnston, J. (1992). Spoken and written language relationships in language/learning impaired and normally achieving school-age children. *Journal of Speech and Hearing Research, 35*, 1303–1315.

Golder, C., & Coirier, P. (1994). Argumentative text writing: Developmental trends. *Discourse Processes, 18*, 187–210.

Golub, L., & Frederick, W. (1971). Linguistic structures in the discourse of fourth and sixth graders. Wisconsin Research and Development Center for Cognitive Learning, Technical Report No. 166. Madison, WI: the University of Wisconsin.

Gombert, J.E. (1992). *Metalinguistic development*. Chicago: University of Chicago Press.

Goodman, Y. (1996). Readers' and writers' talk about language. In C. Pontecorvo, M. Orsolini, B. Burge, & L. B. Resnick (Eds.), *Children's early text construction* (pp. 345–357). Mahwah, NJ: Erlbaum.

Graham, S. (1990). The role of production factors in learning disabled student's compositions. *Journal of Educational Psychology, 82*, 781–791.

Graham, S., & Harris, K. (1993). Teaching writing strategies to students with learning disabilities: Issues and recommendations. In L.J. Meltzer (Ed.), *Strategy assessment and instruction for students with learning disabilities: From theory to practice* (pp. 271–292). Austin, TX: Pro-Ed.

Graham, S., & Harris, K. (1994). The role and development of self-regulation in the writing process. In D.H. Schunk & B.J. Zimmerman (Eds.), *Self-regulation of learning and performance* (pp. 203–228). Hillsdale, NJ: Erlbaum.

Graham, S., Harris, K., MacArthur, C., & Schwartz, S. (1991). Writing and writing instruction for students with learning disabilities: Review of a research program. *Learning Disability Quarterly, 14*, 89–114.

Graham, S., Schwartz, S., & MacArthur, C. (1993). Knowledge of writing and the composing process, attitude toward writing, and self-efficacy for students with and without learning disabilities. *Journal of Learning Disabilities, 26*(4), 237–249.

Graves, D. (1983). *Writing: Teachers and children at work*. Portsmouth, NH: Heinemann.

Graves, D. (1989). *Investigative nonfiction*. Portsmouth, NH: Heinemann.

Gregg, N. (1983). College learning disabled writer: Error patterns and instructional alternatives. *Journal of Learning Disability, 16,* 334–338.

Gundlach, R. (1982). Children as writers: The beginnings of learning to write. In M. Nystrand (Ed.), *What writers know* (pp. 129–148). New York: Academic Press.

Hallenbeck, M. (1996). The cognitive strategy in writing; Welcome relief for adolescents with learning disabilities. *Learning Disabilities Research & Practice, 11(2),* 107–119.

Halliday, M.A.K. (1985). *Spoken and written language*. Oxford: Oxford University Press.

Halliday, M.A.K. (1987). Spoken and written modes of meaning. In R. Horowitz & S.J. Samuels (Eds.), *Comprehending oral and written language* (pp. 55–82). San Diego, CA: Academic Press.

Harrell, L. (1957). A comparison of the development of oral and written language in school-age children. *Monographs of the Society for Research in Child Development, 22,* Serial No. 66, No. 3.

Harris, K., & Graham, S. (1992). Self-regulated strategy development: A part of the writing process. In M. Pressley, K. Harris, & J.T. Guthrie (Eds.), *Promoting academic competence and literacy in school* (pp. 277–309). San Diego, CA: Academic Press.

Hayes, J., & Flower, L. (1980). Identifying the organization of writing processes. In L. Gregg & E. Steinberg (Eds.), *Cognitive processes in writing: An interdisciplinary approach* (pp. 3–30). Hillsdale, NJ: Erlbaum.

Hayes, J., & Flower, L. (1987). On the structure of the writing process. *Topics in Language Disorders, 7,* 19–30.

Houck, C. & Billingsley, B. (1989). Written expression of students with and without learning disabilities: Differences across the grades. *Journal of Learning Disabilities, 22(9),* 561–565.

Hunt, K. (1965). *Grammatical structures written at three grade levels*. Champaign, IL: National Council of Teachers of English, Research Report No. 3.

Hunt, K. (1970). Syntactic maturity in school children and adults. *Monographs of the Society for Research in Child Development, 35,* Serial No. 134, No. 1.

Jensen, J. (1993). What do we know about the writing of elementary school children? *Language Arts, 70,* 290–294.

Johnson, S., Linton, P., & Madigan, R. (1994). The role of internal standards in assessment of written discourse. *Discourse Processes, 18,* 231–245.

Kamhi, A., & Catts, H. (1989). *Reading disabilities: A developmental language perspective*. Boston: Allyn & Bacon.

Knudson, R.E. (1994). An analysis of persuasive discourse: Learning how to take a stand. *Discourse Processes, 18,* 211–230.

Kress, G. (1982). *Learning to write*. London: Routledge & Kegan Paul.

Kroll, B. (1981). Developmental relationships between speaking and writing. In B. Roll & R. Vann (Eds.), *Exploring speaking-writing relationships: Connections and contrasts* (pp. 32–54). Urbana, IL: National Council of Teachers of English.

Langer, J. (1985). Children's sense of genre. A study of the performance on parallel reading and writing tasks. *Written Communication, 2,* 157–187.

Loban, W. (1976). *Language development: Kindergarten through grade twelve*. Champaign, IL: National Council of Teachers of English, Research Report No. 18.

MacArthur, C. (1996). Using technology to enhance the writing processes of students with learning disabilities. *Journal of Learning Disabilities, 29(4),* 344–353.

MacArthur, C. & Graham, S. (1987). Learning disabled students' composing with three methods: Handwriting, dictation, and word processing. *Journal of Special Education, 21,* 22–42.

MacArthur, C., Graham, S., & Schwartz, S. (1991). Knowledge of revision and revising behavior among learning disabled students. *Learning Disability Quarterly, 14.* 61–73.

MacArthur, C., Graham, S., Schwartz, S., & Schafer, W. (1995). Evaluation of a writing instruction model that integrated a process approach, strategy instruction, and word processing. *Learning Disability Quarterly, 18,* 278–291.

Martin, J.R. (1989). *Factual writing: Exploring and challenging social reality*. Oxford University Press.

McCann, T.M. (1989). Student argumentative writing: Knowledge and ability at three grade levels. *Research in the Teaching of English, 23,* 62–76.

McCormick, C., Busching, B., & Potter, E. (1992). Children's knowledge about writing: The development and use of evaluative criteria. In M. Pressley, K. Harris, & J.T. Guthrie (Eds.), *Promoting academic competence and literacy in school* (pp. 311–335). San Diego, CA: Academic Press.

McCutchen, D., & Perfetti, C.A. (1982). Coherence and connectedness in the development of discourse production. *Text, 2,* 113–139.

McFadden, T., & Gillam, R. (1996). An examination of the quality of narratives produced by children with language disorders. *Language, Speech, and Hearing Services in Schools, 27,* 48–56.

Merenda, R. (1996). Writing: An adventure for young children. *Writing Teacher, 9(5),* 12–14.

Morris, N., & Crump, W. (1982). Syntactic and vocabulary development in the written language of learning disabled and non-disabled students at four age levels. *Learning Disability Quarterly, 5,* 163–172.

Morris, N., & Stick, S. (1985, November). *Oral/written language analysis of learning disabled and normal high schoolers.* Paper presented at the annual meeting of the American Speech-Language-Hearing Association, Washington, D.C.

Newcomer, P., & Barenbaum, E. (1991). The written composing ability of children with learning disabilities: A review of the literature from 1980 to 1990. *Journal of Learning Disabilities, 24*(10), 578–593.

Newkirk, T. (1987). The non-narrative writing of young children. *Research in the Teaching of English, 21*(2), 121–144.

Nystrand, M. (1989). A social-interactive model of writing. *Written Communication, 6,* 66–85.

O'Donnell, R., Griffin, W., & Norris, R. (1967). *Syntax of kindergarten and elementary school children: A transformational analysis.* Champaign, IL: National Council of Teachers of English, Research Report No. 8.

Olson, N. Torrance, & A. Hildyard (Eds.), *Literacy, language, and learning* (pp. 389–403). Cambridge, England: Cambridge University Press.

Pappas, C. (1991). Young children's strategies in learning the "book language" of information books. *Discourse Processes, 14,* 203–225.

Pelligrini, A., Galda, L., & Rubin, D. (1984). Context in text: The development of oral and written language in two genres. *Child Development, 55,* 1549–1555.

Perera, K. (1984). *Children's writing and reading.* London: Basil Blackwell.

Perera, K. (1986). Grammatical differentiation between speech and writing in children aged 8 to 12. In A. Wilkinson (Ed.), *The writing of writing* (pp. 90–108). London: The Falmer Press.

Perera, K. (1992). Reading and writing skills in the National Curriculum. In P. Fletcher & D. Hall (Eds.), *Specific speech and language disorders in children: Correlates, characteristics and outcomes* (pp. 183–193). San Diego, CA: Singular Press.

Pontecorvo, C., & Orsolini, M. (1996). Writing and written language in children's development. In C. Pontecorvo, M. Orsolini, B. Burge, & L.B. Resnick (Eds.), *Children's early text construction* (pp. 3–23). Mahway, NJ: Erlbaum.

Popken, R. (1996). A study of the genre repertoires of adult writers. *The Writing Instructor, 15*(2), 85–93.

Read, C. (1985). Effects of phonology on beginning spelling: Some cross-linguistic evidence. In D. Olson, N. Torrance, & A. Hildyard (Eds.), *Literacy, language, and learning* (pp. 389–403). Cambridge, England: Cambridge University Press.

Read, C. (1986). *Children's creative spelling.* London: Routledge & Kegan Paul.

Rubin, D. (1984). The influence of communicative context on stylistic variations in writing. In D.D. Pellegrini & T.D. Yawkey (Eds.), *The development of oral and written language in social contexts* (pp. 213–232). Norwood, NJ: Ablex.

Rubin, D. (1987). Divergence and convergence between oral and written language communication. *Topics in Language Disorders, 7,* 1–18.

Rubin, H., Patterson, P., & Kantor, M. (1991). Morphological development and writing ability in children and adults. *Language, Speech, and Hearing Services in Schools, 22,* 228–235.

Scott, C. (1988). Spoken and written syntax. In M. Nippold (Ed.), *Later language development: Ages nine through nineteen* (pp. 49–95). San Diego, CA: College-Hill Press.

Scott, C. (1989). Problem writers: Nature, assessment, and intervention. In A. Kamhi & H. Catts (Eds.), *Reading disabilities: A developmental language perspective* (pp. 303–344). Boston: Allyn & Bacon.

Scott, C. (1994). A discourse continuum for school-age students: Impact of modality and genre. In G. Wallach & K. Butler (Eds.), *Language learning dis-*

abilities in school-age children and adolescents (pp. 219–252). New York: Merrill.

Scott, C. (1995). Syntax for school-age children: A discourse perspective. In M.E. Fey, J. Windsor, & S.F. Warren (Eds.), *Language intervention: Preschool through the elementary years* (pp. 107–143). Baltimore, MD: Paul H. Brookes.

Scott, C., & Klutsenbaker, K. (1989, November). *Comparing spoken and written summaries: Text structure and surface form.* Paper presented at the Annual Convention of the American Speech-Language-Hearing Association, St. Louis, MO.

Scott, C., & Rogers, L. (1996). Written language abilities of African American children and youth. In A. Kamhi, K. Pollock, & J. Harris (Eds.), *Communication development and disorders in African American children* (pp. 307–332). Baltimore, MD: Paul H. Brookes.

Sheeran, Y., & Barnes, D. (1991). *School writing: Discovering the ground rules.* Philadelphia: Milton Keynes.

Simone, R. (1996). Reflections on the comma. In C. Pontecorvo, M. Orsolini, B. Burge, & L.B. Resnick (Eds.), *Children's early text construction* (pp. 165–175). Mahway, NJ: Erlbaum.

Sulsby, E. (1985). Children's emergent reading of favorite storybooks: A developmental study. *Reading Research Quarterly, 20,* 458–481.

Sulzby, E. (1986). Writing and reading: Signs of oral and written language organization in the young child. In W. Teale & E. Sulzby (Eds.), *Emergent literacy: Writing and reading* (pp. 50–89). Norwood, NJ: Ablex.

Sulzby, E. (1996). Roles of oral and written language as children approach conventional literacy. In C. Pontecorvo, M. Orsolini, B. Burge, & L.B. Resnick (Eds.). *Children's early text construction* (pp. 25–46). Mahway, NJ: Erlbaum.

Sulzby, E., Branz, C. & Buhle, R. (1993). Repeated readings of literature and low socioeconomic status black kindergartners and first graders. *Reading and Writing Quarterly, 9,* 183–196.

Thomas, C., Englert, C., & Gregg, S. (1987). An analysis of errors and strategies in the expository writing of learning disabled students. *Remedial and Special Education, 8(1),* 21–30.

Vygotsky, L. (1978). Mind in society: The development of higher psychological processes. In M. Cole, V. John-Steiner, S. Scribner, & E. Souberman (Eds. & Trans.), *Mind in society: The development of higher psychological processes.* Cambridge, MA: Harvard University Press.

Westby, C. (1994). The effects of culture on genre, structure, and style of oral and written texts. In G. Wallach & K. Butler (Eds.), *Language learning disabilities in school-age children and adolescents* (pp. 180–218). New York: Merrill.

Why Write?, Interview with Stephen & Susan Tchudi (1995). *Writing Teacher, 9(1),* 3–6.

Witte, S. (1983). Topical structure and revision: An exploratory study. *College Composition and Communication, 34,* 313–341.

Writing and Thinking, Interview with Leif Fearn (1996). *Writing Teacher, 9(4),* 3–7.

Writing process: In retrospect, Interview with Donald Graves (1996). *Writing Teacher, 9(5),* 3–7.

Yagelski, R.P. (1995). The role of classroom context in the revision strategies of students writers. *Research in the Teaching of English, 29,* 216–238.

Zimmerman, B. (1989). A social cognitive view of self-regulated academic learning. *Journal of Educational Psychology, 81,* 329–339.

Zuchermaglio, C., & Scheuer, N. (1996). Children dictating a story: Is together better? In C. Pontecorvo, M. Orsolini, B. Burge, & L.B. Resnick (Eds.). *Children's early text construction* (pp. 83–98). Mahway, NJ: Erlbaum.

Chapter 9

The Right Stuff for Writing: Assessing and Facilitating Written Language

CAROL E. WESTBY   *PATRICIA S. CLAUSER*

> *The strongest drive*
> *is not Love or Hate.*
>
> *It is one person's need*
>
> modify *revise*
> to change *another's copy.*
> ^
>   *rewrite amend*
>   *chop to pieces*
>   *change*

Many students have strong feelings about writing, and these feelings, particularly for older students, are frequently not positive. Some, like the graduate student who gave the first author the above quote, are frustrated by their experiences with writing. Even though they may not exhibit any specific reading or writing difficulties, many students do not look

Acknowledgments

Rosario Roman and teachers at Algodones Elementary and Santo Domingo Elementary in the Bernalillo, New Mexico School District, developed and implemented the computer writing activities with students in third through sixth grades.

forward to writing assignments. Like 6-year-old Calvin, in the Calvin and Hobbes comic strip popular in recent years, they find they must be in the right mood to write, and that mood is "last-minute panic." They wish they could jump into a time machine and return after the paper is completed. They complain of writer's block; although unlike Calvin, the block is not a chunk of wood you put on your desk "so you can't write there anymore."

Although more persons than ever possess some literacy skills, the level of literacy that is necessary for functioning within the world has been increasing (Kennedy, 1993). For many years, literacy teaching in schools focused on reading. In recent years, however, increasing attention is being given to writing (Atwell, 1987; Calkins, 1994; Graves, 1983). The majority of students with reading disabilities will also exhibit difficulties with writing. A number of students who exhibit no obvious difficulties with spoken language and reading, however, also exhibit difficulties with writing. Many students, both in regular education and special education classes, have limited writing abilities and spend little time writing (Rueda, 1990).

Increasing interest is being directed to developing methods for assessing and facilitating students' writing (Gentile, 1992). State and national pressure for standards in language arts and for schools to be accountable for the development of ALL students and increased understanding of the role of writing in language and literacy development are resulting in special educators and speech-language pathologists becoming more involved in the evaluation and teaching of writing. In the past, many students could be excluded from taking district-wide or state-wide assessments. Many school districts, in fact, encouraged educators to request exemptions for students who were not good readers and writers so that overall district scores were not lowered. As a consequence, many students with reading and writing problems and second language learners who were not English proficient have been excluded from testing. Currently, efforts are being made at both national and state levels to include all students in assessments. Consequently, more students with reading and writing problems are being assessed. In addition to including ALL students in educational assessments, there is increased interest in methods for evaluating and developing students' writing abilities. In the past, it was believed that successful reading had to precede successful writing. More recently, researchers have claimed that listening, talking, reading, and writing can all develop simultaneously and that, in fact, writing can assist in the development of other language abilities (Nippold, 1988).

Writing education has typically been carried out in the regular education classroom. Special educators may have been involved in developing students' handwriting and emergent writing skills, but they were generally not involved in assisting students in writing extended texts for a variety of purposes or in a variety of genres. Speech-language pathologists have had even less involvement with writing and, in fact, in some school districts they were not permitted to work on written language skills. Many states now mandate a formal writing assessment at several grade levels, and in some states students' performance on these writing assessments and other tests are used to evaluate teacher effectiveness. As a consequence of the extensiveness of writing assessment and the use of assessment for evaluation of teachers and school districts, some states are witnessing increased numbers of students being referred for special services to develop their written language skills. Students who, in the past, may not have received special services because their oral language appeared adequate are now being identified as having written language learning disabilities. The first author of this chapter conducted a workshop in Kentucky not long after state-wide writing assessments were mandated. Speech-language pathologists reported a marked change in the type of students being referred to them. Within a year, a majority of students being referred for speech-language services exhibited writing problems. Special educators and speech-language pathologists are assisting regular education teachers in conducting writing activities within regular education classrooms and are providing support for students who exhibit particular deficits in writing. For students with severe deficits, special educators and speech-language pathologists may work with small groups of students in pull-out programs to develop the writing skills necessary to participate in the regular classroom activities.

This chapter will provide educators, including special education teachers and speech-language pathologists, with information on current philosophies and frameworks for assessing and facilitating written language development. These frameworks consider both the written *product* and the *process* that leads to the product. Attention to the product no longer focuses on the acquisition of spelling and syntax alone, but also on the ability to produce organized, cohesive texts for varying purposes (Bartlett & Scribner, 1981; Pappas, 1985; Scott, 1989). Each purpose or genre has a particular type of text that requires specific vocabulary, syntactic structures, and text structure or organization (Westby, 1994). Attention to the process focuses on the motivational attitudes toward writing and the strategies that students employ in the writing process.

The chapter is organized into two sections: an assessment section and a facilitation/intervention section. In the assessment section we present a model for the writing process that provides a framework for assessing and facilitating the types of student knowledge and behaviors that are critical for successful writing. We then discuss the types of writing assessments and scoring procedures currently used in regular education. Finally, we present three developmental scoring systems for evaluating students' narrative, expository, and persuasive writing and suggestions for evaluating students' motivation and beliefs about the writing process.

In the facilitation section we describe the current writing teaching philosophy and questions raised about the philosophy for students with writing disabilities. We then present suggestions for facilitating writing at the microstructure or sentence level and at the macrostructure or overall organizational level. Finally, we discuss strategies designed to enable students to manage their own writing.

Assessing Student Writers

A Framework for Writing

Current ideas for assessing and facilitating written language have arisen from two sources: the philosophy of the writing process approach to writing education and cognitive information processing research. Beginning with the publication of Janet Emig's (1971) study of the composing process of twelfth graders and Donald Graves' (1975) work with 7-year-olds, the last twenty-five years have witnessed a paradigm shift from product to process in reading and writing (Irwin & Doyle, 1992). Like the whole language philosophy, the writing process approach has been widely and often uncritically adopted in schools across the nation. Cognitive research in the writing process has provided important insights into what expert and novice writers do when they write (Bereiter & Scardamalia, 1987; Flower & Hayes, 1981; Hayes & Flower, 1980; Scardamalia, 1981). Knowledge gained from these two sources has been incorporated into classrooms using the writing process approach. Teachers in regular education classrooms across the nature discuss prewriting, drafting, revising, editing, publishing, and evaluating. Aims of the writing process approach are not simply to get students to write, but also to develop positive attitudes toward writing. When evaluating students with writing problems, it is useful to consider what difficulties they exhibit at each step of the process. Some students exhibit difficulty with all the steps; others may have difficulty with some but not all of the components. Students with writing difficulties may have difficulty coming up with topics to write about (prewriting); with the act of putting words and ideas on paper (drafting); with recognizing unclear or unsupported ideas in their papers and making the necessary modifications to facilitate reader understanding (revising); with correcting grammatical, spelling, and punctuation errors (editing); or with reflecting on feedback given by others (evaluating).

Hayes (1996) presented a model for the writing process that is useful in conceptualizing what should be evaluated when assessing a student writer and what students need to develop to become effective writers (see Figure 9-1). This model frames the writing process in terms of the *task environment* and *the individual*. The task environment has both *social* and *physical* aspects. The social aspect includes the *audience* for the writing and any *collaborators* in the writing process. The physical aspect includes the *text itself* (the writing task) and the *medium for composing* (handwriting or computer). Writing assessments should provide students with a specific audience for their product (a parent or teacher, a penpal, another student). Careful thought should be given to the nature of the task—must the student write about a personal experience, an imaginative story, an explanation of how to do a task, and so on; and will the student handwrite the paper or use a computer?

The individual aspects of the model include *motivation/affect, working memory, long-term memory*, and *cognitive process* components. Students must be motivated to write—they must have positive attitudes toward the writing process, specific goals in writing, and the belief that writing is worth the effort. They must be able to draw on a variety of resources from long-term memory. They must understand the nature of the task and have the necessary topic, linguistic, and genre knowledge to produce the written product. In addition, they must be aware of their audience and how to adjust the topic, linguistic, and genre knowledge in response to the audience. The knowledge from long-term memory underlies the three aspects of the cognitive process component that represent the elements of the writing process discussed earlier. *Text production* involves drafting; *reflection* involves prewriting/planning activities; and *text interpretation* involves revision.

Effective functioning of the cognitive processes are dependent on the *working memory* component. Efficient working memory facilitates management of the multiple simultaneous processes that a student must engage in while writing (retrieving multiple types of information from memory [graphemes, syntax, ideas] while organizing the information and putting it on paper). Changes in working memory can account for some aspects of development across all writing genres and specifics of development within genres. The concept of working memory can be used to characterize developmental changes that impact particularly the structural organizational complexity of texts students write (Case, 1985; McKeogh, 1991; Scardamalia, 1981). Working memory may affect other aspects of the writing task that are not yet automatic for the student. For example, if students attend to organization and content when spelling and syntax are not automatic, spelling and syntax may suffer; or if students are attending too much to spelling and syntax, they will not have sufficient processing capacity to also attend to organization of content. As children mature, their working memory capacity increases.

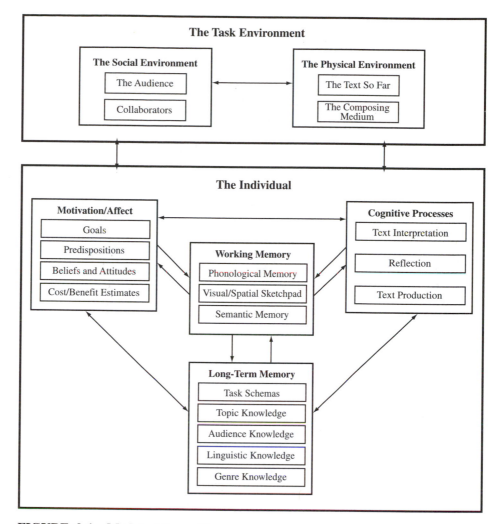

FIGURE 9-1   Model of the writing process.

Reprinted with permission from Hayes, J.R. (1996). A new framework for understanding cognition and affect in writing. In C.M. Levy & S. Ransdell (Eds.), *The science of writing* (pp. 1–27). Mahwah, NJ: Erlbaum.

Types of Writing Assessments

Educational personnel should be aware of the types of writing assessments frequently used in schools. The types of assessments can affect the ways educators or speech-language pathologists prepare students for a writing assessment or the types of assistance they can provide in the process. Special educators and speech-language pathologists are familiar with individualized standardized writing assessments such as the *Test of Early Written Language*

(Hresko, 1988) for children between 3 and 8 years of age and the *Test of Written Language-3* (Hammill & Larsen, 1996) for children between 7 and 17 years of age. These commonly used assessments employ a variety of discrete tasks that measure students' knowledge of microstructure elements of writing, such as phoneme/grapheme awareness, spelling, vocabulary, punctuation, and syntactic structures. These tests provide no information about how a student organizes an extended written text. The *Writing Process Test* (Warden & Hutchinson, 1992) provides a standardized system for evaluating the processes students use in composing a personalized expository text as well as for evaluating the microstructure and macrostructure aspects of the product. This assessment is more comprehensive but it does not provide an authentic writing task, and the tasks (writing about spending a million dollars or boring/exciting experiences) are not ones that have clear genre structures.

Two types of writing assessments are common in regular education classrooms—direct writing assessment and portfolio writing assessment. These assessments generally make use of more authentic activities that reflect tasks common to the curriculum. The purpose of these assessments is to provide teachers and parents with an understanding of how students compare with one another and against a standard for writing. In addition, they provide a mechanism for documenting students' writing development. Ideally, information gained from these types of writing assessments guide teachers as they teach writing to students of varying ability levels. For students with writing disabilities, such assessments provide the best estimate regarding students' ability to manage regular classroom assignments as well as provide special educators and speech-language pathologists with knowledge of the types of assistance they should offer to students.

Direct Assessment

In a direct assessment, students are given a prompt or task and a class period to respond. If they have been working on particular syntactic structures, punctuation, or genres, they will be reminded to incorporate what they have learned. For example, if students have been working on narrative writing in class, they will be reminded to include all the parts of the story in their writing. Papers are collected at the end of the period and scored. Direct writing activities are useful for pre- and posttesting as a means of evaluating what students have integrated from material that has been presented over time.

Direct writing allows educators to see what students are able to do without support on a specific task. For example, teachers and speech-language pathologists may use direct writing assessment before and after conducting narrative interventions. Students may be asked to write a story in response to a verbal prompt, a poster picture, a wordless picture book, or a video. Generally, the verbal prompt for a narrative is a story starter, although prompts for story middles and endings can also be used. Students with learning disabilities produce shorter, less complex stories than students without learning disabilities in all prompt conditions, but score significantly lower when offered middle prompts (Graves, Semmel, & Gerber, 1994).

When to collect the direct writing assessment should be considered carefully. Because writing performance is easily affected by motivation, one should ensure that students are not distracted by other events and that they will have adequate time to complete the writing. Consequently, the writing assessment should generally not be done before recess, an assembly, field trip, or the day before a holiday.

Portfolio Writing

With portfolio assessment, evaluation is not based on a single product produced at one point in time. Portfolio writing assessment usually involves responding to several writing tasks over time. Students are given a writing prompt or task. Then over a period of days or weeks, the teacher takes the students through the writing process. Portfolio assessment allows the educator to evaluate not only the students' written products, but also the process they use in selecting topics, brainstorming ideas, planning drafts, evaluating the product, and revising the piece (Belanoff & Dickson, 1991; Calkins, 1994; Glazer & Brown, 1993; Tierney, Carter, & Desai, 1991). Educators assist students in the process by coaching or scaffolding.

Many writing portfolio assessments provide teachers with several writing prompts for different genres early in the year. (See sample prompts in Appendix A). Teachers are to provide opportunities for students to work on the prompts over several weeks or months. Ideally, teachers should integrate the writing prompts into curricular activities, providing background experiences to motivate students to write and to provide students with content information. For example, for the narrative writing prompt, *One day in science class, you look through a microscope and see strange creatures living in a strange land. Write a story about what you see when you look into the microscope and what might happen*, teachers can provide students with the opportunity to view slides of various things under a microscope (pond water is great for viewing tiny living organisms). They can also use the *Planet Dexter Instant Creature* (1995) book. This book comes with eggs for instant creatures (triops). Triops have been referred to as "living dinosaurs." These crustaceans look like miniature horseshoe crabs. Their desiccated eggs can exist for twenty years. When placed in an aquarium with water, the eggs hatch and the triops live for between 20 to 90 days. The book provides information about triops and how to care for and observe them. Maintaining and observing triops can provide students with ideas for their stories.

In portfolio assessment, teachers are to coach students through the process, but are not to make specific corrections. As coaches, they give positive feedback on specific elements of students' writing (*I really like this paragraph because . . .*), expand writers' thoughts and ideas by having them respond to *who, what, where, when, why*, and *how* questions, and hold peer conferences or *author's chair* in which students share their writing with classmates and receive feedback and questions to encourage clarity of thought. If teachers note that students are experiencing difficulty with sentence structures, punctuation, or paragraphing, for example, they are not to tell the student what to do on their papers. They can, however, provide mini-lessons in which they teach a specific writing skill such as paragraphing, use of quotation marks, use of homophones, and so forth. They can then ask the students to think about what they have learned in the mini-lesson when they work on their writing.

Scoring Systems

These approaches to direct and portfolio assessment generally use scoring rubrics to evaluate the quality of students' work. Rubrics are sets of rules or benchmarks describing different levels of performance. They provide guidelines for what to look for in a student's production. Rubrics are being developed to evaluate all types of performances in all types of narrative, expository, and persuasive genres and in all types of domains—science, math, art, music, oral language, reading, and writing. Rubrics used to evaluate writing may be used for *holistic scoring*, in which a number of factors may be considered, but one single score is given for the writing. Rubrics are also available for *analytic* or *trait scoring* that define the components or traits of good writing and describe each of the traits in terms of relevant strengths and weaknesses. Many scoring systems use numbers from 1 to 4, 1 to 5, or 1 to 7 to rank papers. Others, such as the Kentucky rubric, use terms that have positive connotations at all levels—for example, novice, apprentice, proficient, distinguished. Some holistic scoring rubrics such as those used by Kentucky and New Mexico use the same scoring rubric for narrative, descriptive, and persuasive genres (see Appendix B for an example); while others such as the Illinois Writing Assessment, Oregon Writing Assessment, and the National Assessment of Education Progress use a different rubric for each genre. Educators need to be able to use the rubrics and interpret the scores students receive if they are to facilitate students' writing development.

Few of the scoring rubrics are based upon what is known about students' development of narrative, expository, and persuasive genres. The rubrics tend to depend on what adults perceive as increased organization and development. Descriptions for each stage in the rubrics often use vague terms such as "inconsistencies in coherence," "minor lapses in coherence," "partially developed argument," "developed argument," and so on. Educators must learn the rubric by studying multiple samples of scored texts. A major problem with the present rubrics is that they do not provide educators with specific guidelines of what to teach to facilitate a student's writing development, and they do not provide students with specific information regarding what they must do to improve their writing.

Analytic scoring seeks to define the elements of good writing. Some analytic scoring systems focus primarily at the microstructure level, evaluating aspects of word use, punctuation, and grammar (Appendix C). Others are broader, considering traits at both the microstructure level (word choice, sentence fluency, conventions, or mechanics) and the macrostructure (organizational structure) level (ideas, organization, voice). A summary of a trait scoring system developed by Spandel and Stiggins (1990) is presented in Appendix D. The majority of trait scoring systems are variations of the Spandel and Stiggins system. Holistic scoring provides a general idea of which students are having problems and about how well students are writing overall. It is somewhat quicker than trait scoring, and, consequently, when many students must be assessed, it is somewhat cheaper. Analytic or trait scoring takes longer to learn and to use. Raters can score twenty to thirty papers per hour holistically and ten to twenty per hour analytically. Analytic scoring provides a means of reflecting on the relative strengths and weaknesses in a given piece of writing and hence is more diagnostic.

When educators or speech-language pathologists use scoring rubrics, they need to be aware that these scoring systems are subject to rater bias:

- Some raters tend to score high or low consistently.
- Paper appearance can impact raters' judgments. Poor handwriting and tattered papers are more likely to be misjudged regarding their content.
- Short is not necessarily poor and long is not necessarily good. A short paper may be well structured. A long paper may ramble and not come to the point.
- If the evaluator has many papers on the same topic to score, the papers begin to look

alike. There is a tendency for readers to begin to skim papers and, as a consequence, the scores become less reliable.

- Over time, there is a tendency for readers to unintentionally redefine scoring criteria.
- Each of us may have aspects of writing that we like or do not like that may affect our ratings. Raters need to be aware of their pet peeves. Do you become irritated by wordiness; writing that is too light or too tiny; beginning sentence with *and, and then, but;* inappropriate use of *its* and *it's*; or sloppiness?

Although rubrics can be used to score any written sample, reliability of both holistic and analytic scoring is best achieved when students write on the same topic rather than on topics of their own choosing. If educators or speech-language pathologists use rubrics for scoring written language samples, they should select several stimuli that are appropriate for the ages and ability levels of students they serve and collect all samples to be scored for formal evaluations with these stimuli.

Appropriate and successful use of portfolio writing assessment requires well-trained personnel (Valencia, 1991). Unlike standardized tests, which are scripted and require evaluators to follow precisely defined procedures, portfolio writing assessment requires more knowledge and decision making on the part of evaluators. Educational personnel must be expert assessors of students' capabilities. They must know the students' present skill levels, what students require to develop to higher levels, and what strategies they can use to facilitate students' writing development. To date, the push for portfolio assessment has moved faster than the training of personnel to use it.

Adequate assessment of students' writing abilities cannot be accomplished by evaluation of a single writing sample. Students must write on a variety of topics for assignments requiring a variety of different genres. Three major genres include narrative, expository, and persuasive writing. Each of these genres has a variety of subgenres. Narrative genres include personal and historical recounts, fairy tales, myths, fables; expository genres include technical descriptions, scientific procedures, information reports, and reviews; persuasive genres include evaluations, debates, advertisements, and interpretations. Knowing how to write in one genre does not necessarily mean that a student can write in other genres.

Developmental Rubrics

Educators working with students with writing problems need to know what they can do to facilitate the development of students' writing skills. Trait scoring has the potential to provide direction for writing instruction, particularly for those students who have writing difficulties. The majority of the rubrics presently in use, however, are not based on developmental information. Consequently, they do not provide educators with specific direction in teaching; they provide educators only with information about a student's ranking in comparison to other students. An objective of Project WrITE (Writing Integrative Texts Effectively), a federally funded program carried out by the authors of this chapter, was to draft developmental trait rubrics for narrative, expository, and persuasive texts. Shortly after the project began, we found a comprehensive narrative trait rubric, the Writing What You Read (WWYR) rubric (Wolf & Gearheart, 1993a, 1993b, 1994). The WWYR was incorporated into Project WrITE, and attention was devoted to developing the expository and persuasive rubrics. Information from the literature on writing development and from student papers and journals was synthesized to produce a prototypic developmental rubric for expository and persuasive texts (Clauser & Westby, 1996).

Narrative Assessment
Numerous studies are available that document specific developmental changes in narrative organization and cohesion (see Hedberg & Westby, 1993 for detailed summary). The emphasis in narrative studies has been on the development of plot, as reflected by story grammar levels (see Chapter 7). Story grammar analysis, however, provides only a single holistic score on one trait.

Writing What You Read Rubric.   This rubric is the most thorough trait analysis system for narratives (Wolf & Gearheart, 1993a, 1993b, 1994). It uses a developmental trait analysis that considers theme, character, setting, and communication in addition to development of plot (Table 9-1). Each component has dual dimensions. Note the dimensions listed under each narrative component in Table 9-1, for example, explicit/implicit and didactic/revealing for theme. These dimensions represent continua, but one side is not necessarily more effective than the other. The appropriateness and effectiveness of each dimension must be determined in relationship to a narrative subgenre. For example, fables tend to use the left-hand side of the continua. They have didactic themes with flat, static characters; simple settings that are seldom critical to the story; and simple plots. In contrast, mysteries tend to favor the right-hand side. Characters are rounded and dynamic, settings are often critical to the unfolding of the story, and plots are complex with multiple sources of conflict among characters. Students should be exposed to the full range of narrative genres in their reading. The dimensions work in tandem with the six-level scales. Details of how to score narratives using the WWYR rubric are available in *Writing What You Read: A Guidebook for the Assessment of Children's Narratives* (Wolf & Gearhart, 1993a). The guidebook is available from the National Center for Research on Evaluation, Standards, and Student Testing (CRESST). It can be downloaded from the CRESST home page on the internet (http://cresst96.cse.ucla.edu).

Narrative Landscapes.   If students are to develop characterization and plot in their narratives, they must be aware of the thoughts, feelings, and intentions of characters. As discussed in Chapter 7, most narratives unfold simultaneously on two levels, the *landscape of action,* which represents the events within story time, and the *landscape of consciousness* or of human perception of those events (what those involved in the action know, think, or feel, or do not know, think, or feel) (Bruner, 1986). Maximally coherent narratives create a landscape of consciousness, developing plot as events unfold against a backdrop of alternative possible worlds created through diverse character perspectives. Landscapes of consciousness can be created in a variety of ways. Adjectives referring to emotions (e.g., *sad, angry, jealous, relieved, disappointed*) and metacognitive verbs (e.g., *think, guess, plan, remember*) create a landscape of consciousness. Counting the emotion and metacognitive words in a written narrative can provide a relatively quick measure of the landscape of consciousness. If one wants to develop students' level of plot or characterization, one must develop students' understanding of emotions and metacognition. Children under age 9 may

TABLE 9-1 Narrative Rubric

Theme	Character	Setting	Plot	Communication
explicit/didactic ↔ implicit/revealing	flat/static ↔ round/dynamic	backdrop/simple ↔ essential/multi-functional	simple/static ↔ complex/conflict	context-bound/literal ↔ reader considerate/symbolic
Not present or not developed through other narrative elements	One or two flat, static characters with little relationship between characters; either objective (action speaks for itself) or first person (author as "I") point of view	Backdrop setting with little or no indication of time and place ("There was a little girl. She liked candy.")	One or two events with little or no conflict ("Once there was a cat. the cat liked milk.")	Writing bound to context (You have to be there) and often dependent on drawing and talk to clarify the meaning; minimal style and tone
Meaning centered in a series of list-like statements ("I like my mom. And I like my dad. And I like my . . .") or in the coherence of the action itself ("He blew up the plane. Pow!")	Some rounding, usually in physical description; relationship between characters is action-driven; objective point of view is common	Skeletal indication of time and place often held in past time ("once there was . . ."); little relationship to other narrative elements	Beginning sequence of events, but occasional out-of-sync occurrences; events without problem or problem without resolution	Beginning awareness of reader considerations; straightforward style and tone focused on getting the information out; first attempts at dialogue begin
Beginning statement of theme—often explicit and didactic ("The mean witch chased the children and she shouldn't have done that.")	Continued rounding in physical description, particularly stereotypical features ("wart on the end of her nose"); beginning rounding in feeling, often through straightforward vocabulary ("She was sad, glad, mad.")	Beginning relationship between setting and other narrative elements (futuristic setting to accommodate aliens and spaceships); beginning symbolic functions of setting (often stereotypical images—forest as scary place)	Single, linear episode with clear beginning, middle, and end. ("Once upon a time there were two friends named Frog and Toad. One sunny day when they were tree climbing, Frog got stuck. He was scared. So Toad helped him down. Toad was a good friend.")	Writer begin to make use of explanations and transitions ("because" and "so"); literal style centers on description ("sunny day"); tone explicit
Beginning revelation of theme on both explicit and implicit levels through the more subtle things characters say and do ("He put his arm around the dog and held him close.")	Beginning insights into the motivation and intention that drives the feeling and the action of main characters often through limited omniscient point of view; beginning dynamic features of change and growth	Setting becomes more essential to the development of the story in explicit ways: characters may remark on the setting or the time and place may be integral to the plot	Plot increases in complexity with more than one episode; episodes contain four critical elements of problem, emotional response, action, outcome; beginning relationship between episodes	Increased information and explanation for the reader (linking ideas as well as episodes); words more carefully selected to suit the narrative's purpose (particularly through increased use of detail in imagery)
Beginning tied to overarching theme, but not often tied to overarching theme; main theme increasingly revealed through discovery rather than delivery ("You can't do that to my sister!" Lou cried, moving to shield Tasha with her body.)	Further rounding (in feeling and motivation); dynamic features appear in the central characters and in the relationships between characters; move to omniscient point of view (getting into the minds of characters)	Setting may serve more than one function and the relationship between functions is more implicit and symbolic—for example, setting may be linked symbolically to character mood ("She hid in the grass, clutching the sharp, dry spikes, waiting.")	Stronger relationship between episodes (with the resolution in one leading to a problem in the next); beginning manipulation of the sequence through foreshadowing, and subplots	Some experimentation with symbolism (particularly figurative language), which shows reader considerations on both explicit and implicit levels; style shows increasing variety (alliteration, word play, rhythm . . . etc.) and tone is more implicit
Overarching theme multi-layered and complex; secondary themes integrally related to primary theme or themes	Round, dynamic major characters through rich description of affect, intention, and motivation; growth occurs as a result of complex interactions between characters; most characters contribute to the development of the narrative; purposeful choice of point of view	Setting fully integrated with the characters, action, and theme of the story; role of setting is multi-functional—setting mood, revealing character and conflict, serving as metaphor	Overarching problem and resolution supported by multiple episodes; rich variety of techniques (building suspense, foreshadowing, flashbacks, denouement) to manipulate sequence	Careful crafting of choices in story structure as well as vocabulary demonstrate considerable orchestration of all the available resources; judicious experimentation with variety of stylistic forms that are symbolic in nature and illuminate the other narrative elements

Reprinted with permission from:

Wolf, S., & Gearhart, M. (1994). Writing what you read: Narrative assessment as a learning event. *Language Arts, 71,* 425–444.

make some use of landscape of consciousness, but this aspect of narratives tends to develop after age 9, once students have mastered a basic plot structure involving a goal.

Certain types of predicate constructions and transformations of those constructions also create a landscape of consciousness (Todorov, 1977). Table 9-2 displays examples of the two types of predicate transformations that convey a landscape of consciousness: simple transformations and complex transformations. Simple transformations have auxiliary verbs that modify the action of the main verb, rendering the action or event as psychologically in progress rather than as a completed act. Rather than simply presenting information, these transformations add an element of subjectivity. For example, a pure informational statement about the video *Snail Needs a Shell*, in which Max the Mouse accidentally runs

TABLE 9-2   Measuring Landscape of Consciousness

Simple Transformations

Mode: Modal verbs express the possibility, necessity, impossibility, or prohibition of an action.	X must commit a crime.
Intention: Character plans and motivations frame the action of a verb.	X plans to commit a crime.
Result: The action is presented as accomplished, presupposing intent and crime-raising interest in the process of accomplishment.	X succeeds in committing a crime.
Manner: Specification of the manner of realization of the verb. Linguistically performed by auxiliary verbs (*eager, dare, strive*), adverbs of manner, and comparatives and superlatives.	X is eager to commit a crime.
Aspect: Could be subsumed under manner, but used the aspects of verbs to evoke status of action in time; adverbs of manner also achieve this marking of temporal status.	X is beginning to commit a crime.
Status: Replacing the positive form of a predicate by the negative form manipulates the status of the action, suggesting other possibilities.	X does not commit a crime.

Complex Transformations

Appearance: The initial predicate is not realized, but the derived action in the second predicate allows action to proceed as if the initial predicate was realized; the verbs *feign, pretend, claim, appears* function in this way.	X or Y pretends that X is committing a crime.
Knowledge: Verbs that denote change in the consciousness of an action, signaled by verbs such as *observe, learn, guess, know, ignore.*	X or Y learns that X has committed a crime.
Description: The verbs of speech, including the illocutionary verbs as described by Astington (1990) function to present knowledge indirectly.	X or Y reports that X has committed a crime.
Supposition: The action is predicted in the future.	X or Y foresees that X will commit a crime.
Subjectification: The action of the initial predicate is attributed to the mental attitude of a character: the presupposition of the initial predicate may be true or false.	Y thinks that X has committed a crime.
Attitude: Similar to transformations of manner that modify the predicate, transformations of attitude modify the state of the subject of the action. X enjoys committing a crime; or Y is disgusted that X committed a crime.	X enjoys committing a crime; or Y is disgusted that X committed a crime.

his bicycle over a snail's shell and breaks it, would be, "Max got a new shell for the snail." Simple predicate transformations could include:

Max **must** get a new shell for the snail.

Max **wants** to get the snail a new shell.

Max **is trying** to find the snail a new shell.

Max **cannot** find the snail a new shell.

Each of these sentences conveys information from Max's point of view, and hence reflects a landscape of consciousness.

Complex transformations are two clause structures in which a sentence is altered by adding a verb or verb phase that modifies the original verb. The complex verb phrases add an element of mental activity (or landscape of consciousness) to the main verb, for example,

Max **imagines** he is putting on a show for the snail.

Max **realizes** that he has shattered the snail's shell.

The snail **thinks** that Max is leaving him.

The snail **enjoys** crawling along the road with Max.

Max is **disgusted** that the snail will not stop crying.

Simon-Ailes (1995) explored the development of the landscape of consciousness through use of Todorov's predicate constructions in written narratives of fourth, sixth, and eighth grade students. Children saw the silent video *The Red Balloon* and wrote the story. Use of these constructions increased across this age range, with use of complex predicate constructions particularly increasing between sixth and eighth grades. See Appendix E for samples of the coded written *Red Balloon* transcripts.

Expository Rubric

Compared to narratives, less is known about the development of expository texts. The National Assessment of Educational Progress (NAEP) uses holistic scorings of narrative, informative, and persuasive texts that are developmental. The focus of the NAEP scoring is on the content and organization of the texts. There is a need for developmentally based trait scoring rubrics for a variety of genres. The expository rubric we developed includes developmental considerations of five facets or traits: organization, content, written language style (syntax, cohesion, vocabulary), written conventions, and sense of audience (Table 9-3). In the next sections, development in each of the traits will be described. When first using the rubric, we suggest scoring one trait at a time. Read through a student's paper, then read through the levels of one of the traits and determine which level best describes the writing.

Organization.   Organization of expository texts requires coordination of ideas with the topic and a simultaneous sequencing of ideas. Expository texts should have opening statements that make clear the topic or purpose of the text. Several paragraphs should provide information to support and elaborate the introductory concept. A conclusion should tie the

TABLE 9-3 Developmental Rubric—Expository Writing

Organization (Text Structure)	Content/Theme (Coherence)	Written Language (Development of syntax, cohesion strategies, vocabulary)	Written Conventions* (Mechanics)	Sense of Audience
May be extremely brief or confused	Tendency to write either partially or completely in the narrative mode; associated ideas; much content extraneous to the topic or indirectly related to topic	Use of simple sentences (N+V+O); sentences juxtaposed; if connectors between sentences are used, they are primarily "and," and "then," may use pronominal reference with numerous ambiguous pronouns (referent not retrievable from text); use of simple vocabulary	Beginning differentiation of drawing and printing; use of recursive letter-like shapes when printing; some phoneme-grapheme awareness for initial sounds; text not readable by others	No sense of audience; writes for self from own perspective; often references based on personal experiences that are not retrievable from text
May attempt to structure, attempting to center or chaining ideas, but it may be difficult to determine the structure; Many ideas included in one paragraph or each idea written as a paragraph, or the response may be so brief that its organization cannot be evaluated	May have misleading introductions and/or conclusions; first-hand experiences; some content extraneous to the topic; ideas are quite disjointed	Compound subjects; compound predicates; within text pronominal reference; coordinating conjunctions — primarily "and," "then," "but," "because" (used for motivational, not logical reasons); use of adequate vocabulary	Printing/writing recognizable letters; use of invented spelling with most sounds represented; no spacing between words or inconsistent spacing; incomplete sentences; a variety of grammatical errors; errors likely to affect readers' comprehension	Writes with knowledge that others will read text; does not adjust writing for specific audiences
Structure is somewhat unclear; centers or chains, but has difficulty doing both; lack of clear opening; some of the support and elaborations are paragraphed correctly; most ideas relate to main topic or issue with no specific connections; may include major rambling from the main topic	Topic knowledge developing; some content extraneous to the topic may be present; may have misleading introductions and conclusions; moderately disjointed misleading statements	Adverbial subordinate clauses, particularly with conjunctions "when," "while," "because" (now used for logical justification); relative clauses, primarily those that post-modify object nouns; use of appropriate vocabulary	May continue to have some difficulty with handwriting; invented spelling continues; use of capitals on words at beginning of sentences and persons' names, periods, question marks, exclamation points, apostrophes; pronominal reference may be unclear, errors may affect readers' comprehension	Usually writes for teacher; depends on teacher to set organization format

Structure of paper	Development	Sentence structure / Vocabulary	Conventions	Format
Structure of the paper is clear; coordination of centering and chaining; some clusters of ideas are paragraphed appropriately; planned opening and closing to paper when appropriate; use of specific expository structures (e.g., definitions, comparison/contrast, cause/effect, sequences, problem/solution); ideas relate to the topic without specific connections; may include off topic material	Development may be uneven with some clusters of ideas elaborated, others not; lack depth of content	Use of low-frequency adverbials — "though," "although," "even if," manner "as," conditional "unless," "provided that"; nominal clauses as subjects; use of some precise vocabulary	Handwriting automatized; spelling mostly conventional; developing use of a greater variety of punctuation (comma, colon, semicolon, quotation marks); few run-on sentences; subject/verb agreement and tenses consistent; paragraphing developing	Given an assignment, student begins to select independently the organizational format appropriate to task and audience, may not select the most appropriate format or may not be able to maintain the chosen format
Structure of paper is clear; most of the major clusters of ideas are paragraphed effectively; planned opening and closing to paper if appropriate; coherence may be demonstrated by overall structure (topic sentences in paragraphs); cohesion developed by various methods (pronouns, parallel structure, some repetition); may include minor off-topic material	Main ideas developed with appropriate and varied details; some risks may be taken that are mostly successful; may have minor flaws; progresses logically	Use of concordant conjuncts "similarly," "moreover," "consequently," "therefore," "furthermore," "for example"; and discordant conjuncts "instead," "yet," "however," "nevertheless," "conversely"; Use of vocabulary precise and carefully chosen	Spelling mostly automatized and conventional (student self-edits); more consistent use of correct punctuation; appropriate text formatting for different genres; consistently clear pronominal reference	Given an assignment, student begins to select independently the organizational format appropriate to task and audience, selects from several possible structures the one most appropriate for purpose and audience
Structure of paper is clear; all of the major points; opening and closing when appropriate; effectively paragraphed; transitional devices used to develop coherence and cohesion; all ideas are presented logically and are interrelated; no off-topic material; use of a wide variety of organizational structures	Main ideas developed with appropriate and varied details; writer may take compositional risks resulting in effective, vivid response	Use of structures to achieve literary style, e.g., subject-verb split, absolute phrases; Use of vocabulary precise and carefully chosen	Errors in spelling, punctuation, grammar, usage are rare	Response has a coherent sense of purpose and audience; careful consideration of organizational structure from a wide variety of organizational structures that best highlight information for a particular audience

*Separate lists of major and minor errors

ideas together and relate back to the introduction. Initially, students' attempts at expository texts may be so brief that no clear organization can be identified. As students write more, their texts involve either centering (several statements related to a topic) or chaining (several statements related to each other), but not both (Chapman, 1994). Development of the simultaneous coordination of centering and chaining in expository texts occurs in later elementary school and middle school (Scardamalia, 1981). This developing organization is highly dependent on developments in working memory. As discussed earlier, working memory permits simultaneous coordination of information. Initially, children cannot coordinate multiple pieces of information. Consequently, they produce lists of words or organized ideas when asked to produce an expository text. Later students can either produce a logical chain, or they can produce a series of ideas that relate to the topic. They have difficulty, however, in simultaneously producing an inductive/deductive chain of ideas and linking this chain to the overall topic/theme. Consequently, they may seem to become sidetracked, including associative or off-topic information. Later still, students can integrate a logical inductive/deductive series of statements with an overall topic/theme. Eventually, they can manage complex expository texts that require not only the linking of logical inductions/deductions to a theme, but also an evaluation of the statements. As they develop the ability to center and chain ideas in expository text, they also develop the ability to use linguistic connectives to make explicit the relationships among the ideas and the relationship of the ideas to the overall topic.

All expository texts have this basic organizational structure involving a topic with elaborating statements and a conclusion. There are, however, a variety of expository text subgenres (descriptive, enumerative, sequential, cause and effect, comparison and contrast, and problem and solution), each of which has additional aspects of organizational structure (Englert & Hiebert, 1984; Horowitz, 1985a, 1985b). Students must learn to write all these expository patterns or genres. Various semantic and syntactic techniques have been identified that signal which particular expository structure is being used (Piccolo, 1987). Each type of expository text answers different questions and has different cue words (Englert, 1990; Westby, 1989) (e.g., see Table 7-10 in Chapter 7). Graphic organizers support students in visualizing the text structures and in producing their own texts (Tompkins, 1994). Knowledge of text structure acts as a frame for generating, organizing, and editing.

Content.   If students are to produce an organized text, they must have content to organize. How much students know about a topic influences how well they write. The content trait is heavily influenced by students' interests and personal and educational experiences. Writers with high knowledge of a topic have a great deal more information in memory on which to draw, and they can retrieve it more easily (Benton, Corkill, Sharp, Downey, & Khramtsova, 1995; Kellogg, 1987). This allows writers to plan their writing almost automatically because they have more working memory space to use for setting goals and organizing their ideas. Students with high knowledge can exert less effort toward accessing ideas. This frees them to spend more cognitive processing on organizing their ideas around a theme.

The nature of students' writing gives insight into their levels of content knowledge. Rambling and associated ideas reflect little topic knowledge. Reported first-hand experiences reflect some knowledge. Definition of a major aspect of a topic requires more knowledge. At early levels, however, students may include extraneous and misleading information, and even relevant information may be presented in a disjointed manner. Gradually, students become able to elaborate on topics and provide descriptive details. Finally, writers can give a definition with a precise meaning, produce in-depth discussion, and use topical analogies in their text.

Written Language Style (Syntax and Cohesion Strategies). This trait is used to judge the developmental complexity of students' syntax and cohesion strategies. (Chapter 7 presented information on strategies for measuring some aspects of syntactic complexity.) Early studies in the development of written language at grades 4, 8, and 12 (Hunt, 1964) and of language development from kindergarten through grade 12 (Loban, 1976) have provided educators with an extensive information base on children's written syntactic language development. The development of syntax in the age range from 9 to 19 is a gradual acquisition of infrequently used structures (Scott, 1988b). These older students also acquire an ability to make unique combinations of structures. To write expository text using rhetorical devices and advanced sentence constructions, most students must study these forms in information texts and participate in mentored discussion with teachers and peers who successfully use these constructions. They need practice in using the forms to internalize their use. Students do not naturally learn these forms as they read; additional discussion integrated with practice writing is required to become a proficient author of expository and persuasive texts. Feedback from knowledgeable readers is invaluable for the student working to become an advanced writer.

There is considerable variability in student syntactic abilities at the higher levels and because the various syntactic structures and connecting words are used with lower frequency, the teacher must know the student's writing well. The following represents a developmental hierarchy for syntactic structures.

1. Simple sentences (noun + verb + object); sentences juxtaposed; if connectors between sentences are used, they are primarily *and, then*; may use pronominal reference exophorically (i.e., the referent is in the context, not the text); may use numerous ambiguous pronouns

2. Compound subjects; compound predicates; endophoric pronominal reference (referent retrievable from text)—coordinating conjunctions, primarily *and, then, but*; subordinating conjunction *because* (used for motivational reason—*he can't have it, because it's mine*)

3. Adverbial subordinate clauses, particularly with the conjunctions *because, when, while, because* (now used for logical justification), relative clauses, primarily those that postmodify object nouns (*He asked his friend who lives in Ohio*). Quotation (*He said, "Draw a picture of your favorite character"* or *He told us to draw a picture of our favorite character*).

4. Use of low-frequency adverbials (adverbials of concession—*though, although, even if*; manner—*as*; conditional—*unless, provided that*); nominal clauses as subjects (e.g., *Birds that fly south in winter cannot stand cold weather.*)

5. Use of concordant conjuncts (*similarly, moreover, consequently, therefore, furthermore, for example*); and discordant conjuncts (*instead, yet, however, contrastively, nevertheless, conversely*);* use of structures to achieve literary style, for example, absolute phrases, participle phrases, and subject-verb splits

---

*Note: Conjunctions link propositions within a sentence; conjuncts link ideas across sentences (Quirk, Greenbaum, Leech, & Svartvik, 1985).

These literary devices are defined as follows:

a. absolute phrases (a modifier that grammatically resembles a complete sentence; it has a subject and partial verb. Because the verb is only partial and not complete, absolutes are considered phrases and not clauses. Missing in every absolute phrase is an auxiliary verb—almost always a form of the verb to be [*is, are, was, were*]. Another distinguishing characteristic of the great majority of absolute phrases is the kind of word they usually begin with—often a pronoun such as *her, his, their, your, its, our*). Examples: *His head aching, his throat sore, he forgot to light the cigarettes* (from Sinclair Lewis, *Cass Timberlane*); *Six boys came over the hill half an hour early that afternoon, running hard, their heads down, their forearms working, their breath whistling* (from John Steinbeck, *Of Mice and Men*) (Killgallon, 1987).

b. participle phrase as a modifier of a noun or pronoun. The first word in the participle phrase is almost always the participle itself. There are two types of participles—present participles that always end in *ing,* and past participles that almost always end in either *-ed* or *-en.* Example: *Standing there in the middle of the street, Marty suddenly thought of Halloween, of the winter and snowballs, of the schoolyard* (from Murry Heyert, *The New Kid*) (Killgallon, 1987).

c. subject-verb split: any nonrestrictive modifying structure of structures filling the intermediate position. Example: *The twins smeary in the face, eating steadily from untidy paper sacks of sweets, followed them in a detached way* (from Katherine Anne Porter, *Ship of Fools*) (Killgallon, 1987).

Written Conventions (Mechanics).   Mechanics is a catch-all term referring to handwriting and correctness of spelling, punctuation, and grammar. In the developmental rubrics we are emphasizing the quality of ideas expressed on paper; however, it is important that responses can be read easily. Writers should know the written conventions and punctuate as carefully as possible at the writers' level of maturity. This category provides a holistic score for handwriting, spelling, and grammar combined. This may present a problem for some students with writing problems because a student may have excellent handwriting but poor spelling, excellent spelling and grammar but poor handwriting, or any combination of the three skills.

Many students with writing problems exhibit significant deficits in syntactic and metaphonological skills that impact their ability to produce meaningful written tasks. By third to fourth grade, children's spelling should be phonetically accurate and errors should have some pattern to them. Students with writing difficulties frequently exhibit difficulty learning English sound/symbol relationships. The stages of development of spelling skills have been well documented (Clay, 1973; Gentry & Gillet, 1993; Temple, Nathan, Temple, & Burris, 1993). For young children or children with severe spelling problems it is useful to know their spelling stage to plan appropriate interventions (Bolton & Snowball, 1993; Gentry & Gillet, 1993; Moats, 1995). Four stages in the development of spelling have been described:

1. Random letters: The child knows that writing involves the use of letters, rather than drawings, or unnamed marks, but the child shows no awareness of sound/symbol relationships.

Example: M M T S T F (I like my new school).

2. Semiphonemic: Children attempt to represent phonemes in words with letters, but write down only one or two sounds in a word. They may finish words with a random string of letters.

Example: NOID DUSW (No, I didn't. Did you see one).

3. Phonetic (letter-name spelling): Children break a word into its phonemes and represent the phonemes with letters of the alphabet.

Example: MY DaD wun some Mune He wun 1000 dalrs. I was stan at my sestr to hap her weh the baby. (My dad won some money. He won $1,000 dollars. I was staying at my sister to help her with the baby).

At this stage, children may be more sensitive to some sounds than adults, for example, writing CHRE for tree or JRIVE for drive. When one says tree and drive, the pronunciation does have an affricate component, hence resulting in the spelling of CH and J.

4. Transitional: Spellings look like English words, although they are not spelled correctly. Features of standard spelling are employed, but incorrectly.

Example: egghorn   = acorn
younighted = united
redey   = ready
mite   = might
monstur   = monster

Preadolescents are frequently known to produce written texts that are well structured syntactically but incorrectly punctuated (Scott, 1988a). In general, use of periods, question marks, and explanation marks emerges in early elementary school. Use of quotation marks develops in mid to late elementary school. Appropriate use of commas has a long developmental course, and even college students exhibit confusion over their appropriate use.

Sense of Audience. In its present form, the levels of this trait for expository texts are less explicit than the others and may not be scorable from viewing the text alone. Good writers develop the sense of audience and keep their potential readers in mind as they write. Audience is an important consideration for expository writing, even though the writer may not know exactly who will read his or her writing. Initially students write only for themselves. Gradually they develop the awareness that their writing will be read by others, and they begin to write for a specific audience. Initially, they rely heavily on guidance from teachers in determining how to structure the text for a particular audience. Eventually they can independently select the organization, vocabulary, and syntactic structures that will make the text clear to the audience.

Persuasive Rubric

We drafted the prototype of the developmental rubric for persuasive writing in the same manner as the expository rubric—information was synthesized from student papers, journal articles, and writing texts (see Table 9-4). The traits included in this rubric are organization,

TABLE 9-4 Developmental Rubric—Persuasive Writing

Organization (Text Structure)	Argument	Content/theme (Coherence)	Written language (Development of Syntax, Cohesion Strategies, Vocabulary)	Written conventions* (Mechanics)	Sense of audience
May be extremely brief or confused.	No claim is made or claim is made but no reasons are given to support the claim or reasons given are not relevant to the claim.	Tendency to write either partially or completely in the narrative mode; some content extraneous to the claim present.	Use of simple sentences (N+V+O); sentences juxtaposed; if connectors between sentences are used, they are primarily "and," and "then"; may use pronominal reference with numerous ambiguous pronouns (reference not retrievable from the text); use of simple vocabulary.	Displays severe mechanical errors and/or may be so brief that knowledge of mechanics can not be determined (errors may interfere with readers' comprehension).	No sense of audience; writes for self from own perspective; often references personal experiences that are not retrievable from text.
May attempt to structure, but structure is difficult to determine; many ideas included in one paragraph or each idea written as a paragraph, or the response may be so brief that its organization cannot be evaluated.	Claim is made and reasons are given to support it, but the self-centered reasons are not developed or are rambling or disjointed.	May have misleading introductions and/or conclusions; some content extraneous to the claim present.	Compound subjects, compound predicates; within text pronominal reference; coordinating conjunctions primarily "and," "then," "but"; "because" used for motivational reasons; use of adequate vocabulary.	Displays numerous severe errors in mechanics (errors may interfere to a degree with readers' comprehension).	Writes with knowledge that others will read text; does not adjust writing for specific audiences.
Structure is somewhat unclear, some of the support and explanations are paragraphed correctly, most ideas related to claim or issue with no specific connections, may include major rambling from the main topic.	Claim is made and supported by self-centered reasons to support the claim; some further explanations made but not elaborated; may mention briefly an opposite point of view.	May have misleading introductions and/or conclusions; some content extraneous to the claim may be present.	Adverbial subordinate clauses, particularly with the conjunctions "when," "while," "because" (now used for logical justification); relative clauses, primarily those that post modify object nouns; use of age-appropriate vocabulary.	Displays a pattern of errors in mechanics (errors may interfere with readability).	Increasing ability to assume another's perspective; begins to adjust writing for the audience and to identify problems in own writing that may be difficult for others to understand.

Structure	Claim/Support	Development	Language/Style	Mechanics	Perspective
Structure of the paper is clear; some clusters or argument are paragraphed appropriately; planned opening and closing to paper; ideas related to the topic without specific connections; may include minor off-topic material.	Claim is made and supported by a nonself-centered reason; at lease one explanation included with formal development; may have a brief summary of the opposite point of view.	Development may be uneven with some clusters of ideas elaborate, others not.	Use of low-frequency adverbials: "though," "although," "even if," manner "as"; conditional "unless," "provided that"; nominal clauses as subjects; use of some precise vocabulary.	May display errors in mechanics, but there is no consistent pattern.	Can take a third person perspective; recognizes what might be difficult for a reader to understand; makes appropriate changes.
Structure of the paper is clear; most of the major clusters of ideas are paragraphed effectively; planning opening and closing to paper; coherence may be demonstrated by overall structure (topic sentences in paragraphs); cohesion developed by various methods (pronoun, parallel structure, some repetition); may include minor off-topic material.	Claim is made that is supported by general reasons with explanations; includes an attempt to discuss or disprove the opposite point of view.	Main ideas developed with appropriate and varied details; some risks may be taken that are mostly successful; may have minor flaws; progresses logically.	Use of concordant conjuncts "similarly," "moreover," "consequently," "therefore," "furthermore," "for example," and discordant conjuncts "instead," "yet," "however," "nevertheless," "conversely"; use of vocabulary precise and carefully chosen.	Few errors in mechanics.	Considers potential readers' perspective as text is written; presents persuasive information with beliefs and values of readers in mind.
Structure of the paper is clear; all of the major points, opening and closing, are appropriately paragraphed; transitional devices used to develop coherence and cohesion, all ideas are presented logically and are interrelated; no off-topic material.	Claim is made that is supported by general reasons with explanations, including a thorough discussion and/or refutation of the opposite point of view; summarizes this view and discusses why it is narrow or incorrect.	Main ideas developed with appropriate and varied details; writer may take compositional risks resulting in an effective, vivid response.	Use of structures to achieve literary style, e.g., subject-verb splint, absolute phrases; careful crafting in choice of vocabulary.	Minor, if any, errors in mechanics.	Able to consider the opposite point of view, presents it, and discusses the reason it is incorrect.

*Separate list of major and minor errors

argument, content, written language style (development of syntax, cohesion, and vocabulary), written conventions, and sense of audience. The traits of written language style and written conventions are the same as those for expository texts.

The argumentative or persuasive genre is frequently considered the most complex or cognitively demanding genre. Persuasive texts develop children's negotiation strategies that they employ to make a point, assert a right, or negotiate for possessions. Andrews (1995) proposed ten stages in the cognitive development of argumentation beginning with nonverbal strategies.

1. Child uses nonverbal means (e.g., physical struggles) to make a point, defend a position, assert a right, or negotiate territory or possessions.
2. Child uses vocalizations, but not words, to convey argument.
3. Child states an opinion but offers no support.
4. Student asserts an opinion and gives a single reason to support the opinion.
5. Student asserts an opinion and supports it with a number of reasons or proofs.
6. Student takes on opposing arguments and incorporates them into his or her own positions. This might be done simply by saying *I don't think what you say can be true* or *Some people say.* . . .
7. Student is able to sustain an argumentative position at length in speech and writing. Listens/reads others' arguments and reinforces one's own position accordingly, sustaining position by a number of different strategies (e.g., different kinds of proof, use of refutation, logical consistency, etc.).
8. Student is able to consider both sides of an argument, weighing pros and cons of each side and judging quality of reasons provided to support those cases.
9. Student is not only able to weigh two or more sides to an argument, but is also able to make a judgment and determine his or her own position in the light of such deliberation.
10. Student realizes that no argument can be final. Once a position has been established, it can act as basis for further argument and integration of information. Student understands not only the nature of a single argument, but also the whole process of argumentation and its relationship to the advancement of thought and knowledge.

The demands of producing an extended text and taking the perspective of the opposition place a heavy load on working memory. Educators have thought that persuasive writing could only be taught and mastered by older students because of the heavy working memory load required by these written monologues (Applebee, Langer, & Mullis, 1986). Younger students, who have mastered the ability to argue orally, have been able to rely on the other participant in the argument to help structure their discourse and turn taking. The other participant in the discourse also produced the counterargument. The most important processes to understand in studying persuasive writing, or production of argumentative text, are the supporting processes, which involve stating one or more reasons to back a claim or assertion, and the negotiation process, which involves getting the addressee to accept those reasons.

Persuasive writing is not easy for the following reasons (Burkhalter, 1995):

- Students tend to use their knowledge of oral persuasion as a strategy until they develop the schema for the written persuasive genre (Bereiter & Scardamalia, 1982; Crowhurst, 1980, 1986; White, 1989). To write a sound persuasive test, students must learn the organized and abstracted form of persuasive writing (Moffett, 1968). To do this they must reorganize their thoughts substantially (Burkhalter, 1992).

- Students must take a position and defend it by writing sound and convincing reasons (Toulmin, Rieke, & Janik, 1984).
- Students must think about the objections their readers may have to the reasons that they have written.

Effective written arguments have three parts: a claim (an assertion), data, and a warrant (principle by which one gets from data to claim). The most difficult aspects of persuasive writing for the students are warrants, which require an abstract conceptualization of relationship. Table 9-5 shows warrants and data for the claim, *The rainforests should not be cut down to make room for ranches and farms.*

Organization.   Written persuasion requires an organizational structure very different from its oral counterpart. The persuasive essay has a highly organized and abstract organizational form. Organizing the essay compels the student to use synthesis and hierarchical thinking (Freedman & Pringle, 1984). In persuasive writing, students plan different ways to introduce an argument, present their reasons of support, draw conclusions, and influence the reader to take the writer's viewpoint. Normally, in the beginning writers state their position, opinion, or argument plainly. In the middle, writers develop their opinion by selecting three or more reasons to support their position and developing them with data and warrants. In the end, writers influence their readers by using planned devices such as giving a personal state-

TABLE 9-5   Components of an Argument

Claim	Warrant	Data
The rainforests should not be cut down to make room for ranches and farms.	1. Loss of the rainforest will alter weather patterns around the world.	1a. Worldwide rainfall will decrease, creating more deserts.
		1b. It will contribute to global warming, causing icecaps to melt.
	2. Cutting the rainforest will result in loss of valuable resources.	2a. Rare plants that can be used to develop medicines against cancer and AIDS will be lost.
		2b. Unique animals will be destroyed.
	3. There is no need for additional ranch and farmland.	3a. Present farmland could provide better yields if crops are rotated.
		3b. People are eating less beef and more chicken; chickens don't require the large amounts of land required by cattle.

ment, making a prediction, or summarizing the major ideas (Tompkins, 1994). As with expository texts, students must produce clear opening statements that express the topic or issue. They must chain a logical sequence of statements that are linked or centered on the topic. Effective use of chaining and centering requires appropriate use of a variety of connectives.

Argument.   This trait considers the strategies students use in presenting an argument. Students demonstrate an increasing sophistication by grade in knowledge of what works in making a written argument (Knudson, 1994). High school students use different strategies and a wider variety of strategies than elementary school students. Elementary school students make greater use of simple statements and requests than older students and seldom use more than one type of statement or reason. Older students use compromising strategies significantly more than younger students and use a variety of statements or reasons in their arguments. Inclusion of the opposing position in an argumentative text tends to occur at only the most mature levels.

The developmental sequence in the argument trait is based on the work of Andrews (1995) and Golder and Coirier (1994). In their model Golder and Coirier proposed six categories or degrees on a continuum from texts with no claim to texts in which a claim was made and supported with elaborate argumentation.

A. Preargumentative Text

Degree 0 No claim is made. (*Penguins live in Antarctica.*)

Degree 1 A claim is made. (*Pollution is causing global warming. Ice is melting in Antarctica and Greenland. Ocean water is getting warmer.*)

B. Minimally Argumentative Text (the argumentation supports structure)

Degree 2 (Degree 1 + self-centered support): A claim is made and supported by a self-centered argument. (*Music lessons should be given for free in school. Then I could learn to play the guitar and earn money on the weekends playing in a band.*)

Degree 3 A claim is made and supported by a non-self-centered argument. (*Music should be taught in preschool. Learning rhythm and rhyme helps children do better in reading and math.*)

C. Elaborate Argumentative Text

Degree 4 A claim is made and supported by a general argument plus one or more marks of restriction. (*Students should be allowed to choose their own subjects in school. They would be more motivated to work hard in a class if it was something they were interested in. But they might take only easy subjects.*)

Degree 5 A claim is made and supported by a general argument plus a mark of speaker endorsement. (*Many people think that freedom of speech means we should be allowed to say anything we want. I think that there are some things that we should not be allowed to say. We shouldn't be allowed to shout "fire" just because we want to see what will happen because people could get hurt.*)

Golder and Coirier's (1994) data demonstrated that by ages 11 to 12 students could, in writing, express their opinions, support them, and to some degree participate in negotiation with the reader. This establishes their linguistic argumentation behavior but in the following years important changes occur. The ability to use counterarguments increases from 40 percent use at 11 to 12 years to 80 percent use at 15 to 16 years of age. Caution must be used in interpreting this data, however, because there are substantial and numerous within-age differences. Counterarguments are a complex operation from a psycholinguistic standpoint that involve late mastery of connectives and concessive forms (McClure & Geva, 1983). Students must master terms such as *however, nevertheless, inasmuch, conversely.* Elaborate argumentation structure is not acquired by students until the age of 15 or 16 (Coirier & Golder, 1993).

Content. Several of the ideas presented for content in exposition are also valid for persuasion. Students have less knowledge of written persuasive discourse schema than of the corresponding narrative and expository discourse schemas. Two reasons are considered for the students' lack of knowledge: one is that the persuasive schema is further removed from the oral schema, and the second is that students have read fewer, if any, examples of written persuasion. At the earlier grade levels, they are not usually exposed to instruction in this genre because educators have thought that it was too difficult for them. Therefore, students have greater cognitive difficulty with the more demanding problems of persuasion and less experience with persuasion than they have with the easier tasks in narrative and expository writing. The higher level of difficulty and lack of early instructional support appear to be some of the reasons that students revert to narrative writing when they are first requested to write persuasively and write shorter pieces in the persuasive genre than in other genres (Crowhurst, 1980, 1986).

As writers develop greater knowledge of written persuasive discourse schema, they will write richer elaborations of claims, and they will use effective varieties of support. Their greater persuasive knowledge will enable writers to plan and implement successful introductions and influential conclusions.

Sense of Audience. The sense of audience trait measures students' developing ability to modify their texts to fit the needs of differing audiences and to consider opposing views of the audience when producing a persuasive text. This trait is critical to an effective argument. A sense of audience requires social cognitive skills, which involve speakers' and writers' ability to take on the perspectives and roles of their listeners and readers. Quality of students' writing is related to their social cognitive abilities (O'Keefe & Delia, 1979; Rubin, Piche, Michlin, & Johnson, 1984; Simon-Ailes, 1995). Even preschool children are sensitive to listeners' behavior, but only older children are able to use language to deal with difficulties in interaction. For example, 7- and 9-year-olds are more able to reformulate requests after refusals than 5-year-olds (Axia & Baroni, 1985). By age 8, children are often able to anticipate a listener's point of view and will increase politeness of their requests (Axia, 1996).

Studies of students' persuasive writing in grades 2, 4, and 6 reflect increases in sense of audience with increasing age (Atkins, 1983; Knudson, 1989). Young writers can only consider the reader or audience that is present. Adolescent writers can consider their audience even when it is not well-defined. Novice writers negotiate but inconsistently and only in some situations. As they grow older and develop experience in persuasive writing, students begin to negotiate systematically (Golder & Coirier, 1994). Expert writers of persuasion apply the results of their social inferences to predict the effectiveness of their persuasive strategies, the adequacy of their informational content, the appropriateness of syntax, and the effectiveness of organizational cues and patterns (Rubin, et al., 1984). Concerns for audience needs are involved in all phases of writing, during production (Flower & Hayes, 1981) as well as during revision (Sommers, 1980). The ability of writers to conceptualize an audience and to use this conceptualization to develop effective persuasive texts involves the following subskills (Rubin et al, 1984):

1. Perspective differentiation: Writer recognizes that audience may have a different point of view
2. Construct repertoire: Writer knows that there can be different types of audiences who will have different types of backgrounds and beliefs
3. Sense of instrumentality: Writer recognizes that social cognitive activity will contribute to effective persuasion
4. Representation: Writer infers audience's perspective on the basis of available information together with general expectations culled from experience
5. Maintenance: Writer is able to maintain the perspective of the audience even when this perspective is in marked opposition to the writer's beliefs
6. Sense of applicability: Writer attempts to use the knowledge of audience perspective in selecting appropriate communication strategies

These social cognitive subskills essential for a sense of audience become more developed in writers as they mature. They are influenced by feedback from a writer's knowledgeable mentor and by explicit teaching of these social cognitive subskills.

Metacognitive Awareness

Writing assessment should not be limited to assessment of the product. What students produce is directly related to their motivation, goals, and beliefs about the writing process. Consequently, assessment should also consider students' views and knowledge about writing. A variety of questionnaires to assess students' attitudes and knowledge about writing are available (Hill & Ruptic, 1994; Rhodes, 1993). Table 9-6 shows interview questions we have used with fourth and sixth grade regular and special education students participating in the New Mexico Writing Portfolio Assessment. Although similar questions can be used with all students, an ethnographic approach should be used in the process. In using an ethnographic approach, students' responses should not be judged as good or bad, nor should evaluators restate the responses in their own words. Instead, they should use a variety of structural questions to clarify meaning. See Table 9-7 for types of ethnographic questions and examples of when and how to use them.

Students responses' to writing interview questions can be analyzed to determine if they are focusing on the mechanical, product, or process aspects of writing. Ideally, students need to recognize that good writing requires a balanced attention to all three aspects. There is a tendency for students with writing disabilities to focus on the mechanical aspects to the exclusion of the product and process (Graham, Schwartz, & MacArthur, 1993). A table in Appendix F displays a coding system for judging students' focus in the writing interview (Rhodes, 1993).

TABLE 9-6   Student Interview Guide

In the fourth and sixth grades we do some special things with writing called the New Mexico Writing Portfolio. Different kinds of writing go into your portfolio. In schools across the country students are doing writing portfolios. I am looking into the best way to do writing portfolios. I would like to get your ideas about writing and portfolios. The information you provide me will be used by teachers to help students become better writers.

1. What kinds of things do you write?
2. How do you think people learn to write? How did you learn to write?
3. Why do people write?
4. What kinds of things do you write?
5. People have many different feelings about writing. How do you feel when your teacher gives you a writing assignment? Some people really like writing and some people really don't like it. What makes you feel that way? Is it easy or hard for you to write? What makes it easy (hard) for you to write?
6. What do you think a good writer needs to do in order to write well?
7. What do you really like about your writing?
8. What would you like to improve about your writing?
9. When you are writing and you have a problem (or get stuck), what do you do?
10. What kinds of things do you do to write well?
11. What are things that teachers could do to help you learn to write?
12. When you and your teacher look at your writing, what does he or she say about it?
13. What have you told your parents about your writing?
14. What are you learning from doing the writing portfolio?
15. What do you like/dislike about the writing portfolio process?
16. What suggestions do you have to improve the writing portfolio assessment?

Facilitating Writing

The increased time spent on writing instruction across the nation is showing results. In general, students who receive more writing instruction tend to write more proficiently (Applebee, Langer, Mullis, Latham, & Gentile, 1994). In addition, increases in writing proficiency are associated with changes in the nature of writing instruction. Current educational approaches used in writing instruction consider both the written product and the process that leads to that product. Students exposed to a process-oriented approach to writing instruction with an emphasis on planning, writing multiple drafts, and on defining audience and purpose tend to write more proficiently than students exposed primarily to a product-oriented skills approach to writing instruction (Goldstein & Carr, 1996).

Students' writing proficiency, however, varies according to the nature of the writing task or function or genre of the writing, with students exhibiting their most proficient writing on narrative texts and their least proficient on persuasive texts. Students must write for many purposes to become accomplished writers. Writing for different purposes requires that students know distinct forms of texts that may require specific vocabularies, a variety of organizations, and a variety of syntactic structures (Callaghan, Knapp, & Noble, 1993; Coe,

TABLE 9-7   Ethnographic Interviewing Questions

Semantic Relationship: Question Type	Student Statement	Interviewer's Follow-up Question
• Strict inclusion: kinds of things	My mom did lots to teach me to write.	Tell me about some of the things your mom did.
	Lots of people helped me.	Who were some of the people who helped you?
• Spatial/location: part of or places for	I can't write in class. I gotta have a quiet place.	Where are some of the places that you like to write?
• Cause-effect: cause of or result of	I do my best writing in Mr. James' class.	What do you think causes you to do your best writing in Mr. James' class?
		What happens when you do your best writing?
• Rationale: reasons for doing something	I like to use the computer.	What are the reasons you like to use the computer when you write?
• Function: uses for	I really like writing in my diary.	What do you use you diary for?
• Means-end: ways to do something	Ms. Bartlett is helping me be a better speller.	What are the ways Ms. Bartlett tries to help you with your spelling?
• Sequence: steps in doing something	Sometimes I get stuck and I can't figure out what to write about.	What steps do you go through when you're stuck for an idea to write about?
• Attribution: attributes of characteristics of something or someone	My fourth grade teacher was really a good writing teacher.	You told me your fourth grade teacher was a really good writing teacher. What did she do that made her a good teacher?

1994; Westby, 1994). Importance is given to students' meaningful involvement in their writing, with classroom opportunities for them to discuss their writing with peers. Assignments support writing in various genres and link these genres to authentic purposes for student writing such as letters that will be mailed and reports that can be shared with other students in the school, parents, and community members.

Although students' writing proficiency is showing improvement, relatively few students produced "elaborated or better" responses on the National Assessment of Educational Progress (NAEP) tasks (Applebee et al., 1994). In 1996, the National Council of Teachers of English and the International Reading Association released new voluntary national standards for English-language arts (International Reading Association, 1996). Among the twelve standards are four that address relevant written language concerns with knowledge of genres and development of sense of audience. The students should

- Adjust their use of spoken, written, and visual language to communicate effectively with a variety of audiences and for different purposes.
- Employ a range of strategies as they write, and use different writing-process elements appropriately to communicate with different audiences.
- Apply knowledge of language structure, language conventions, media techniques, figurative language, and genre to create, critique, and discuss print and nonprint texts.
- Use spoken, written, and visual language to accomplish their own purposes (learning, enjoyment, persuasion, and exchange of information).

In time these standards may guide writing teachers to fulfill their challenge of teaching the higher order writing skills required for more effective writing achievement.

Many advocates of the writing process approach employ a constructivist approach to teaching in which students are expected to discover how to write by writing. Constructivists view children as active, self-regulating learners who construct knowledge in developmentally appropriate ways within a social context (Harris & Graham, 1996a). The starting point for learning is the child's prior knowledge and experiences. Constructivists also tend to reject the teaching of discrete skills, as well as the belief that mastery of basic skills is a necessary prerequisite for more advanced learning. They believe that teachers are to facilitate the construction of knowledge rather than to provide knowledge explicitly (Tharp & Gallimore, 1988).

The advantages of a constructivist approach over a skill-and-drill or workbook approach are intuitively obvious. The activities are more authentic and if students self-select activities, they are more likely to be motivated to do them well. Difficulties, however, arise in practice. Some advocates maintain that direct explanation and practice are neither necessary nor desirable and may, in fact, be harmful. Children are expected to learn all they need in due time though social interaction and immersion in authentic learning activities. When the purist, constructivist philosophy is applied to writing, teachers are not to assume the role of experts either by requiring particular types of writing or by correcting students' writing. In fact, one researcher involved with the National Writing Project suggested to us that there was no need to teach particular types of writing and that teachers should give only positive comments about students' writing and should not correct students' work before eighth grade. Indeed, guidance from an expert is sometimes looked upon with disdain.

Because of the widespread nature of the constructivist movement and increasing inclusion of students with disabilities into regular education classrooms, children with reading and writing disabilities are experiencing constructivist educational philosophies. Although these practices work for a some students, parents, teachers, and students are voicing concerns about students who do not learn to read naturally and students whose handwriting is illegible and labored and whose spelling remains invented long past the early grades. Although the writing process approach has certainly led to more writing in classrooms and to students generally feeling more comfortable in writing, some researchers working with students from culturally/linguistically diverse and low socioeconomic backgrounds and students with writing disabilities have expressed concern about the writing process. Delpit (1988) suggested that the writing process approach keeps students from nondominant cultures from having access to the mainstream language code. In interviewing students, she discovered that a number of them were confused by what was or was not happening in writing activities. After she explained the writing process approach, an African American student commented about his experience with a teacher:

> I didn't feel she was teaching us anything. She wanted us to correct each other's papers and we were there to learn from her. She didn't teach anything, absolutely nothing . . . When I'm in a classroom, I'm looking . . . for structure, the more formal language. Now my buddy was in a black teacher's class. And that lady was very good. She went through and explained and defined each part of the structure. This white teacher didn't get along with that black teacher. She said that she didn't agree with her methods. But I don't think that white teacher had any methods. Well, at least now I know that she thought she was doing something. I thought she was just a fool who couldn't teach and didn't want to try (Delpit, 1988, p. 287).

Similarly, de la Luz Reyes (1991) reported that a group of Hispanic sixth grade students did not understand the nature of the writing process approach. De la Luz Reyes noted over the course of the year that students were not making changes in their writing. When she questioned the students about this, they responded that the teacher must like what they were doing because she didn't make any corrections.

Harris and Graham (1996a) have expressed concern about the use of a pure writing process or constructivist approach with students with learning disabilities. As discussed by Scott (Chapter 8), students with learning disabilities exhibit a wide range of difficulties in writing. They are likely to have difficulty generating ideas and content, translating the ideas into graphemes and sentence structures, organizing the ideas, monitoring their performance, and identifying errors and knowing how to correct them. Simply allowing these students opportunities to write is not likely to result in improvements in their writing. Many of these students will require more extended, structured, and explicit instruction to develop the skills and strategies essential for writing. Harris and Graham (1996a, 1996b) advocate integrating explicit writing strategy instruction within the writing process. There is no reason that one cannot use the process stages (prewriting, drafting, revising, editing, publishing, and evaluating) while also providing students with writing disabilities with direct teaching of components essential to carry out the writing process. This requires attention to the individual strengths and needs of the students and the requirements of the writing tasks. To be successful writers, students need

- Motor skills to write or type
- Knowledge of phoneme-grapheme relationships
- Knowledge of a variety of literate syntactic structures
- Knowledge of a variety of genre macrostructures
- Knowledge of and ability to use a variety of self-regulatory strategies in the writing process

Students with writing disabilities exhibit deficits at multiple levels that impair their ability to produce cohesive, coherent written texts. Intervention programs to facilitate development of writing should address each of these components. Many writing intervention programs are beneficial for all students and can be carried out within regular education classrooms. Many students with writing disabilities, however, will generally require more time and more explicit instruction than can generally be given within the regular classroom (Scanlon, Deshler, & Schumaker, 1996). Such students will require support from speech-language pathologists and special educators to develop their writing abilities.

Facilitating Skills and Knowledge

Handwriting

Many students with writing disabilities have difficulty with the motor act itself of putting pencil to paper. For these students, the physical act of writing—putting graphemes on paper—disrupts the writing process before it begins. Attending to mechanics of writing may interfere with higher order writing in several ways (Graham, 1992):

- Causing writers to forget already developed intentions and meanings.
- Disrupting the planning process, resulting in writing that is less coherent and complex.
- Taking time away from the time necessary to find expressions that precisely fit their intentions.
- Preventing students from writing fast enough to keep up with their thoughts, thus causing them to lose ideas and plans.
- Affecting students' persistence, motivation, and sense of confidence for writing.

If students are to be able to attend to the process and products of writing over the mechanics, the motor act of writing must become automatic or at least easier. Some children will benefit from instruction and practice in handwriting. Computers can also reduce the motoric effort, although attention will need to be given to keyboarding skills. For early elementary school children the program *Read, Write & Type* (The Learning Company, 1996) provides practice in keyboarding and letter/sound relationships in the context of a story. For students from mid-elementary through high school, the program *Mavis Beacon Teaches Typing* (Mindscape, 1996) provides training in keyboarding skills using a series of arcade games to increase accuracy and speed.

Syntactic Structures

To write effectively, students must also be capable of a range of syntactic and cohesive strategies. By middle elementary school children must be capable of producing a variety of independent and dependent clause structures (see examples in Chapter 7) linked by coordinating and subordinating conjunctions. Table 9-8 lists and defines these coordinating and subordinating conjunctions. May (1994) suggested a variety of strategies for facilitating students' comprehension of and ability to use a variety of connective words. For example, for the connector *while* students can practice conversations that require use of *while* (meaning *during the time* that).

Student 1: What will you be doing while I _____ (action word)?

Student 2: While you're (action word), I'll _____ (state alternative activity)

TABLE 9-8   Clausal Connecting Words

Connecting Words	Definition	Words with Similar Meaning
Coordinating connectors: Link independent clauses		
and	plus together with occurring at the same time	in addition as well as
or	tells us we have a choice	no true synonyms; in some contexts optionally, alternatively, or on the other hand may be substituted
but	contrary to expectations	on the contrary however yet still nevertheless except that
hence	as a result from this time	therefore as a result from now on
therefore	for that reason	consequently hence
yet	means the same as but	but however nevertheless still except that
Subordinating connectors: Link dependent clauses		
after	following the time that	
although/though	in spite of the fact	even though even if supposing that
as	to the same degree that in the same way that	while because
because	for the reason that since	for in view of the fact inasmuch as taking into account that
before	in advance of the time when	prior to
if	in the case that in the event that whether	granting that on condition that
meanwhile	during or in the intervening time at the same time	
since	from the time that (preferred meaning) continuously from the time when as a result of the fact that	inasmuch because for

TABLE 9-8   Continued

Connecting Words	Definition	Words with Similar Meaning
Subordinating connectors: Link dependent clauses		
so that/in order that	for the purpose of	so with the wish that with the purpose that with the result that
than unless until	compared to the degree that except on the condition that up to the time that to the point or extent that	
when/whenever	at the time that	as soon as if while (although not synonymous)
where/wherever	at what place in a place that to a place that	
while	during the time that at the same time that although	as long as

Example:

Student 1: What will you be doing while I wash the dishes?

Student 2: While you're washing the dishes, I'll play tennis.

or

Student 1: Yesterday I _____ (state an appropriate activity for the pictured item) with this. What did you do yesterday?

Student 2: While you (restate activity), I _____ (state an alternative activity).

Example:

Student 1: Yesterday I took pictures with this camera. What did you do yesterday?

Student 2: While you took pictures, I cleaned house. (May, 1994, p. 228)

Stories can be selected that emphasize a particular conjunction. Students can be asked questions about the story that requires their comprehension and production, for example:

It was the job of Ray and Pete to take care of the yard work at their house.

They made up a list of jobs. While Ray did the top half of the list, Pete did the bottom half.

Who did what? or What did Ray do? (May, 1994, p. 232)

Students can also be presented with story starters using specific connectives, for example,

While I slowly backed away, I watched it closely.

The bridge shook *while* I walked across it.

Sentence combining is another strategy that has been recommended for facilitating development of more complex syntactic patterns (Strong, 1986). The goal of sentence combining is to make sentence construction in writing more automatic, less labored, and at same time to make students more conscious of sentence options because text revision requires such awareness. One can begin by providing students with support for the combining. In the following examples, connecting words are put in parentheses following the sentences in which they appear; the word SOMETHING is a placeholder word for noun constructions; words or phrases that will be embedded (inserted) into a sentence are underlined; word ending cues, for example, (-ING, -LY) can be introduced after students get comfortable with the basic cues.

I like diving.	I like diving because it is very exciting.
It is very exciting. (BECAUSE)	
I can see SOMETHING.	
You're skilled in diving	I can see that you're skilled in diving.
Please tell me SOMETHING.	Please tell me how you acquired your
You acquired your skill. (HOW)	skill.
I would say SOMETHING.	
My intelligence was the key. (THAT)	I would say that my natural intelligence is
My intelligence is natural.	the key.
Please tell me more.	Please tell me more because I am
I am fascinated by this. (BECAUSE)	completely fascinated by this.
My fascination is complete. (-LY)	

Students can also be given a series of sentences and encouraged to work in groups to see how many different ways they can be combined, for example:

Titania was working hard on her test.

Kaylene slipped her a note.

Titania unfolded the paper carefully.

She didn't want her teacher to see.

Examples:

Titania was working hard on her test when Kaylene slipped her a note. Not wanting the teacher to see it, Titania unfolded the paper carefully.

or

While Titania was working hard on her test, Kaylene slipped her a note that Titania unfolded carefully because she didn't want the teacher to see.

Or the teacher or speech-language pathologist can take complex sentences from literature and textbooks, reduce them to simple sentences, have students recombine them and then compare their combined sentences with the original texts.

Macrostructure Knowledge

Story-Grammar Strategies.   Many teachers and speech-language pathologists are familiar with teaching story macrostructures. The Story-Grammar Marker (Moreau & Fidrych-Puzzo, 1994) is one system that has been used to increase students' awareness of narrative structure. Students use a braided yarn "critter" with small charms attached to it. A pompom head represents the story characters, a star below the head represents other elements of the setting (time, place), a boot represents the story kickoff or initiating event, a heart the reaction to the initiating event, a hand represents a character's goal or plan to respond to the event, beads represent a series of attempts, bows near the end of the braid represent the consequences, and small hearts at the very end of the braid represent characters' reactions to the consequences. The marker provides students with a physical reminder of the story elements.

In preparing to write a story, students can be encouraged to outline the elements of the story on a sheet that lists each of the story elements. Westby and Roman incorporated the symbols from the story-grammar marker with the circular presentation of story elements proposed by Esterreicher (1994). A circle or wheel was divided into seven equal pies, representing the setting, initiating event, internal response, internal plan, attempt, consequence, and ending for a story. The story-grammar marker symbols were drawn in their respective pies. The circular format reminded the students that the end of the story should tie back to the beginning—a story should *come full circle*. A small version of this wheel was taped (using wide plastic tape) to the upper left-hand side of all third through sixth grade students' desks for reference when reading stories. When students were to write stories, they were given large wheels on 8 1/2 by 11 inch sheets of paper. They planned or outlined their stories on these sheets before writing them.

Genre-Based Writing Approach.   Academic success in later elementary school and beyond requires more than the ability to read and write narrative texts. Students must be able to produce texts representing a variety of functions or genres. A genre-based approach to the teaching of writing arose in Australia influenced by Halliday's work in functional linguistics (Halliday, 1985). Halliday's work brought educators and linguists together in a transdisciplinary manner to enable teachers to see linguistics as a practical tool in their everyday work. The genre-based approach employs a pedagogy in which teachers adopt an authoritative negotiating role as opposed to what was viewed as a benevolent inertia in the writing process approach. A genre is defined as *a staged, goal-oriented social process* achieved primarily through language (Martin, 1987, cited in Coe, 1994). Genres are ways that people make meaning with one another in stages to achieve their goals. Stages represent the components or structure of the genres (e.g., the beginnings, middles, and ends). Genres are considered social processes because members of a given culture have learned particular ways to use them in particular settings. Genres are designed for a variety of goals: to inform, to entertain, to argue a point, to persuade, to complain, to consult, and so on.

The interest in the genre-based approach increased in Australia in the 1980s as concern arose that the progressive constructivist curriculum was marginalizing working-class, migrant, Aboriginal, and other disadvantaged children. The argument for teaching genres in school is that society has a typology of genres that are more highly valued than others; these valued genres need to be made explicit and taught so that all students have equal access to the means for learning. The same concerns have been raised in the United States by persons working with students from culturally/linguistically diverse and low socioeconomic backgrounds. Genre-based teaching addresses there three content areas:

- Making connections between content knowledge and language (developed through experiences, reading, research)
- Using generic genre structures to provide a scaffold for student writing (modeling the generic structures/text organizations and scaffolding with content)
- Grammar-editing

Three phases are employed in genre-based teaching.

Phase 1: Modeling.   In the first phase, teachers introduce the genre to be studied. They discuss the social function of the genre, the schematic stages or components of the genre, and the linguistic characteristics of the genre. A model of the genre is introduced that is tied to a thematic unit in the curriculum. The text is displayed on an overhead, and macrostructure elements and linguistic characteristics are highlighted and the components of stages of the text are discussed (see an example of an persuasive text from an eighth grade student in Figure 9-2). The first stage thesis presents the case or issue. After the thesis, each argument is dealt with in a paragraph. There is only one thesis, but there can be any number of arguments. The final stage, restatement of thesis, sums up the case as forcefully as possible. The teacher points out that it is through these stages that the writing accomplishes its purpose to persuade or convince. The teacher also notes particular grammatical structures and technical vocabulary that are also important in building the case. It can also be useful for students to compare a good model with a model that fails to meet the criteria of the genre. See an example of a poor persuasive text also written by an eighth grade student in Figure 9-3.

Phase 2: Joint construction of a text.   During this phase the teacher and students work together to produce a text. The teacher guides the students by asking questions that focus on the stages of the genre. Initially the students research the topic through reading, interviewing others, watching videos, using library books and computer resources, or going on field trips.

After they collect data, the class is brought together to summarize their information on the chalkboard/whiteboard. The teacher may assist the students to organize the information they have gathered in a semantic web. Once all the information has been gathered and organized, the teacher guides the students as a group in producing the text. The teacher asks

Written in response to the prompt: Your teacher has asked you to write a letter to the President of the United States telling him about one change that you think would make this country a better place. Be sure to tell what the change is and give convincing reasons why the president should make the change.

Dear President:

Thesis

> I think the thing that, if changed, would most improve out nation would be education. This means changes in schools as well as in the home if it will truly be effective.

Position

Preview

Argument

> First the attitude toward education in poor and uneducated communities must change. I know that in my community there are many intelligent children who choose not to do well in or put effort into school because their families do not encourage them or give them reason to think that a good education is valuable. It is bad to see a perfectly good mind wasted for lack of use.

Point

Elaboration

Argument

> Second, courses should not be taught toward the mediocre. We should challenge all students because they will rise to the level of expectation. if a student is only expected to be average that is all they will achieve, but if we make each and every child feel that they can and should achieve higher goals, they will. a teacher who makes their class less challenging in hopes of more students passing and making them look better, is only cheating the students who actually care about their education.

Point

Elaboration

Argument

> Third, I say that teachers should not be baby sitters. If a person cares so little about their education that they cannot follow the rules and do their work, they should not be in school. These students are not only hurting themselves but are taking away from those who actually care. Instead of forcing kids into staying in school, we should let the serious ones stay and let the rest do the dirty jobs. All of this struggle could be avoided if society instilled a higher value for education in young people.

Point

Elaboration

Argument

> Fourthly in the year 2000 plan for education, music and art are not mentioned once. It will be a sad, sad day when all of us are math wizards and nuclear physisists but cannot recall hearing Shakespeare or Beethoven. what is the point of life if you can't enjoy it.

Point

Re-statement of theses

> If we are to continue being a great country and a leader of nations, things must change.

Sincerely,

FIGURE 9-2   Example of good persuasive text.

Dear Mr. Clinton

As far back as 1992 when you were running for President I could have cared less. You were just another face. Now that I know you have the power to change our country I hope you will take into deep consideration what I have to say.

If there is one bad thing about this country on plauge. That plauge is poverty and homelessness. I know you and your staff have addressed these issues but still they remain as deadly as ever. I know as well as you do that you are trying very hard to eliminate poverty but more remains. It the only was to cure this plauge is to raise taxes I know my family would gladly pay a higher tax if they knew these issues could be stopped.

I know I'm not an adult and I don't vote or pay taxes and you probally won't even get this letter. But please listen to me listen to your heart and put an end to the misery. Please your this country only hope.

FIGURE 9-3   Example of a poorly structured persuasive text.

---

questions and makes comments that point to the structure of the text or the possibility or reasonableness of a statement. The teacher writes the text on the board or overhead transparency so that the children can concentrate on the meanings they are formulating. Table 9-9 shows a group-generated story by several elementary school students in a classroom for children with severe language learning disabilities. The children had read two of the Miss Nelson books (*Miss Nelson is Missing* [Allard, 1977] and *Miss Nelson Is Back* [Allard, 1982]). The teacher presented a poster with a picture of Miss Viola Swamp (the mean, ugly teacher who had appeared in the two Miss Nelson books). She is dressed in a sweatsuit with the words, "Coach and Don't You Forget It," on her shirt. The teacher tacked this poster to the board and asked the students to generate a story. She was seeking not only a narrative, but a narrative that maintained the characteristics of the Miss Nelson books. As the children offered ideas, she asked them if the idea could go in a Miss Nelson story. For example, when the children suggested they would get even with the Swamp, the teacher asked, "Could you really do that?" As students struggled with ideas, she suggested they act out the story, and then describe what they were doing. The children's resulting narrative displays an understanding of the genre of Miss Nelson books.

Phase 3: Independent construction of a text.   Students choose a new topic for their writing. Students must conduct their background research more independently. They write a draft, referring to the model and jointly constructed text that had been presented. The students then consult with the teacher about their draft. The teacher's questions and comments focus in a constructive way on what the students have done and what they can do to further develop their piece. This strategy is different from simply telling the students what they did right or wrong. The feedback is explicit. It is not simply encouraging; it also offers advice or guidance on how to make the text more effective.

TABLE 9-9   Group-Generated Story

The Swamp Is Back

Anthony, David, and Rene decided to get suspended so they could play all day. When the boys went to the gym, they painted on the walls with crayons and paint. They threw the basketballs, footballs, all kinds of balls all over the gym. When the Swamp opened the door, balls fell all over her. she fell down!. She got mad. Her face was all red. She got up and chased those boys all around the gym. She yelled, "STOP!" She blew her whistle. Her feet sounded like hammers hitting the floor.

Miss Swamp threw a ball and hit the boys on the back of their knees and made them fall down. The boys were embarrassed because everyone in the whole school knew that the Swamp caught them.

"Now," yelled Miss Swamp, "You guys get busy cleaning up this mess! Scrub the walls! Put the balls away."

They worked very hard cleaning the gym. The Swamp watched the whole time. When they finished cleaning, the kids were so tired they fell on the floor.

"Anthony, David, Rene, wake up!"

The boys jerked up and stood shaking. "Now, you boys may do 50 push-ups!"

After the push-ups the boys were really pooped. They fell on the floor. "Now run 50 laps," said Miss Swamp.

When the boys finished their laps, they were breathing loud and sweating hard. They fell to the floor again. Just then, the principal's voice came over the speaker, "Miss Viola Swamp, please come to the office."

Minutes later, coach came into the gym. "Yea, coach is here," yelled the boys. "Do you forgive us for being mean?" We promise we'll behave. Please don't call Miss Swamp again.

Coach just smiled.

Gearhart and Wolf (1994) proposed some specific guidelines that can be used in this phase. The comments should be very specific to the text genre (rather than general), they should be specific to the child's work, and they should be significant to the task. Table 9-10 gives examples of the types of comments that can be made. The examples given are for a narrative text. The comments should also address the components or specific features of the genre. For example, in Gearhart and Wolf's narrative work, they draw children's attention to the theme, setting, characters, plot, and communication aspects of narratives. Because these are aspects of the narrative on which they are being evaluated, teachers should provide comments on these components. Gearhart and Wolf suggest using a feedback sheet of the type in Figure 9-4. So as not to overwhelm a student, however, they recommend initially commenting on only two aspects—one positive comment about a strength and one comment on how to improve an element.

Many students with writing disabilities lack a knowledge base from which to write. Advocates of the writing process methodology often recommend that novice writers write from their personal experience. Yet expert writers draw richly from a wider knowledge base acquired through reading. Using the Writing What You Read rubric, Wolf and Gearhart (1994) advocated exploring literature with students to give them backgrounds and frameworks for writing. See Table 9-11 for the types of information to be discussed in developing understanding of narratives. Many students who are poor writers are also poor readers. Consequently, they have difficulty researching topics and gathering information to write about. CD-ROM computer programs provide poor readers with a means of gathering information. Many of the programs will read the information to students. The programs can be incorporated into thematic curricular units that will form the basis for writing. The *Magic School Bus* series (*Solar System, Inside the Earth, Inside the Human Body, Rainforest, Dinosaurs, Ocean*) are attractive science programs for elementary school children. Even the most reluctant student is willing to explore them. In a story format with arcade-like games, students are exposed to scientific vocabulary, problem-solving, and model informational reports. As they interact with the computer, they also can gather information that they can use in developing their own projects.

TABLE 9-10   Commenting on a Student's Text

Appropriateness to Narrative

Value Specific: Praise that pinpoints a particular aspect of the child's story (*You've given a vivid description of the rainforest setting and why the peccaries were exhausted.*)

Value General: Praise that is global in nature (*This is well written.*)

Guidance Specific: Guidance that offers a particular direction regarding what the child is to think about or to do (*I know the jaguar destroyed two of the peccaries' houses, but I don't know how. Tell me how the jaguar found the peccaries and what he did to each of the houses.*)

Guidance General: Guidance that is global in nature, often a generalized request simply "add more." (*I would like you to tell me more about the jaguar.*)

Links to the Child's Text

Linked to text: Comment could only be applied to this text (summary or direct quote) (*Having the peccaries get a restraining order against the jaguar was a surprising way to end your story.*)

Not linked to text: Comment could be applied to text, or any example of the genre (*You gave your story a good ending.*)

Significance of the Comment

Significant: Comment that is significant to the component, genre, particular story, or child's development (*You did a good job explaining how the jaguar tried to trick the peccaries into letting him in their houses*).

Insignificant: Comment that focuses on a minor detail or is relatively subgenre inappropriate. (*What piece of clothing did the second peccary use for his house?*) Or, for example, congratulating a child on a happy ending may be appropriate for a fairy tale but not for a fable.

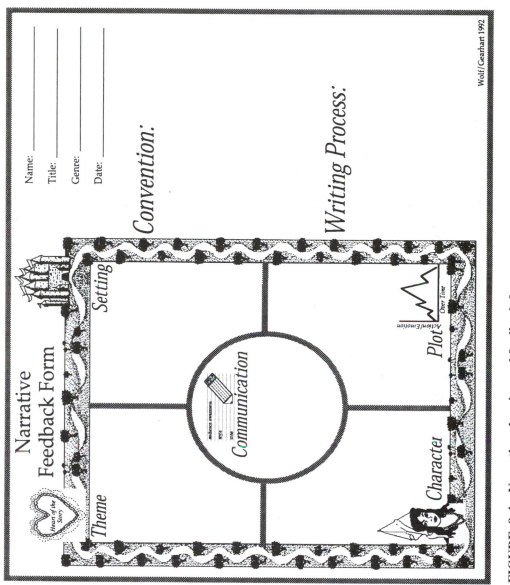

Name: _____
Title: _____
Genre: _____
Date: _____

Narrative
Feedback Form

Heart of the Story

Theme

Convention:

Setting

Communication

audience awareness
style
tone

Plot
Action/Emotion
Over Time

Character

Writing Process:

Wolf/Gearhart 1992

FIGURE 9-4 Narrative planning and feedback form.
Reprinted with permission from:
Wolf, S., & Gearhart, M. (1994). Writing what you read: Narrative assessment as a learning event. *Language Arts, 71,* 425–444.

TABLE 9-11 Components of Narrative

	Genre	Theme	Character	Setting	Plot	Point of View	Style	Tone
Define the Terms	Genre is a classification system for organizing literature. It chunks stories with common elements together, although the categories are the subject of much debate.	Theme is the message of the story: an idea or comment about life. Theme illuminates the emotional content of the human condition.	The character is an actor in the story. The character can be a person, an animal, or an personified animal, object, or creature.	The basic elements of the setting are the place, time, and situation of the story.	The plot is a series of events that occur in a specific order. Not necessarily linear, the sequence represents the author's decisions for moving the story along.	Point of view is the view of the action the reader follows. It is often signalled by insights into thoughts and feelings.	Style is the use of language that reflects the spirit and personality of the writer through specific devices.	Tone is the manner of expression which conveys (through stylistic choices) the author's attitude toward his or her subject.
Develop a Common Language	Fantasy: Traditional Folk, Myth, Fable High Fantasy Science Fiction Reality: Problem Realism Historical Fiction Animal Realism	Universal Moral Implicit & Explicit Primary & Secondary	• Major/Minor • Protagonist/Antagonist • Features: emotional, physical, intellectual • Character development, revelation	Time Place Situation Historical context Mood	• Story Graph • Episode Analysis: Problem Emotional Response Action Outcome • Flashback, Conflict, Suspense, Foreshadowing, Climax	First person (often the protagonist) Omniscient (spread across characters) Focused (usually on one character) Objective (actions reveal motivation)	Imagery Allusion Puns Hyperbole Figurative Language Metaphor Personification Sound Devices Alliteration Assonance Rhythm	Humor Warmth Condescension Didacticism
Explore the Text	• Identify elementary characteristics of particular genres. • Identify the genre you prefer and analyze why you like it. • Recognize that each genre tends to follow certain patterns. For example, fairy tales tend to have stock characters. Historic fiction relies heavily on the development of setting. Fables offer specific rules to live by. • Defend the author's choice of genre for delivering the theme of the story.	• Identify the theme(s) in the text. • Describe the relationship of the theme to your life. • Compare/contrast other pieces of literature with similar theme(s). • Describe how your understanding of character, setting, & plot enhance your understanding of the theme(s). • Decide on the universality of the theme(s): Who is most affected by the theme's message?	• Identify the major and minor characters in a story. • Compare/contrast the story characters to you or people you know. • Trace the development of a character through the story. • Trace the relationship between characters. • Analyze how the character is revealed through other characters' eyes.	• Explain the relationship of the setting to the story. • Relate the time, place, & situation to your own. • Explore the historical and cultural significance of the setting. • Describe how the setting reflects the character. • Compare/contrast two or more settings in the story (e.g. How do the different settings affect the character?)	• Compare the plot to events that have occurred in your own life. • Identify an episode in terms of problem, emotional response, action, and outcome. • Outline several episodes relating the outcome of one episode to the problem of the next episode. • Explain the effect of the character's motivation on the plot or vice versa.	• Identify who's telling the story. • Analyze how the point of view reveals the character(s) motivations, intentions, and feelings. • Justify the effectiveness of the point of view. • Criticize the author's choice of point of view. Would the story have been better served by an alternative?	• Describe the stylistic choices of the author and how they enhance the story. • Describe how the author's style reveals character, setting, and plot. • Compare/contrast stylistic choices within one author's work or between authors. • Reflect on the stylistic choices you will incorporate in your own speech and writing.	• Evaluate the tone(s) of the narrative voice. • Describe the influence of the narrative voice in relation to the major characters (e.g. sympathetic, condescending). • Analyze how the stylistic choices reflect the tone. • Compare/contrast choices in tone within one author's work or between authors.

Reprinted with permission from:
Wolf, S. & Gearhart, M. (1994). Writing what you read: Narrative assessment as a learning event. *Language Arts, 71,* 425–444.

A number of computer programs focus on the act of writing. Many of them, however, also provide considerable information and ideas for writing. *The Amazing Writing Machine* (Broderbund, 1995) provides students with genre frames that permit students to change words within the frames. Students can type in a word of their choice or select from several other optional words. The story, with pictures, can be printed. With limited spelling and writing skills, students can have the sense of producing a story. The *Ultimate Writing & Creativity Center* (The Learning Company, 1996) provides a cartoon setting for learning about the writing process, gathering information about four environments (rainforest, desert, ocean, and space), creating and printing pictures of the four environments, getting ideas for writing in a variety of genres, taking notes, and producing a novel piece of writing. Penny Pencil coaches students through each step of the writing process. In each of the four environments, students can click on items to see them move and talk. *Creative Writer II* (Microsoft, 1996) has fewer of the bells and whistles of other programs. It is primarily a user-friendly word processing program that permits students to use a variety of fonts, formats, and pictures to produce writing in a variety of genres. It defines a wide variety of genres such as report, editorial, thank you letter, apology letter, obituary, play script, and many story sub-genres (adventure, mystery, fantasy, science fiction, fairy tale, and tall tale). Samples of the beginnings of each of these genres are provided that students can complete.

A number of computer programs are useful at both the second and third phases of the genre-based writing approach. A word of caution: The nature of the writing program or word processing program can affect the quality of the students' writing. Halio (1990) analyzed the first-year English papers of college students assigned to IBM or Macintosh computer writing labs. Compared to IBM users, Mac writers wrote on less complex, more personal themes (fast food, dating, television, foam popcorn as opposed to essays on capital punishment, teenage pregnancy, and drunk driving), used fewer complex sentences, and averaged more misspellings per essay (15 compared to 4 for IBM writers). Halio observed that Mac writers spent more time playing with the graphics and formatting styles that were available on the Macintosh. Although Macintosh and PCs with Windows have become quite similar in their capabilities, there are considerable variations in the types of software available to teach writing skills and process.

Effects of writing software programs have been observed in students with learning disabilities (Bahr, Nelson, & Van Meter, 1996; Bahr, Nelson, Van Meter, & Yanna, 1996). Learning disabled students (ages 9;8 to 13;10) spent more time typing and wrote longer stories with programs that had fewer options. Such research might suggest that when selecting computer writing programs for learning disabled students, one should select programs that emphasize the writing itself, rather than those that provide a lot of topical information and opportunities to play with the topical information (e.g., clicking on animals or people to have them do or say something) or offer opportunities to produce elaborate colorful pictures. In deciding what program to select for a particular students, teachers or speech-language pathologists need to think about students' present writing skills and attitudes toward writing.

Recently, the first author of this chapter has been working with third through sixth grade Native American students who are English language learners and who have limited literacy skills. Many of these students did not have a positive attitude toward school and resisted writing activities. These students could be enticed into writing by using programs such as the *Imagination Express Rainforest* and *Ocean* programs. The rainforest program provides information on the Kuna Indians in the Panama rainforest and gives examples of their stories. The Ocean program gives information about the Native Americans who originally inhabited the Channel Islands off the coast of California and samples of their stories. Both programs provide information about the plants and animals in the environments, suggest a variety of story starters, and permit students to create and print elaborate colored scenes and write the story below the scenes they create.

The rainforest computer writing program was incorporated into an ecology unit for fifth and sixth grade students. In addition to the rainforest program, the teachers and speech-language pathologist read a number of narrative and factual books about the rainforest. Earlier in the year, the students had completed a unit on pigs, reading a variety of the Three Little Pig stories (a traditional version, *The Three Little Hawaiian Pigs and the Magic Shark* [Laird, 1981]; *The Three Little Javelinas* [a Southwest version] [Lowell, 1992]; *The Three Little Wolves and the Big Bad Pig* [Trivizas, 1993]; and *The True Story of the Three Little Pigs* [Scieszka, 1989]). The speech-language pathologist then suggested that the students write a rainforest version of the story. Because there are no pigs and wolves in the rainforest, the students had to research what animals might replace pigs and the wolf and what they might use for building materials. Appendix G shows a story written by a sixth grader. The student has replaced with pigs with peccaries, the wolf with a jaguar, and has used leaves, vines, cloth, and logs for building materials. He has also put a twist in the ending, perhaps based an idea triggered by *The True Story of the Three Little Pigs*. The student has used the genre structure of Three Little Pig stories.

Facilitating Self-Regulatory Writing Strategies

Just having information on a topic and knowing a variety of vocabulary, sentence structures, and genres offers no guarantee that students will independently use the information when they write. Lack of self-regulated learning is common in a large percentage of students with writing disabilities, language-learning disabilities, and attention-deficit hyperactivity disorder (Barkley, 1990; Pressley & Woloshyn, 1995; Westby & Cutler, 1994). For these students, teaching of vocabulary, syntax, and genre must be integrated with teaching of writing strategies. Each aspect of the writing process requires metacognitive strategies:

- Prewriting planning strategies: Students must consider the purpose of writing (the why), the audience (the who), and the knowledge they have or need to have.
- Organizational strategies: Students must have strategies for considering the genre structure, putting ideas into related groups, labeling groups of ideas.
- Drafting strategies: Students must have strategies for ordering ideas, translating ideas into syntactic units and print, expanding/supporting ideas.
- Editing/revising strategies: Students must have strategies for monitoring if the plan was met; monitoring organization and meaningfulness.

Cognitive strategy instruction has become a rich area of research in recent years, although strategy instruction has been slow to be integrated into classroom curricula. The goal of teaching strategies is to increase the likelihood that students will use the strategies independently in a self-regulated way. The focus of many of the current writing strategies is teaching students to monitor how they are doing—checking their performance, tracking progress, and remediating problems. Just knowing strategies is not sufficient—students must also know when and how to use the strategies. Students must be motivated to use strategies. Thus, strategy instruction should include explicit information regarding the usefulness of the strategies. Without effective strategy instruction, Pressley and Woloshyn (1995) suggested that:

- Students often fail to establish a goal for their writing.
- They do not generate enough content; they fail to search their long-term memory for relevant information and they do not make effective use of information available in the environment.
- Rather than planning and organizing, they tend to *knowledge tell* (Bereiter & Scardamalia, 1987) or *knowledge dump,* simply writing down anything that comes to mind about the topic.
- Because their sentence construction, spelling, handwriting, and keyboarding skills are weak, they spend so much effort on low-level skills that they fail to attend to making the writing make sense.
- They treat their first draft as their final draft, having little or no idea of how to revise it to improve communication.

General Principles of Strategy Instruction

Strategy instruction should match the writing tasks with the characteristics of the students and provide activities that promote active involvement of the students. Characteristics of effective strategy instruction include (Pressley, 1992):

- Introducing strategies by directly explaining to the person the purpose of the strategies and how to execute them.
- Showing students how their goals can be achieved by using strategies.
- Discussing the cognitive nature of tasks by using terms like strategies and prior knowledge.
- Repeatedly explaining, reexplaining, modeling, and remodeling the strategies.
- Prompting students to model and explain the strategies to others.
- Teachers/clinicians acting as coaches who scaffold instruction.

The majority of strategy instruction programs encourage the use of self-verbalizations that include comments such as:

- Problem definition: "What do I have to do? I've got to write a story about how something came to be, a story like the one the teacher read to us about *Why Ducks Sleep on One Leg*" (Garland & Tseng, 1993).
- Focusing attention and planning: "The teacher read a bunch of stories about problems animals had. I gotta come up with some kind of problem."
- Self-instructions: "I need to remember to put in all the parts of the story. I have to begin with a setting."

- Self-evaluating coping skills and error correcting: "People won't believe it if I just say the skunk woke up smelly one day. Maybe I could have him fall in a smelly place when he's trying to get away from a wolf."
- Self-reinforcement: "I know, I could tell about how skunks got smelly. That would work."

Writing Strategies

Strategy instruction should address the phases of the writing process. The phases should be viewed as recursive, not linear. That is, one plans before one begins to write, but one may adjust plans as one translates and revises. Similarly, revision may occur in all phases; it need not be limited to the final phase. One can revise as one plans and as one is producing the text. During the last ten years, three programs of research have developed and evaluated the effectiveness of explicitly teaching writing strategies and self-regulation procedures with general education students and with students with learning difficulties. Englert and her colleagues (Englert, Raphael, Anderson, Anthony, Stevens, & Fear, 1991) designed the *Cognitive Strategy Instruction Writing Program* (CSIW) for elementary school students to learn to write explanation and comparison/contrast texts. Harris and Graham (1996b) developed a wide range of self-regulatory writing strategies for students of all ages—*Self-Regulated Strategy Development* (SRSD). With SRSD, student learn specific strategies for accomplishing tasks along with strategies for regulating their use and undesirable behaviors (such as impulsivity) that impede performance. They use acronyms to facilitate students' memory for the strategies. The *Kansas Strategies Instruction Model* (Schumaker & Deshler, 1992) has been the most extensively researched and validated program. The Kansas Model was specifically designed for students with learning disabilities and hence is the most detailed. The Kansas focus, however, tends to be on strategies for more basic writing such as sentence writing and paraphrasing, rather than production of extended texts.

As with strategies for effective reading comprehension, strategies for effective writing must consider *declarative, procedural*, and *conditional* knowledge. Students must know what is expected at each stage of the writing process (declarative knowledge); they must have strategies for how to perform each stage (procedural knowledge), and then must know when and where to employ particular strategies (conditional knowledge). For example, one must know that narratives have particular elements (story grammar components) and that one can use knowledge of these elements to generate a story. One must also realize that these elements cannot be used to generate a comparison/contrast text.

Strategies for Planning.   Many students, at all age levels, do no planning when they write. When given a topic, they employ *knowledge telling,* simply writing down anything that comes to mind (Bereiter & Scardamalia, 1987). In order to plan, students must have adequate background information on a topic, and they must have declarative knowledge about the structural components of the genre. A planning strategy can be as simple as having a student outline the components of a text, as described in the use of the story wheel for developing narratives. The CSIW employs "think-sheets" that function like the story wheel. They are designed to make the strategies for each of the text structures explicit (Englert et al., 1991). In a generic plan-think sheet, the students indicate:

Topic:

Who: Who am I writing for?

Why: Why am I writing?

What: What do I know? (Brainstorm a list of what is known about the topic)

How : How can I group my ideas?

A plan-think sheet for an explanatory text may include:

What is being explained?

Materials/things you need?

Setting?

What are the steps?

First,

Next,

Third,

Then,

Last.

Harris and Graham (1996b) use the mnemonic, TREE, with elementary school children to plan an opinion or persuasive essay:

- Note **T**opic sentence
- Note **R**easons
- **E**xamine reasons—will my reader buy this?
- Note **E**nding

Older students use the STOP strategy. When using this strategy, students first think about their audience and their purpose for writing, then they:

- **S**uspend judgment
- **T**ake a side
- **O**rganize ideas
- **P**lan more as you write

In the first step, students generate all the ideas they can that support each side of an issue. In the second step they evaluate the ideas and take a side. In the third step they organize their ideas by putting a star next to ideas they want to use, an X next to arguments they want to dispute, and then number the ideas in the order they will use them.

The final step is a reminder to continue to plan throughout the writing process. During the writing process, students consult a cue card with the acronym DARE that reminds them to check that they are including all the structural components of the argument:

- **D**evelop your topic sentence
- **A**dd supporting ideas
- **R**eject possible arguments for the other side
- **E**nd with a conclusion

The planning strategies described so far are intended for use on assignments that have specific product goals. For such assignments, students are asked to write on a specific topic, for a specific purpose, using a specific genre. As students progress through school, however, they are often given minimally defined writing assignments—for example, do a science project or write a paper for social studies. Such assignments require that students independently decide on topics and goals for their papers. For such assignments, Harris and Graham (1996a) proposed the PLANS strategy:

- Do PLANS: **P**ick goals
  List ways to meet the goals
  And make
  Notes
  Sequence notes
- Write and say more
- Test goals

Goals for papers may be quite varied, including the general purpose of the paper (convince audience that the rainforest should not be cut), the length of the paper (300 words, 2 pages, etc.), completeness (include all the parts of an argument), sentence variety (write at least five sentences with dependent clauses), and so on. For each goal, the student should also develop an action plan for reaching the goal. Goals should be specific and product oriented. For example, a goal to convince readers that the rainforest should not be cut is a goal for a specific product; a goal to write an interesting science paper would not be specific.

Strategies for Production.   During the translating or actual writing, students are encouraged to use self-verbalizations to make certain they are following their plans and self-regulating their performance, for example,

- Focusing attention and planning: "I've got to come up with a topic sentence. Maybe I could say, 'The world cannot exist without rainforests.' "
- Self-evaluating and error correcting: "I've given two reasons. but I haven't really said why they are important; this isn't long enough—I've got to write some more."
- Coping and self-control: "I'm not going to crumple the paper and start over."
- Self-reinforcement: "I know a lot about rainforests. This last sentence is good."

For elementary school children, Harris and Graham (1996a) recommend working with them to develop self-regulatory statements in categories such as: things to get me started (problem definition and focusing/planning), things to say while I work (focusing/planning, strategy, self-evaluating/error correcting, coping, and self-reinforcement), and things to say when I'm done.

Strategies for Revising.   Students frequently resist revising, and when they do revise, they tend to confine their revisions to proofreading for spelling errors rather than revising to improve meaning and organization. Revising is a difficult, complex activity that taxes working memory. Students must be able to compare what they have written with their goals, evaluate the degree to which they have achieved their goals, and, when the text does not meet the goals, modify the text. Bereiter and Scardamalia (1987) proposed a compare-diagnose-operate (C-D-O) strategy that reduces the working memory or executive demands on students. Students are given cards with the following evaluative statements:

1. People won't see why this is important.
2. People may not believe this.
3. People won't be very interested in this part.
4. People may not understand what I mean here.
5. People will be interested in this part.
6. This is good.
7. This is a useful sentence.
8. I think this could be said more clearly.
9. I'm getting away from the main point.
10. Even I'm confused about what I'm trying to say.
11. This doesn't sound quite right.

Students read a sentence in their drafts, then choose one of these evaluative statements. If students select evaluative statements such as "This is a useful sentence," they go on to the next sentence and choose another evaluative card. If they choose a statement such as, "Even I'm confused about what I'm trying to say," they then choose a directive statement to facilitate tactical choice:

1. I think I'll leave it this way.
2. I'd better give an example.
3. I'd better leave this part out.
4. I'd better cross this sentence out and say it a different way.
5. I'd better say more.
6. I'd better change the wording.

If they chose a statement such as "I'd better change the wording," they make a wording change and then go on to the next sentence.

The C-D-O strategy may be a good way to get students to begin to think about revision; however, because it focuses on sentence level revision, it may not influence higher text level issues related to content and organizational structure. One may want to add another series of statements that students use for the overall text:

1. I've included too few ideas.
2. Part of the essay doesn't belong with the rest.
3. This is an incomplete idea.
4. I've ignored the obvious point someone would bring up against what I'm saying.

5. This is a weak reason.
6. This is choppy—ideas are not connected to each other very well.
7. It's hard to tell what the main point is.
8. This part doesn't give the reader reason to take the idea seriously.
9. I've given too much space to an unimportant point.

Harris and Graham (1996b) use a very simplified version of this procedure, which they term SCAN:

SCAN each sentence:
> Does it make Sense?
> Is it Connected to my central idea?
> Can I Add more detail?
> Note errors.

Writing process classrooms often use peer revising strategies. Students may come to an author's chair where they read their papers to a small group of other children. The children:

1. Listen to the text.
2. Comment on something they like about the text and why they like it.
3. Comment on something they think could be done better and how the text could be revised.

Effective use of the author's chair and peer revision requires modeling by adults of types of statements that can be helpful. Otherwise, students give vague responses such as "I liked it 'cause it's a story" or "Make it look neater."

Summary

Expert writers are made not born. Some current process approaches to the teaching of writing assume that students learn to write simply by writing a lot; they do not need explicit teaching of form and style. Although it may be true that some students do learn to write simply by writing, many students require more specific teaching or mentoring. Such assistance is particularly important for students such as those with language learning disabilities who have difficulty acquiring the written language code or those from culturally/linguistically diverse backgrounds who have had less exposure to the English written language code. More explicit teaching and careful scaffolding of teacher-student interactions around writing would probably be beneficial for all students. Coe (1994) suggested:

> People learned to swim for millennia before coaches explicitly articulated our knowledge of how to swim, but kids today learn to swim better (and in less time) on the basis of that explicit knowledge. The same can be said about most athletic and craft skills. Might it be true for writing as well? (Coe, 1994, p. 159).

If teachers and speech-language pathologists are to provide explicit teaching to develop students' writing, they must know how writing develops in a variety of genres. They must be able to assess students' present writing abilities, provide meaningful activities for writing, and provide both scaffolded support and direct instruction in the components of writing (handwriting, keyboarding, punctuation, spelling, sentence construction, genre organization). Finally, they must ensure that students acquire cognitive strategies and the motivation and ability to use these strategies to become independent writers.

References

Allard, H. (1977) *Miss Nelson is missing*. Boston: Houghton Mifflin.

Allard, H. (1982) *Miss Nelson is back*. Boston: Houghton Mifflin.

Andrews, R. (1995). *Teaching and learning argument*. New York: Cassell.

Applebee, A.N., Langer, J.A., & Mullis, I.V.S. (1987). *Learning to be literate in America: Reading, writing, and reasoning*. National Assessment of Education Progress. Princeton, NJ: Educational Testing Service.

Applebee, A.N., Langer, J.A., Mullis, I. V. S., Latham, A.S., & Gentile, C.A. (1994). *NAEP 1992 writing report card*. Washington, DC: U.S. Department of Education.

Astington, J.W. (1990). Narrative and the child's theory of mind. In B.K. Britton & A.D. Pelligiani (Eds.), *Narrative thought and narrative language* (pp. 151–171). Hillsdale, NJ: Erlbaum.

Atkins, C.L. (1983). Examining children's sense of audience on a persuasive writing task: grades two, four, and six. *Dissertation abstract international, 44*, 2351a.

Atwell, N. (1987). *In the middle: Reading, writing and learning from adolescents*. Portsmouth, NH: Heinemann.

Axia, G. (1996). How to persuade mum to buy a toy. *First Language, 16, 301–317*.

Axia, G., & Baroni, M.R. (1985). Linguistic politeness at different age levels. *Child Development, 56, 918–927*

Bahr, C.M., Nelson, N.W., & Van Meter, A. (1996). The effects of text-based and graphics-based software tools on planning and organizing stories. *Journal of Learning Disabilities, 29*, 355–370.

Bahr, C.M., Nelson, N.W., Van Meter, A., & Yanna, J.V. (1996). Children's use of desktop publishing features: Process and product. *Journal of Computing in Childhood Education, 7*, 149–177.

Barkley, R.A. (1990). *Attention-deficit hyperactivity disorder: A handbook for diagnosis and treatment*. New York: Guilford Press.

Bartlett, E.J., & Scribner, S. (1981). Text and context: An investigation of referential organization in children's written narratives. In C.H. Frederiksen & J.F. Dominic (Eds.), *Writing: The nature, development, and teaching of written communication*. Hillsdale, NJ: Erlbaum.

Belanoff, P., & Dickson, M. (1991). *Portfolios: Process and product*. Portsmouth, NH: Boynton/Cook.

Benton, S. L., Corkill, A. J., Sharp, J. M., Downey, R. G., & Khramtsova, I. (1995). Knowledge, interest, and narrative writing. *Journal of Educational Psychology*, 87, 66–79.

Bereiter, C., & Scardamalia, M. (1982). From conversation to composition: The role of instruction in a developmental process. In R. Glaser (Ed.), *Advances in instructional psychology* (Vol. 2). Hillsdale, NJ: Erlbaum.

Bereiter, C., & Scardamalia, M. (1987). *The psychology of written composition*. Hillsdale, NJ: Erlbaum.

Bolton, F. & Snowball, D. (1993). *Ideas for spelling*. Portsmouth, NH: Heinemann.

Bruner, J. (1986). *Actual minds, possible worlds*. Cambridge, MA: Harvard University Press.

Burkhalter, N. (1992). *Persuasive writing: Analyzing why and where students have problems*. Unpublished manuscript.

Burkhalter, N. (1995). A Vygotski-based curriculum for teaching persuasive writing in the elementary grades. *Language Arts, 72*, 192–199.

Callaghan, M., Knapp, P., & Noble, G. (1993). Genre in practice. In B. Cope & M. Kalantzis (Eds.), *The powers of literacy: A genre approach to teaching writing*. Pittsburgh, PA: University of Pittsburgh Press.

Calkins, L.M. (1994). *The art of teaching writing*. Portsmouth, NH: Heinemann.

Case, R. (1985). *Intellectual development*. Orlando: Academic Press.

Chapman, M.L. (1994). The emergence of genres: Some findings from an examination of first-grade writing. *Written Communication, 11*, 348–380.

Clauser, P., & Westby, C.E. (1996, April). *Developmental writing rubrics for expository and persuasive texts*. New York: American Educational Research Association, New York.

Clay, M. (1973). *Reading: The patterning of complex behavior*. Portsmouth, NH: Heinemann.

Coe, R.M. (1994). Teaching genre as process. In A. Freedman & P. Medway (Eds.), *Learning and teaching genre* (pp. 157–169). Portsmouth, NH: Heinemann.

Coirier, P., & Golder, C. (1993). Production of supporting structure: Developmental study. *European Journal of Psychology of Education, 2*, 1–13.

Crowhurst, M. (1980). Syntactic complexity in narration and argument at three grade levels. *Canadian Journal of Education, 5*, 6–13.

Crowhurst, M. (1986). Revision strategies of students at three grade levels. *English Quarterly, 19,* 217–226.

Crowhurst, M. (1991). Interrelationships between reading and writing persuasive discourse. *Research in the Teaching of English, 25*, 314–338.

de la Luz Reyes, M. (1991). A process approach to literacy instruction for Spanish-speaking students: In search of a best fit. In E.H. Hiebert (Ed.), *Literacy for a diverse society*. New York: Teachers College Press.

Delpit, L.D. (1988). The silenced dialogue: Power and pedagogy in educating other people's children. *Harvard Educational Review, 58*, 280–298.

Emig, J. (1971). *The composing processes of twelfth graders*. Urbana, IL: National Council of Teachers of English.

Englert, C.S. (1990). Unraveling the mysteries of writing through strategy instruction. In T. E. Scruggs & B. Y. L. Wong (Eds.), *Intervention research in learning disabilities* (pp. 186–223). New York: Springer-Verlag.

Englert, C.S. (1992). Writing instruction from a socio-cultural perspective: The holistic, dialogic, and social enterprise of writing. *Journal of Learning Disabilities, 25*, 153–172.

Englert, C.S., & Hiebert, E.H. (1984). Children's developing awareness of text structures in expository materials. *Journal of Educational Psychology, 76*, 65–74.

Englert, C.S., Raphael, T., Anderson, L., Anthony, H., Stevens. D., & Fear, K. (1991). Making writing strategies and self-talk visible: Cognitive strategy instruction in writing in regular and special education classrooms. *American Educational Research Journal, 28*, 337–373.

Esterreicher, C.A. (1994). *Scamper strategies*. Eau Claire, WI: Thinking Publications.

Flower, L., & Hayes, J.R. (1981). Plans that guide the composing process. In C. Frederiksen & J. Dominic (Eds.), *Writing: Process, development and communication* (pp. 39–58). Hillsdale, NJ: Erlbaum.

Freedman, A., & Pringle, I. (1984). Why students can't write arguments. *English Education, 18*, 2, 73–84.

Garland, S., & Tseng, J. (1993). *Why ducks sleep on one leg*. New York: Scholastic.

Gearhart, M., Herman, J.L., Novak, J.R., Wolf, S.A., & Abedi, J. (1994). *Toward the instructional utility of large-scale writing assessment: Validation of a new narrative rubric*. CSE Technical Report No. 10. Los Angeles: National Center for Research on Evaluation.

Gearhart, M., & Wolf, S. (1994). Engaging teachers in assessment of their students' narrative writing: The role of subject matter knowledge. *Assessing Writing, 1*(1), 67–90.

Gearhart, M., & Wolf, S. (1995). *Teachers' and students' roles in large-scale portfolio assessment: Providing evidence of competency with the purposes and processes of writing*. CSE Technical Report 406. Los Angeles: National Center for Research on Evaluation.

Gearhart, M., Wolf, S., Burkey, B., & Whittaker, A. (1994). *Engaging teachers in assessment of their students' narrative writing: Impact on teachers' knowledge and practice*. CSE Technical Report 377. Los Angeles: National Center for Research on Evaluation.

Gentile, C. (1992). *Exploring new methods for collecting students' school-based writing: NAEP's 1990 portfolio study*. Washington, DC: Office of Educational Research and Improvement.

Gentry, J.R., & Gillet, J.W. (1993). *Teaching kids to spell*. Portsmouth, NH: Heinemann.

Glazer, S. M., & Brown, C.S. (1993). *Portfolios and beyond: Collaborative assessment in reading and writing*. Norwood, MA: Christopher-Gordon.

Golder, C., & Coirier, P. (1994). Argumentative text writing: Developmental trends. *Discourse Processes, 18*, 187–210.

Goldstein, A.A., & Carr, P. (1996). Can students benefit from process writing? *NAEP Facts, 1*, 1–6.

Graham, S. (1992). Issues in handwriting instruction. *Focus on Exceptional Children, 25*, 1–16.

Graham, S., Schwartz, S.S., & MacArthur, C.A. (1993). Knowledge of writing and the composing process, attitude toward writing, and self-efficacy for students with and without learning disabilities. *Journal of Learning Disabilities, 26*, 237–249.

Graves, D.H. (1975). An examination of the writing processes of seven-year-old children. *Research in the Teaching of English, 9*, 227–241.

Graves, D.H. (1983). *Writing: Teachers and children at work*. Portsmouth, NH: Heinemann.

Graves, A., Semmel, M., & Gerber, M. (1994). The effects of story prompts on the narrative production of students with and without learning disabilities. *Learning Disability Quarterly, 17*, 154–164.

Halio, M.P. (1990). Student writing: Can the machine maim the message? *Academic Computing*, 16–19, 45.

Halliday, M.A.K. (1985). *An introduction to functional grammar*. London: Edward Arnold.

Hammill, D.D., & Larsen, S.C. (1996). *Test of written language-3*. Austin, TX: Pro-Ed.

Harris, K.R., & Graham, S. (1996a). Constructivism and students with special needs: Issues in the classroom. *Learning Disabilities: Research and Practice, 11*, 133–137.

Harris, K.R., & Graham, S. (1996b). *Making the writing process work: Strategies for composition and self-regulation*. Cambridge, MA: Brookline Books.

Hayes, J.R. (1996). A new framework for understanding cognition and affect in writing. In C.M. Levy & S. Ransdell (Eds.), *The science of writing* (pp. 1–27). Mahwah, NJ: Erlbaum.

Hayes, J.R., & Flower, L.S. (1980). Identifying the organization of writing processes. In L. Gregg & E.R. Steinberg (Eds.), *Cognitive processes in writing* (pp. 3–30). Hillsdale, NJ: Erlbaum.

Hedberg, N., & Westby, C. (1993). *Analyzing storytelling skills: From theory to practice*. Tucson: Communication Skill Builders.

Hill, B.C., & Ruptic, C. (1994). *Practical aspects of authentic assessment*. Norwood, MA: Cristopher Gordon.

Horowitz, R. (1985a). Text patterns: Part I. *Journal of Reading, 28*, 448–454.

Horowitz, R. (1985b). Text patterns: Part II. *Journal of Reading, 28*, 534–541.

Hresko, W.P. (1988). *Test of early written language*. Austin, TX: Pro-Ed.

Hunt, K.W. (1964). *Differences in grammatical structures written at three grade levels, the structures to be analyzed by transformational methods* (Cooperative Research Project #1998). Washington, DC: U.S. Department of Health, Education, and Welfare.

Illinois State Board of Education (1994). *Write on, Illinois*. Springfield, IL: Illinois State Board of Education.

International Reading Association (1996). IRA/NCTE standards released. *Reading Today, 13*, 1.

Irwin, J.A., & Doyle, M.A. (Eds.). (1992). *Reading/writing connections: Learning from research*. Newark, DE: International Reading Association.

Kellogg, R.T. (1987). Effects of topic knowledge on the allocation of processing time and cognitive effort to writing processes. *Memory & Cognition, 15*, 255–266.

Kennedy, P. (1993). *Preparing for the twenty-first century*. New York: Random House.

Killgallon, D. (1987). *Sentence composing: The complete course*. Portsmouth, NH: Heinemann.

Knudson, R.E. (1989). Effects of instructional strategies, grade, and sex on students' persuasive writing. *Journal of Experimental Education*, 141–152.

Knudson, R.E. (1994). An analysis of persuasive discourse: Learning how to take a stand. *Discourse Processes 18*, 211–230.

Laird, D. (1991). *The three little Hawaiian pigs and the magic shark*. Honolulu, HI: Barnaby Books.

Langer, J., & Applebee, A. (1987). *How writing shapes thinking: A study of teaching and learning*. Urbana, IL: National Council of Teachers of English.

Licht, B.G., & Dweck, C.S. (1984). Determinants of academic achievement: The interaction of children's achievement orientations with skill area. *Developmental Psychology, 20*, 628–636.

Loban, W. (1976). *Language development: Kindergarten through grade twelve*. (NCTE Research Report No. 18). Urbana, IL: National Council of Teachers of English.

Lowell, S. (1992). *The three little javelinas*. Flagstaff, AZ: Northland.

Martin, J.R. (1985). *Factual writing: Exploring and challenging social reality*. Victoria, Australia: Deakin University Press.

May, C.H. (1994). *Conversations with conjunctions*. Tucson, AZ: Communication Skill Builders.

McClure, E., & Geva, E. (1983). The development of the cohesive use of adversative conjunctions in discourse. *Discourse Processes, 6*, 411–432.

McKeough, A. (1991). A neo-structural analysis of children's narrative and its development. In R. Case (Ed.), *The mind's staircase*. Hillsdale, NJ: Erlbaum.

Moats, L.C. (1995). *Spelling: Development, disabilities, and instruction*. Baltimore: York Press.

Moffett, J. (1968). *Teaching the universe of discourse*. Boston: Houghton Mifflin.

Moreau, M.R., & Fidrych-Puzzo, H. (1994). *The story grammar marker*. Easthampton, MA: Discourse Skills Productions.

National Council of Teachers of English (1996). *Standards for the English language arts*. Urbana, IL: National Council of Teachers of English.

New Mexico State Department of Education (1992). *New Mexico portfolio writing assessment: Teacher's guide grade 4, 6, & 8*. Santa Fe, NM: New Mexico State Department of Education.

Nippold, M.A. (1988). *Later language development ages nine through nineteen*. Boston: College Hill.

O'Keefe, B., & Delia, J.G. (1979). Construct comprehensiveness and cognitive complexity as predictors of the number and strategic adaptations of arguments and appeals in a persuasive message. *Communication Monographs, 46*, 231–240.

Pappas, C.C. (1985). The cohesive harmony and cohesive density of children's oral and written stories. In J.D. Benson & W.S. Greaves (Eds.), *Systemic perspectives on discourse*. (Vol. 2). Norwood, NJ: Ablex.

Piccolo, J. (1987). Expository text structure: Teaching and learning strategies. *The Reading Teacher*, 838–847.

Planet Dexter (1995). *Instant creatures*. Reading, MA: Addison-Wesley.

Pressley, M. (1992). Teaching cognitive strategies to brain-injured clients: The good information processing perspective. *Seminars in Speech and Language, 14*, 1–17.

Pressley, M., & McCormick, C.B. (1995). *Cognition, teaching, and assessment*. New York: Harper Collins College Publishers.

Pressley, M., & Woloshyn, V. (1995). *Cognitive strategy instruction that really improves children's academic performance*. Cambridge, MA: Brookline Books.

Quirk, R., Greenbaum, S., Leech, G., & Svartvik, J. (1985). *A comprehensive grammar of English*. London: Longman.

Rhodes, L.K. (1993). *Literacy assessment: A handbook of instruments*. Portsmouth, NH: Heinemann.

Richardson, P.W. (1994). Language as personal resource and as social construct: Competing views of literacy pedagogy in Australia. In A. Freedman & P. Medway (Eds.), *Learning and teaching genre*. Portsmouth, NH: Heinemann.

Rosen, L. J., & Behrens, L. (1994). *The Allyn & Bacon handbook* (2nd ed.). Boston: Allyn & Bacon.

Rubin, D.L., Piche, G.L., Michlin, M.L., & Johnson, F.L. (1984). Social cognitive ability as a predictor of the quality of fourth-graders' written narratives. In R. Beach & L.S. Bridwell (Eds.) *New directions in composition research*. New York: Guilford Press.

Rueda, R. (1990). Assisted performance in writing instruction with learning-disabled students. In L.C. Moll (Ed.), *Vygotsky and education*. New York: Cambridge Press.

Scanlon, D., Deshler, D.D., & Schumaker, J.B. (1996). Can a strategy be taught and learned in secondary inclusive classrooms? *Learning Disabilities: Research & Practice, 11*, 41–57.

Scardamalia, M. (1981). How children cope with the cognitive demands of writing. In C. H. Frederiksen & J. F. Dominic (Eds.) *Writing: The nature, development, and teaching of written communication*. Hillsdale, NJ: Erlbaum.

Schumaker, J.B., & Deshler, D.D. (1992). Validation of learning strategy interventions for students with learning disabilities: Results of a programmatic research effort. In B. Y. Wong (Ed.), *Contemporary intervention research in learning disabilities: An international perspective.* (pp. 22–46). New York: Springer-Verlag.

Scieszka, J. (1989). *The true story of the three little pigs.* New York: Puffin.

Scott, C. M. (1988a). A perspective on the evaluation of school children's narratives. *Language, Speech, and Hearing Services in Schools, 19,* 67–82.

Scott, C. M. (1988b). Spoken and written syntax. In M. A. Nippold (Ed.), *Later language development.* Boston: College Hill.

Scott, C.M. (1989). Problem writers, assessment, and intervention. In A. Kamhi & H. Catts (Eds.), *Reading disabilities: A developmental language perspective* (pp. 303–344). Boston: Allyn & Bacon.

Simons-Ailes, S.J. (1995). *Children's developing abilities to author fictional narratives.* Unpublished doctoral dissertation, University of New Mexico, Albuquerque.

Sommers, N. (1980). Revision strategies of student writers and experienced adult writers. *College Composition and Communication, 31,* 278–388.

Spandel, V., & Stiggins, R.J. (1990). *Creating writers: Linking assessment and writing instruction.* New York: Longman.

Spradley, J. (1979). *Ethnographic interviewing.* New York: Holt, Rinehart & Winston.

Strong, W. (1986). *Creative approaches to sentence combining.* Urbana, IL: National Council of Teachers of English.

Temple, C., Nathan, R., Temple, F., & Burris, N. (1993). *The beginnings of writing.* Boston: Allyn & Bacon.

Tharp, R.G., & Gallimore, R. (1988). *Rousing minds to life.* Cambridge, England: Cambridge University Press.

Tierney, R.J., Carter, M.A., & Desai, L.E. (1991). *Portfolio assessment in the reading-writing classroom.* Norwood, MA: Christopher-Gordon.

Todorov, T. (1977). *The poetics of prose.* Ithaca, NY: Cornell University Press.

Tompkins, G. E. (1994). *Teaching writing: Balancing process and product* (2nd ed.). New York: Merrill.

Toulmin, S., Rieke, R., & Janik, A. (1984). *An introduction to reasoning* (2nd ed.). New York: Macmillan.

Trivizas, E. (1993). *The three little wolves and the big bad pig.* New York: Aladdin.

Valencia, S.W. (1991). Portfolios: Panacea or Pandora's box? In F.L. Finch (Ed.), *Educational performance assessment.* Chicago: Riverside Press.

Vygotsky, L. S. (1978). *Mind in society: The development of higher psychological processes.* In M. Cole, V. John-Steiner, S. Scribner, & E. Souberman (Eds.). Cambridge, MA: Harvard University Press.

Warden, M.R., & Hutchinson, T.A. (1992). *Writing process test.* Riverside.

Westby, C.E. (1989). Assessing and facilitating text comprehension. In A. Kamhi & H. Catts (Eds.), *Reading disabilities: A developmental language perspective.* (pp. 199–259). Boston: Allyn & Bacon.

Westby, C.E. (1994). Communication refinement in school age and adolescence. In W.O. Haynes & B.B. Shulman (Eds.), *Communication development: Foundations, processes, and clinical applications.* Englewood Cliffs, NJ: Prentice Hall.

Westby, C.E., & Cutler, S. (1994). Language and ADHD: Understanding the bases and treatment of self-regulatory behaviors. *Topics in Language Disorders, 14*:4, 58–76.

White, J. (1989). Children's argumentative writing: A reappraisal of difficulties. In F. Christie (Ed.), *Writing in schools: Reader* (ECT 418) (pp. 9–23). Geelong, Victoria: Deakin University Press.

Wolf, S., & Gearhart, M. (1993a). Writing what you read: A guidebook for the assessment of children's narratives. *CSE Resource Paper No. 10.* Los Angeles: National Center for Research on Evaluation.

Wolf, S., & Gearhart, M. (1993b). *Writing what you read: Assessment as a learning event* (CSE Tech. Rep. No. 358). Los Angeles: University of California, Center for the Study of Evaluation.

Wolf, S., & Gearhart, M. (1994). Writing what you read: Narrative assessment as a learning event. *Language Arts, 71,* 425–444.

Computer Programs

Creative Writer II (1996), Microsoft
Imagination Express, Edmark
 Castle
 Neighborhood
 Ocean
 Pyramids
 Rainforest
 Time Trip USA
Mavis Beacon Teaches Typing (1996), Novato, CA: Mindscape
Read, Write & Type (1996), Cambridge, MA: The Learning Company
The Amazing Writing Machine (1995), Novato, CA: Broderbund
The Magic School Bus Explores, Microsoft
 Inside the Earth
 The Age of Dinosaurs
 The Human Body
 The Ocean
 The Rainforest
 The Solar System
Ultimate Writing & Creativity Center (1996), Cambridge, MA: The Learning Company

Appendix A: Example Writing Prompts

4th Grade Prompts

Expository Prompts

Everyone has a hero or someone he or she admires. Think of ONE person who is your hero or that you admire. Write an essay for your classmates explaining why this person is your hero or someone you admire. Be sure to include supporting details.

Think of a place you would like to visit. Write an essay for your teacher explaining why you would like to visit this place.

Narrative Prompts

Pretend that you wake up one morning and you are only six inches tall. Write a story about the adventures you would have during the day.

Suppose a time machine could take you to any place at any time in the past or future. Where and what time period would you choose? Write a story about your adventure in the time and place you have chosen.

One day in science class, you look through a microscope and see strange creatures living in a strange land. Write a story about what you see when you look into the microscope and what might happen.

Think about a time you had fun. It could have been with a grown up, a friend, a relative, or even a pet. Remember what you did that was so much fun. Write a story for your friend telling what you did that was so much fun.

6th Grade Prompts

Expository Prompts

There is always something that can be done to make a place safer. Think about your school—the grounds, the hallways, the parking area. What one thing could be done to make your school a safer place? Write an essay telling the ONE thing that needs to be done to make your school a safer place and explaining why it should be done. Be sure to include supporting details.

Many things have been invented or discovered that have made the world a better place. Think about one invention or discovery and write an essay telling what the invention or discovery is. Explain how it has made the world a better place.

Narrative Prompts

Think of a time you were proud of yourself. Remember what happened that made you proud. Write a story for your classmates telling what happened the time you were proud of yourself.

Suppose a time machine could take you to any place at any time in the past or future. Where and what time period would you choose? Write a story about your adventure in the time and place you have chosen.

One day in science class, you look through a microscope and see strange creatures living in a strange land. Write a story about what you see when you look into the microscope and what might happen.

Many times we wonder how something happens or why it happens. People think up stories to explain why things happen in nature. Use your imagination and have fun writing a story for your friends about one of the topics mentioned below. Choose one of the following "happenings" or pick one of your own and write a story to explain how it came to be.

How people came to have wrinkles

How leopards came to have spots

How giraffes came to have long necks

How cats came to have nine lives

How tears came to be salty

How the sea became salty

Persuasive Prompts

Write a letter to the school principal to convince him or her that there should be more school holidays.

Write a letter to the school principal to convince him or her that American children should go to school six days a week.

8th Grade Prompts

Expository Prompts

There is always something that can be done to make a place safer. Think about your school — the grounds, the hallways, the parking area. What one thing could be done to make your school a safer place? Write an essay telling the ONE thing that needs to be done to make your school a safer place and explaining why it should be done. Be sure to include supporting details.

Many things have been invented or discovered that have made the world a better place. Think about one invention or discovery and write an essay telling what the invention or discovery is. Explain how it has made the world a better place.

Narrative Prompts

Everyone needs help sometimes. Think about a time when you needed help or when you helped someone else. Write a story about that time. Tell what happened in the order that it happened and how it turned out.

Pretend you are spending the summer with a family in another country. Think about what you see, what you do, and what you learn there. Select a country and write a story about the adventures you have while living in that country for the summer.

Persuasive Prompts

School officials at some schools have the right to search students' personal property (lockers, book bags, purses) whether the students agree to the search or not. Think about whether you are FOR or AGAINST school officials having the right to conduct such searches. Write an essay for the school newspaper to convince students that these searches are a good idea OR a bad idea. Be sure to include supporting details.

Think of ONE school rule you believe should be changed. Write a letter convincing your principal to make the change. Be sure to use details to support your position.

Appendix B: *Portfolio Writing Assessment*

Strong Command of Genre	Generally Strong Command of Genre	Command of Genre	Partial Command of Genre	Limited Command of Genre	Inadequate Command of Genre
Score Point 6	Score Point 5	Score Point 4	Score Point 3	Score Point 2	Score Point 1
Has an effective opening and closing that ties the piece together	Has an opening and a closing	Generally has an opening and closing	May not have an opening and/or closing	May not have an opening and/or closing	May not have an opening and/or closing
Related to the topic and has a single form	Related to the topic and has a single focus	Related to the topic and has single focus	Relates to the topic and usually has a single focus; some responses may drift from the focus	Some responses relate to the topic but drift or abruptly shift focus	May state a subject or a list of subjects; may have an uncertain focus that must be inferred
Well-developed, complete response that is organized and progresses logically; writer takes compositional risks resulting in highly effective vivid response	Key ideas are developed with appropriate and varied details; some risks may be taken and are mostly successful; may be flawed, but has sense of completeness and unity	Development may be uneven with elaborated ideas interspersed with bare, unelaborated details	Some responses are sparse with clear, specific details but little elaboration; others are longer but ramble and repeat ideas	Details are a mixture of general and specific with little, if any, elaboration, producing a list-like highlight response	Details are general, may be random, inappropriate, or barely apparent
Very few, if any, errors in usage	Few errors in usage	Some errors in usage, no consistent pattern	May display a pattern of errors in usage	May display numerous errors in usage	May have several problems with usage including tense formation, subject-verb agreement, pronoun usage and agreement, word choice
Variety of sentences and/or rhetorical modes demonstrates syntactic and verbal sophistication, very few if any errors in sentence construction	Syntactic and verbal sophistication though a variety of sentences and/or rhetorical modes	May demonstrate a generally correct sense of syntax; avoids excessive monotony in syntax and/or rhetorical modes; may contain a few errors in sentence construction	May demonstrate excessive monotony in syntax and/or rhetorical modes; may display errors in sentence construction	Excessive monotony in syntax and/or rhetorical modes; may contain numerous errors in sentence construction	May contain an assortment of grammatically incorrect sentences; may be incoherent or unintelligible
Very few, if any, errors in mechanics	Few errors in mechanics	May display some errors in mechanics but no consistent pattern	May display a pattern of errors in mechanics	May display numerous errors in mechanics	May display severe errors in mechanics
			NOTE: Errors may interfere with readability	NOTE: Errors may interfere somewhat with comprehension	NOTE: Errors may interfere with comprehension

Adapted from: NM Writing Portfolio

Appendix C: Analytic Scoring Guidelines

	Sentence Formation	Mechanics	Word Usage	Development
1	Sentences are generally complete and often varied in length and structure.	Punctuation and capitalization are consistently appropriate for grade level. There are few or no spelling errors in words appropriate to grade level.	Vocabulary is carefully or imaginatively used. There are few or no problems with subject-verb agreement, correct forms of verbs, selection of pronouns, possessives, etc.	Response is clearly elaborated, well-organized, detailed enough to enhance clarity, follows from a main idea to a logical conclusion.
2	There is basically a good sentence structure with occasional awkward, confusing, or repetitive constructions. There may be several run-ons or fragments.	Use of punctuation and capitalization is adequate but will contain certain errors. Several spelling mistakes may be present, or the same mistake may be repeated.	Vocabulary is acceptable in scope and appropriateness. Some difficulties with agreement, verbs, pronouns, possessives, etc., may be manifest.	Details are clear and specific, but they may be unevenly elaborated or disorganized.
3	There may be many problems with sentence structure. Simple sentence patterns are used. Sentences are short and repetitious. Run-ons and fragments are common.	Capitalization is erratic and basic punctuation is omitted or haphazard. There are too many errors in mechanics that interfere with communication.	Vocabulary is quite limited: the essay evidences too many errors in agreement, verb forms, pronoun choice, possessives, etc., that interfere with communication.	The response includes only a few details, which may be vague, sketchy, or confusing.

Appendix D: Analytic Trait Scoring

Ideas and Content

Score of 5: This paper is clear, focused, and interesting. It holds the reader's attention. Relevant anecdotes and details enrich the central theme or story line.

Score of 3: The paper is clear and focused, even though the overall result may not be especially captivating. Support is attempted, but it may be limited or obvious, insubstantial, too general, or out of balance with the main ideas.

Score of 1: The paper lacks a central idea or purpose or forces the reader to make inferences on very sketchy details.

Organization

Score of 5: The organization enhances and showcases the central idea of theme. The order, structures, or presentation is compelling and moves the reader through the text.

Score of 3: The reader can readily follow what's being said, but the overall organization may sometimes be ineffective or too obvious.

Score of 1: Organization is haphazard and disjointed. The writing lacks direction, with ideas, details, or events strung together helter-skelter.

Voice

Score of 5: The writer speaks directly to the reader in a way that is individualistic, expressive, and engaging. Clearly, the writer is involved in the text and is writing to be read.

Score of 3: The writer seems sincere but not fully involved in the topic. The result is pleasant, acceptable, sometimes even personable, but not compelling.

Score 1: The writer seems wholly indifferent, uninvolved, or dispassionate. As a result, the writing is flat, lifeless, stiff, or mechanical. It may be (depending on the topic) overly technical or jargonistic.

Word Choice

Score of 5: Words convey the intended message in an interesting, precise, and natural way. The writing is full and rich, yet concise.

Score of 3: The language is quite ordinary, but it does convey the message; it's functional, even if it lacks punch. Often, the writer settles for what's easy or handy, producing a sort of "generic paper" stuffed with familiar words and phrases.

Summarized from Spandel, V., & Stiggins, R. (1990). *Creating writers: Linking assessment and writing instruction.* New York: Longman.

Score of 1: The writer struggles with a limited vocabulary, groping for words to convey meaning. Often the language is so vague and abstract or so redundant and devoid of detail that only the broadest, most general sort of message comes through.

Sentence Fluency

Score of 5: The writing has an easy flow and rhythm when read aloud. Sentences are well built, with consistently strong and varied structure that makes expressive oral reading easy and enjoyable.

Score of 3: Sentences tend to be mechanical rather than fluid. The text hums along efficiently for the most part, though it may lack a certain rhythm or grace, tending to be more pleasant than musical. Occasional awkward constructions force the reader to slow down or reread.

Score of 1: The paper is difficult to follow or to read aloud. Sentences tend to be choppy, incomplete, rambling, irregular, or just very awkward.

Conventions

Score of 5: The writer demonstrates a good grasp of standard writing conventions (e.g., grammar, capitalization, punctuation, usage, spelling, paragraphing) and uses them effectively to enhance readability. Errors tend to be so few and so minor that the reader can easily skim right over them unless specifically searching for them.

Score of 3: Errors in writing conventions, while not overwhelming, begin to impair readability. While errors do not block meaning, they tend to be distracting.

Score of 1: Numerous errors in usage, sentence structure, spelling, or punctuation repeatedly distract the reader and make the text difficult to read; in fact, the severity and the frequency of errors tend to become so overwhelming that the reader finds it very difficult to focus on the message and must reread for meaning.

Appendix E: Predicate Transformations Reflecting Landscape of Consciousness

Low Transformation Use (Sixth Grade Male)

One day a little third grade boy, named Pascal, was walking to school when he found a red balloon. It was tied to a pole, and he climbed the pole and got it. Then he <u>went to get</u> $_{aspect}$ on the bus, but the balloon was <u>not</u> $_{status}$ allowed on the bus. So he ran to school. When he got there, the doors were locked, but he rang the buzzer and got in. Before he went into the classroom, he gave his balloon to the custodian and went in. After school, he got his balloon but it was raining. So he walked home under other people's umbrellas. When he got home, his mom threw the balloon out. But when she <u>wasn't</u> $_{status}$ looking, he went out and got it. The next day, he got his balloon and he <u>found out that it was alive</u> $_{knowledge}$. It followed him everywhere he went! So, when he got on the bus, he just _{manner/adverb} let the balloon go and it followed him. When he got to school, all the kids wanted the balloon but no one could _{modal} catch it, including the principal and the vice principal, so they left it out. But Pascal opened a window, and the balloon got in. Then the principal led Pascal to the Detention Room. Then the balloon followed the principal till he let Pascal out of the Detention Room. After school he and his balloon went to the store, where they looked at stuff. Then the bullies chased him and lost him. When he went to church he was chased out by the guard. Then he went to the baker and left his balloon outside and the bullies stole it. Then they popped it. A whole fleet of balloons came to Pascal and they were all his.

High Transformation Use (Sixth Grade Female)

Pascal a little boy from France was on his way to school <u>when he saw a balloon tied</u> _{knowledge} to a lamp post and <u>decided to get</u> _{intent} it. It was hard for him to climb the pole but when he was done he <u>was sure it was worth it</u> _{attitude}. Pascal <u>usually</u> _{aspect} took the trolley to school but that day he was <u>not</u> _{status} allowed because of his wonderful red balloon. The trolley conductor <u>told Pascal that balloons were not</u> _{status} <u>allowed and he should</u> _{modal} <u>leave</u> _{description}. <u>Quickly</u> _{manner/adverb} Pascal ran to school <u>trying not</u> _{status} <u>to be late</u> _{intent}, but he was <u>not</u> _{status} fast enough, when he got there the door was locked and he <u>had to</u> _{modal} <u>wait to be let</u> _{manner} in. Pascal <u>knew he would</u> _{modal} <u>never</u> _{aspect} <u>be allowed to take</u> _{knowledge} his balloon into class so he left it with the janitor until he was released from school. As Pascal was walking home it <u>started to rain</u> _{aspect} and he <u>didn't</u> _{status} <u>want to get</u> _{intent} his balloon wet he <u>would</u> _{model} walk with people that had umbrellas. He walked with nuns, old men and women, and just about anyone who <u>would</u> _{modal} let him.

As Pascal's mother <u>watched him walking</u> _{knowledge} up the sidewalk, she saw the balloon and <u>decided right then</u> _{aspect/adverbial} <u>it was not</u> _{status} <u>going to be</u> _{subjective} a long-term visitor. In fact <u>as soon as</u> _{aspect/adverbial} Pascal entered the house, she <u>let the balloon soar up</u> _{modal} and out of the house into the wind, but it <u>didn't</u> _{status}. It lingered outside the balcony until Pascal came out and snuck the red balloon back in.

The next day Pascal had <u>already</u> _{aspect/adverbial} <u>realized this was not</u> _{status} <u>an ordinary balloon</u> _{subjective}. If he let go it did <u>not</u> _{status} float away. The balloon <u>would</u> _{modal} <u>just</u> _{manner/adverbial} walk with him side by side to wherever he was going. This made many hide and seek games possible for Pascal and the balloon. It <u>would</u> _{modal} run and he <u>would</u> _{modal} <u>try to catch</u> _{intent} it <u>by hiding</u> _{manner} in doorways and around corners. Today Pascal did <u>not</u> _{status} <u>have to</u> _{modal} run. He <u>simply</u> _{manner} let the balloon go and got on the trolley, sat back and <u>watched it follow</u> _{knowledge} <u>closely</u> _{manner/adverbial} behind. School was <u>not</u> _{status} <u>as easy as it</u> _{manner} <u>could</u> _{modal} have been because the balloon <u>caused</u> many children <u>to become</u> _{result} rowdy and <u>also</u> _{manner/adverbial} <u>want to catch</u> _{intent} the balloon.

Appendix F: Coding Chart for Writing Interview

Mechanical Focus

Level	Logistics	Appearance	Skill	Format
1	Time of class Location of class Use paper/pencil/computer Seat work	I (we) do printing I (we) do cursive ABCs Writing looks good Erase & start over Size, spacing Looks neat or sloppy Speed, fast, slow	Tracing Copy off board Copy words/letters Write or copy name Dictation by teacher (what teacher says) Drawing (w/ emphasis on artistic skill)	Write words Layout of paper (e.g., name at top) Write sentences
2	Do worksheet Complete assignment Follow directions	Letter formation (print cursive) Practicing letters Writing letters accurately/poorly Any reference to practice Penmanship Easy to read (writing/ printing clear)	Specific skill: • capitals • punctuation • divide words • spelling • grammar Use of dictionary Sound out words • phonetic skill	Write sentences Write paragraphs Do outline Layout of paper w/ more requirements

Product Focus

Level	Topic/Content	Amount/Type Information	Type of Writing	Recognition of Product
1	General/vague/limited reference (e.g., snow, my dog, summer vacation, football, etc.) Name/title of product Name character(s)	Length • number of words • number of products • number of pages Word selection looking for word; can't think of word	Story Poem Essay Autobiography Short Story	Teacher (other) said it was good Received good grade
2	Elaboration of topic or content (e.g., description of characters, events, or more detail re: topic)	Style Vocabulary Illustrator (make better, produce) Use more than one language Story sounds real	Nature of writing funny, sad, interesting clarity/detail Some elaboration of types listed above	Reference to completed work Parts of book/work (chapters, table of contents, etc.) Book in library or book fair Using product as model

Process Focus

Level	Step in Process	Reaction to Doing Writing	Interact with Others	Reference to Self
1	General reference to step (choose topic, do draft, revise) Do drawing, then tell story Do drawing to illustrate story Edit	It's fun to do It's interesting I enjoy it Simple, brief, no elaboration	Implied interaction w/o specific reference (talk about it) Listen to stories Working w/ friend	Vague or general reference w/o specifics or elaboration (write what I want)
2	Describe process strategy(ies) (write down several ideas, use imagination, read work over, use invented spelling, keep going, plan story) List steps	Elaboration of reaction to doing writing Writing outside of school/assignment Finish one story/piece, do another	Explicit interaction w/ reference to specific type of interaction (ask for suggestions or ideas, or others' questions about their story, etc.) Communication function of writing	Reference to self w/more detail (write about how I feel, helps me to think, like/ask to read my stories) Reliance on self as source of information Unique/different

Each response is scored in terms of the degree of emphasis in three areas:

MT: Mechanical/technical focus

PDT: Product focus

PCS: Process focus

Mechanical/Technical Focus

0 = None; no indication of any focus in this area.

1 = Reference to a general nonspecific skill; to general appearance; to physical items/tools used; or to location, class, or time (e.g., do cursive; writing looks good; use paper & pencil; copy off board; follow directions; ABCs; practice).

2 = Reference to a specific skill(s) or to a specific characteristic(s) of the writing (e.g., finger spaces, spacing, spelling, penmanship, punctuation, divide words, use dictionary, practice letters).

Product Focus

0 = None, no indication of any focus on this area.

1 = Reference to any topic/content; to amount or type of information; to type of writing (e.g., story, poem); to length; to completing product.

2 = Reference to quality; to language or words used; description of characters, events or nature of writing (e.g., funny, interesting); to books published, books completed, or book fair; to parts of book (e.g., chapters, table of contents); to impact of writing.

Process Focus

0 = None, no indication of any focus on this area.

1 = Implied interaction (e.g., talk about it, ask for help); reaction to doing writing (e.g., it's fun, interesting, enjoy it); general reference to step in process (e.g., choose topic, get started).

2 = Explicit interaction (e.g., listen to others, ask others for ideas or suggestions); describe working strategies (e.g., write down several ideas, use my imagination, read work over); reaction elaborated.

From:

The writing interview: A writer's view of the writing process by Catherine M. Felknor, PhD, Education Evaluation Consultant, Boulder, Co. Reprinted with permission.

Appendix G: The Three Little Peccaries and the Big Bad Jaguar

There once were three little peccaries that were walking though the humid rain forest of Bolivia. They were walking north towards Brazil to cool off in the Amazon River. They went the wrong way. They reached Argentina. The peccaries were exhausted of the heat, the snakes, the vines. They were fed up with almost every thing about the rain forest. So they decided that they had to postpone their trip until they were more organized.

The first peccary decided to make his house out of vines and large leafs. He was successful in building himself a nice large mansion with a moon around it. The second little peccary, Joe was proud of his younger brother, Al. Joe gradually decided to walk along and built himself a nice shelter until they would start their journey again.

After a few days the first little peccary felt safe sleeping at his house alone. The first night nothing happened except for a little noise outside. But the second night, he woke up because he heard something at the door and it wasn't his imagination. There was the jaguar at the door and he said: "Please open the door peccary. I'm a poor jaguar and I need some food for my journey."

While all this was happening, the second little peccary was building his own little house out of all his cloths. It was even bigger than the first little peccary's house. Al was still in trouble with the jaguar. Some how the jaguar destroyed Al's house.

As Joe was outside, admiring the beautiful flower, Al bumped into him yelling hysterically. Joe slapped him and said: "Get a hold of your-self. what's wrong?"

"The big bad jaguar has been chasing me for miles."

"Well, I just finished my house come inside and have some coffee. Don't worry. You are safe inside my house."

The next day the jaguar went to Joe's house disguised as an old lady. The jaguar asked for sugar. But Joe knew, he was the jaguar. So he said: "I haven't gone to the Market yet. I have no groceries.

"May I pease come in? It's cold out here. My house is two days away, and I'm so tired to go on for today."

"There is a motel five miles west."

"Let me in or I'll bleach your house down." And so he did. And the house fell down just like that. The two peccaries were able to get out in time to get a really good head start.

While all this was happening. The oldest peccary was making his house out of logs from the huge trees in the rain forest. He had started since the first day they settled, but he still was not finished. He decided not to stop working, even thought he had blisters in his hands, legs, and arms. He was so tired from carrying the logs. Later that day he finished his house.

Not long after that his brothers had managed to find him along the trail of the Amazon. They were yelling about how scary the jaguar was and how he was going to eat them. They went inside the log house for shelter.

The jaguar found them. The jaguar decided to ring the door bell. They let him in even thought they knew who he was. Right when he was about to attacked, the oldest peccary pulled out a paper in front of him. It was restraining order against him. The jaguar was shocked. He started to cry and decided to leave, but the peccaries decided to hug him good bye. After that they went on the trail for their long journey.

The End

Index